THE
SOCIETY OF
AUTHORS

Entered for the Society of Authors'

Medical Book Awards 1999

Sponsored by the Royal Society of Medicine

84 DRAYTON GARDENS, LONDON SW10 9SB

TELEPHONE 0171 373 6642   FACSIMILE 0171 373 5768

email: authorsoc@writers.org.uk

Video-Assisted Thoracic Surgery

Edited by

William S. Walker MA FRCS FRCS(Ed)

Consultant Surgeon, Department of Cardiothoracic Surgery,
Royal Infirmary of Edinburgh, Edinburgh, UK

I S I S
MEDICAL
MEDIA

© 1999 by Isis Medical Media Ltd.
59 St Aldates
Oxford OX1 1ST, UK

First published 1999

British Library Cataloguing in Publication Data.
A catalogue record for this title is available from
the British Library.

ISBN 1 899066 09 8

Walker, W.
Video Assisted Thoracic Surgery
William S. Walker (ED)

Always refer to the manufacturer's Prescribing
Information before prescribing drugs cited in this book.

Commissioning Editor: John Harrison
Editorial Project Manager: Sarah Mawditt
Production Controller: Peter Gresford
Artwork: Dee McLean

Typeset by
Creative Associates Ltd., UK

Colour reproduction by
Track Direct, UK

Printed by
Bookprint, S.L. Spain

Distributed in the USA by
Books International, Inc., PO Box 605,
Herndon, VA 20172, USA

Distributed in the rest of the world by
Plymbridge Distributors Ltd., Estover Road,
Plymouth PL6 7PY, UK

Contents

List of contributors

Stefano A. Artuso MD
Staff Surgeon, Division of Thoracic Surgery, Ospedale Maggiore, Bologna, Italy

Alain Batisse MD
Paediatric Cardiologist, Cardiovascular Department, L'Institut Mutualiste Montsouris, Centre MÈdico-Chirurgical de la Porte de Choisy, Paris, France

Paul Blenkinsopp
Formerly, Smith and Nephew Dyonics, UK; currently, Autosuture, UK

Maurizio A. Boaron MD
Professor and Chief, Division of Thoracic Surgery, Ospedale Maggiore, Bologna, Italy

Patrick J. Broe MCh FRCS(I)
Consultant Surgeon, Department of Surgery, Beaumont Hospital, Dublin, Ireland

Thomas A. Burdon MD
Assistant Professor, Stanford University Medical School, Chief of Surgical Services, Department of Veterans Affairs, Stanford University Medical Center, Stanford, USA

Daniel Carbognani MD
Intensivist, Cardiovascular Department, L'Institut Mutualiste Montsouris, Centre MÈdico-Chirurgical de la Porte de Choisy, Paris, France

Gabriela B. Corneli MD
Staff Surgeon, Department of Thoracic Surgery, Ospedale Maggiore, Bologna, Italy

Stewart R. Craig FRCS(Ed)
Senior Registrar, Department of Cardiothoracic Surgery, Royal Infirmary of Edinburgh, Edinburgh, UK

Sir Alfred Cuschieri MD ChM FRCS(Ed & Eng) FRCPS(Glas)
Professor and Head, Department of Surgery, Ninewells Hospital and Medical School, Dundee, UK

Eduardo Dacruz MD
Paediatric Cardiologist, Cardiovascular Department, L'Institut Mutualiste Montsouris, Centre MÈdico-Chirurgical de la Porte de Choisy, Paris, France

Alain Dibie MD
Cardiologist, Cardiovascular Department, L'Institut Mutualiste Montsouris, Centre MÈdico-Chirurgical de la Porte de Choisy, Paris, France

James I. Fann MD
Clinical Assistant Professor, Department of Cardiothoracic Surgery, Stanford University Medical Center, Stanford; Staff Cardiac Surgeon, Veterans Administration, Paulo Alto, California, USA

Thierry Folliguet MD
Cardiovascular Department, L'Institut Mutualiste Montsouris, Centre MÈdico-Chirurgical de la Porte de Choisy, Paris, France

S. William Fountain FRCS
Consultant Surgeon, Thoracic Surgical Unit, Harefield Hospital, Harefield, Middlesex, UK

Justin G. Geoghegan MCh FRCS(I)
Department of Surgery, Beaumont Hospital, Dublin, Ireland

Stephen R. Hazelrigg MD
Associate Professor and Chair, Division of Cardiothoracic Surgery, Southern Illinois University School of Medicine, Springfield, Illinois, USA

Rolf G. C. Inderbitzi MD
Chief, Department of Surgery, Spital Limmattal, Schlieren-Zurich, Switzerland

Edmund S. Kassis MD
University of Pittsburgh Medical Center and Cancer Institute, Pittsburgh, USA

François Laborde MD
Chief, Cardiovascular Department, L'Institut Mutualiste Montsouris, Centre MÈdico-Chirurgical de la Porte de Choisy, Paris, France

Nicola V. Lacava MD
Staff Surgeon, Department of Thoracic Surgery, Ospedale Maggiore, Bologna, Italy

Emanuel Le Bret MD
Staff Surgeon, Cardiovascular Department, L'Institut Mutualiste Montsouris, Centre Médico-Chirurgical de la Porte de Choisy, Paris, France

James D. Luketich
Director, Thoracic Surgery Oncology and Co-Director, Minimally Invasive Surgery, University of Pittsburgh Medical Center; Co-Director, Lung Cancer Center, University of Pittsburgh Cancer Institute, Pittsburgh, USA

Michael J. Mack MD
Assistant Clinical Professor, Cardiothoracic Surgery, Cardiothoracic Surgery Association, Dallas, Texas, USA

Mitchell J. Magee MD
Assistant Professor, Division of Cardiothoracic Surgery, Southern Illinois University School of Medicine, Springfield, Illinois, USA

Oliver J. McAnena MCh FRCS(I)
Consultant Surgeon and Lecturer in Surgery, Surgical Department, University College Hospital, Galway, Cork, Ireland

Graham N. Morritt FRCS
Consultant Surgeon, Department of Cardiothoracic Surgery, South Cleveland Hospital, Middlesbrough, UK

Jean Pétri MD
Anaesthesiologist, Cardiovascular Department, L'Institut Mutualiste Montsouris, Centre Médico-Chirurgical de la Porte de Choisy, Paris, France

Mario F. Pompili MD
Clinical Assistant Professor, Department of Cardiothoracic Surgery, Stangeon, Department of Cardiothoracic Surgery, Royal Infirmary of Edinburgh, Edinburgh, UK

Bruce A. Reitz MD
Professor and Chairman, Department of Cardiothoracic Surgery, Stanford University Medical Center, Stanford, California, USA

Nichola A. Santelmo MD
Practicien Hospitalier, Thoracic Surgery Service, Centre Hospitalier d'Avignon, France

John H. Stevens MD
Consultant, Stanford University Medical Center, Stanford, California, USA

William S. Walker MA FRCS FRCS(Ed)
Consultant Surgeon, Department of Cardiothoracic Surgery, Royal Infirmary of Edinburgh, Edinburgh, UK

David A. Waller BMedSci FRCS
Consultant Surgeon, Groby Road Hospital, Leicester, UK

Preface

Video-Assisted Thoracic Surgery (VATS) developed amid an explosion of interest in the autumn of 1991 and spring of 1992 following the application of laparoscopic video imaging technology to the chest. Thoracoscopy is often presented as the forerunner of VATS but in reality although VATS encompasses all that was once accomplished by direct thoracoscopy, it is a truly new field of operative surgery. This book is intended to stimulate further interest in VATS by providing collected reviews of current practice which discuss practical considerations in selection and technique as well as presenting overall results.

Those of us who attended the 1st International Symposium on Thoracoscopic Surgery in San Antonio, Texas, in January 1993 will recall the immense interest that gripped thoracic surgery at this time. Here for perhaps the first time in 30 years was a field of development at the leading edge of technology where thoracic surgery was at the forefront. I well recall attending that meeting and listening to the presentation given by Professor Giancarlo Roviaro of Milan on VATS lobectomy. There might have been 300 people in the auditorium but there was absolute silence as the video of his procedure played and at the end there was a spontaneous outbreak of applause.

In the seven or so years since those heady days, almost all thoracic surgical procedures and an increasing number of cardiac operations have been performed using VATS techniques. Many of the more straightforward procedures have now become standard operations and even on the basis of these alone it seems likely that perhaps one third to one half of all thoracic interventions will eventually be performed in this way. Development of major VATS procedures has, rightly, been far more cautious. Some of these may not stand the test of time and may prove to be examples of that which is possible rather than desirable. Others, however, continue to be developed by a few responsible centres and some of these may also become standard procedures when the techniques, indications and results are fully established.

It is interesting to speculate why the uptake of VATS has been so limited in regard to major procedures. There is a difference between scientific scepticism and the almost emotional opposition to any form of major VATS procedure which has been advocated by some surgeons. It must be debatable to what extent this reflects genuine scientific concern as opposed to an anxiety that the currency of their surgical practice and their own skills could be challenged. A separate impediment to the further development of VATS could also be that it exposes and questions underlying unresolved issues in thoracic surgery such as the argument concerning mediastinal lymph node clearance or sampling, the curative or palliative nature of major oesophageal resection and the many shibboleths relating to minutiae of orthodox operative practice.

The key to the responsible development of VATS techniques is the detailed and accurate reporting of objective data. In the initial phase this will inevitably be derived from pilot series but randomised comparative trials are ultimately necessary. Such trials must, however, compare mature techniques and not underdeveloped VATS procedures against established open surgery. They must also ask pertinent questions. One trial of VATS lobectomy, for example, failed to enquire into postoperative pain — surely one of the most cogent reasons for undertaking a VATS procedure in the first place. Similarly, if cost benefit analyses are to be included these should be assessed with great care. For instance, in the UK discharge is limited more often by social considerations than by medical ones whereas in the USA early discharge might represent cost transference to a secondary health care provider rather than a true absolute reduction in overall costs. It is unfortunate that VATS has developed against the backdrop of financial stringency that has characterised health care in this decade. One might question how cardiac surgical development, for example, would have fared if such considerations had applied 20 years ago.

Ultimately, VATS approaches simply provide another way of performing established open procedures. The techniques are different and new skills do have to be learned but the principles of therapy are unchanged. It is to be hoped that further development in imaging technology, instrumentation and VATS surgical technique will allow thoracic surgery to evolve from current traumatic and destructive open procedures towards a style of surgery appropriate to the 21st century.

W.S. Walker

The evolution of thoracoscopic surgery

S.R. Craig

1

Several authors have reviewed aspects of the early development of thoracoscopy.[1,2,3] This account seeks to place that process in context and to describe in greater detail the contribution and original observations made by Jacobaeus.

Background

In 1882, Forlanini (Fig. 1.1) noticed that tuberculous cavities sometimes healed when they collapsed, usually as a result of either a spontaneous pneumothorax or the development of a large pleural effusion. He subsequently reproduced this collapse in patients with pulmonary tuberculosis by injecting air or nitrogen under water pressure into the pleural space through a needle inserted in the anterior axillary line thereby creating a *pneumotorace artificale*.[4] This technique, in conjunction with rest, became widely adopted in the management of tuberculosis cases. Lung collapse therapy was often unsuccessful, however, because of intrapleural adhesions which prevented the creation of a satisfactory pneumothorax. The available alternative procedures were often drastic and included thoracoplasty, open division of the adhesions, phrenic nerve crush and, latterly, extrapleural pneumothorax or plombage.[5] The development of thoracoscopic division of the intrapleural adhesions allowed an artificial pneumothorax to be created and was, therefore, a major step forward in the then current management of pulmonary tuberculosis. This technique of 'closed pneumonolysis' became widely practised in the first half of the twentieth century.

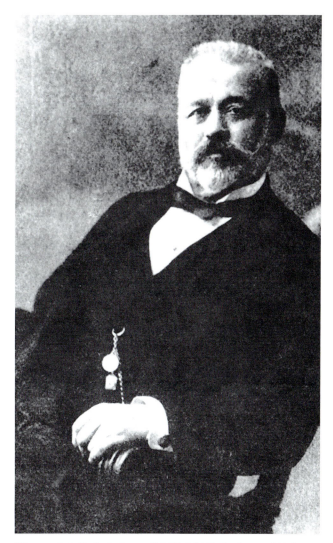

Figure 1.1 *Carlo Forlanini (1847–1918), Professor of Medicine, University of Pavia, Italy.*

Early thoracoscopy

Jacobaeus (Fig. 1.2) described the first direct visual inspection of the pleural cavity when, in 1910, he used a cystoscope to examine the pleural spaces of two patients with exudative pleuritis, a procedure which he termed 'thorakoskopie'.[6] He had previously pioneered the development of 'laparoskopie', using the same instrument, to investigate the aetiology of ascites in a series of patients. In this technique he allowed air to enter the peritoneal cavity after tapping the ascites, allowing him to directly inspect the abdominal organs with the cystoscope. He later extended the indications to patients without ascites and diagnosed conditions such as cirrhosis, benign and malignant tumours, Pick's disease, syphilis and peritoneal tuberculosis. In an address (Fig. 1.3) to the Clinical Congress of the American College of Surgeons, Philadelphia in October 1921, he stated however that 'the most interesting use of the endoscope is for the examination of the pleural cavity — so-called thoracoscopy'.[7] The early technique of thoracoscopy used by Jacobaeus involved the insertion of a straight cystoscope through an equally sized trocar (Fig. 1.4) which was introduced into the pleural space under sedation. If he encountered pleural exudate he relied upon expiration to allow drainage through the trocar, which was often hastened by turning the patient. Once the exudate was removed he used a right-angle lens system to inspect the thoracic cavity in great detail. In a summary of his experience in 1925 he described what could be seen at thoracoscopy.[8] He observed that the normal pleura was best seen in patients undergoing collapse therapy for tuberculosis in which there was no pleuritis. He also described the appearance of the parietal pleura, ribs, intercostal muscles and vessels, heart and diaphragm, though his main interest was in the examination of the lungs and pleura. He recognized this technique as being of particular value in the identification of pulmonary neoplasms and tuberculosis, but thought that the most important aspect of thoracoscopy lay in the therapeutic

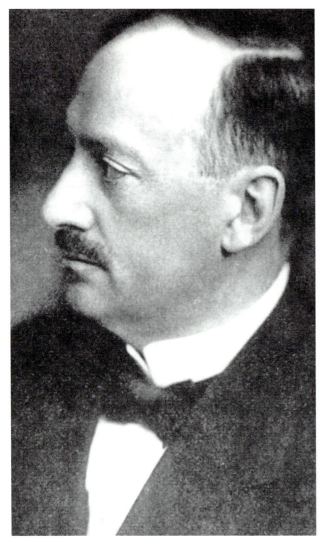

Figure 1.2 *Hans Christian Jacobaeus (1879–1937), Professor of Medicine, University of Stockholm, Sweden.*

SURGERY, GYNECOLOGY AND OBSTETRICS

AN INTERNATIONAL MAGAZINE PUBLISHED MONTHLY

VOLUME XXXIV   MARCH, 1922   NUMBER 3

THE PRACTICAL IMPORTANCE OF THORACOSCOPY IN SURGERY OF THE CHEST[1]

By Dr. H. C. JACOBAEUS, Stockholm, Sweden
Professor of Medicine, University of Stockholm

FOR the last 10 years I have been using the endoscope in studying the peritoneal and pleural cavities. At first I was interested only in the diagnostic advantages that could be gained with such a method. For instance in cases with ascites, after tapping and replacing the ascitic fluid with air, I could obtain by means of the endoscope a clear and comprehensive picture of the abdominal organs. It was thus easy to study the different conditions of the liver and to diagnose cirrhosis, benign tumor, malignant tumor, Pick's disease, syphilis, etc.; in cases of carcinoma and tuberculosis of the peritoneum, the endoscope revealed the characteristic changes. At first I used endoscopy and laparoscopy only on patients with ascites, but I have recently used it to a great extent in examining patients without

Without doubt, however, the most interesting use of the endoscope is for the examination of the pleural cavity —so-called thoracoscopy. For, as we know, we have nothing for examining the chest cavity which corresponds to the exploratory laparotomy for examining the abdominal cavity. Furthermore, thoracoscopy is such a simple method that it can be performed without inconvenience in every case of exudative pleurisy in which thoracocentesis can be done. The ocular examination of the pleural surfaces can in most cases be made relatively complete. In most cases of so-called idiopathic pleurisy I have also succeeded in finding distinct tuberculous nodules. In making a differential diagnosis between tumors and pleurisy of other origin, thoracoscopy is of no small value. After some practice it is

Figure 1.3 *Address given by Jacobaeus to the Clinical Congress of the American College of Surgeons in Philadelphia in 1921.*

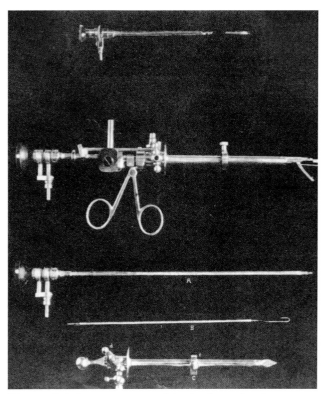

Figure 1.4 *Instrument set used by Jacobaeus for thoracoscopic pneumonolysis.*

applications that could be performed under direct visualisation and guidance.

Jacobaeus was aware of the limitations of artificial pneumothorax therapy in the presence of pleural adhesions and set about developing ways of dividing them thoracoscopically. Under fluoroscopic control he was able to mark the exact position of an adhesion on the chest wall and using local anaesthesia, thereby insert his thoracoscope, close to the adhesion, allowing it to be directly visualised and categorised. He classified adhesions by their position (apical, lateral and diaphragmatic), shape and their surgical difficulty. Apical adhesions were frequently short, technically difficult to reach with the galvanocautery and often resulted in pain when they were divided, due to their proximity to the parietal pleura. Lateral adhesions, the most frequent, were usually associated with a good clinical outcome, but diaphragmatic adhesions presented their own difficulties. Although division of diaphragmatic adhesions was usually painless, movement of the diaphragm required the patient to hold his or her breath, otherwise the adhesion was in constant

movement. Having identified the adhesions, he then used a second trocar to insert the galvanocautery (Fig. 1.5), which consisted of a small metal rod with a platinum loop through which an electrical current could be passed, thereby cauterising, or dividing, the adhesion (Figs. 1.6, 1.7). The galvanocautery was introduced in the line of the scapula in the fifth or seventh interspace when the adhesions were near the apex, and further down when they were at the middle or base of the lung. He generally divided the narrowest part of an adhesion although, if there were an underlying tuberculous cavity, he stayed as close to the chest wall as possible in an attempt to prevent postoperative air leak. Cauterisation of adhesions often took one to two hours and there was the ever-present danger of haemorrhage, especially if the galvanocautery was too strong and the adhesion divided too quickly.

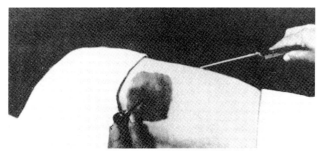

Figure 1.5 *Two cannula thoracoscopy technique used by Jacobaeus. The thoracoscope is inserted posteriorly and the cautery anteriorly.*

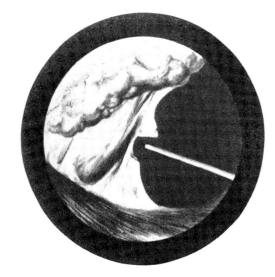

Figure 1.6 *Original Jacobaeus illustration showing the use of his cautery to divide a pleuro-pulmonary adhesion.*

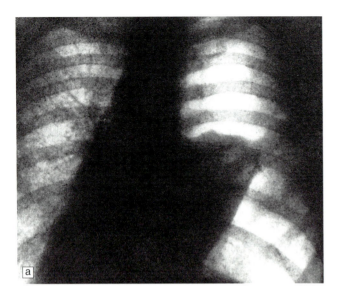

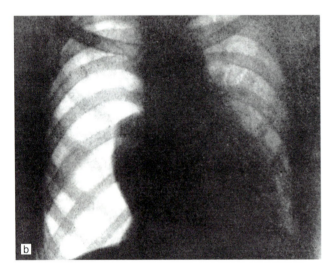

Figure 1.7 *(a) Original Jacobaeus chest X-ray showing a right lateral adhesion prior to thoracoscopic pneumonolysis. (b) The same patient, following division of the adhesion.*

Jacobaeus published the results of his work in 1921 and 1927,[9] but the definitive article appeared in the *Proceedings of the Royal Society of Medicine* in London in 1922–3,[10] in the section Electrotherapeutics. This work was reproduced in the USA in the *Archives of Radiology and Electrotherapy* in 1923.[11] In his report of 1922, published in *Surgery, Gynaecology and Obstetrics*,[7] he summarised his experience of intrapleural thoracoscopic pneumonolysis. In the 50 patients operated on by him personally at the Serafimerlasarettet Hospital, Stockholm, he achieved complete collapse of the tuberculosis cavities in over three-quarters of his patients who had no or little pleural exudate, though only 70% were described as having a good clinical result. The remaining 11 patients were described as having 'incomplete cauterisation' and had either early or late pleural exudate usually in combination with persisting infection.

Thoracoscopic pneumonolysis became widely accepted throughout Europe and the USA although the two cannula technique was later modified by Davidson[12] and then Cutler[13] who used a single instrument in an attempt to limit the number of 'port-holes', at the expense however of a limited view of the pleural cavity. A later and disastrous development was the use of a bronchoscope to perform thoracoscopy, which, because of the high incidence of complications such as surgical emphysema and haemorrhage, occasionally with fatal results, meant that it was soon abandoned.[14] The last large series of patients undergoing closed thoracoscopic intrapleural pneumonolysis was published in 1947 by Day and colleagues. This report testified to the safety of the procedure with only two post-operative deaths in 1000 cases.[15]

Post tuberculosis era

Thoracoscopic pneumonolysis and pulmonary collapse therapy remained the mainstay of treatment for cavitating pulmonary tuberculosis until the introduction of chemotherapy with streptomycin in 1945.

Thereafter, thoracoscopy was performed relatively infrequently. It found most use in the investigation of pleural effusion stimulated in part by the increasing incidence of malignant mesothelioma experienced in Western industrialized countries. Pulmonary and mediastinal mass biopsy were rarely practised with most surgeons preferring a limited open thoracotomy for this purpose, although thoracoscopic pulmonary biopsy for interstitial lung disease was described in the context of immunocompromised patients.[16,17] Therapeutic use continued in the hands of a few interested exponents who described removal of intrathoracic foreign bodies and management of pneumothorax.[18–20] Perhaps the most successful continued applications, however, were the use of thoracoscopy to interrupt the thoracic sympathetic chain[21] and in the irrigation and debridement of empyema.[22,23]

The advent in about 1990 of video imaging techniques and minimal access surgical instrumentation adopted from laparoscopic practice hugely expanded the interest in and applicability of minimal access techniques to thoracic surgery. Initial reports confirmed not only the facilitated performance of previously undertaken procedures but also described entirely novel and significantly complex surgical operations including major pulmonary resection.[25-28] The majority of intrathoracic procedures, including most recently cardiac surgery, have now been performed either clinically or experimentally as videothoracoscopic or video-assisted procedures. The ultimate role of many of these procedures is controversial but it is clear that the horizons of thoracoscopic surgery can only expand as instrumentation continues to improve and both economic forces and public demand increase the push towards minimal access thoracic surgical techniques.

References

1   Davis CJ. A history of endoscopic surgery. *Surg Laparosc Endosc* 1992; **2**: 16–23.

2   Braimbridge MV. The history of thoracoscopic surgery. *Ann Thorac Surg* 1993; **56**: 610–14.

3   Thomas PA. A thoracoscopic peek: What did Jacobaeus see? *Ann Thorac Surg* 1994; **57**: 770–1.

4   Forlanini C. A contribuzioni della terapia chirurgica della tisi-Ablazione del polmone? Pneumotorace artificiale? *Gazz Osp* 1882; **3**: 537–707.

5   Forsee JH. Collapse therapy. In: *The Surgery of Pulmonary Tuberculosis*. London: Kimpton, 1954: 47–69.

6   Jacobaeus HC. Ueber die Moglichkeit die Zystoskopie bei untersuchung seroser hohlungen anzuwenden. *Munchen Med Wochenser* 1910; **57**: 2090–2.

7   Jacobaeus HC. The practical importance of thoracoscopy in surgery of the chest. *Surg Gynaecol Obstet* 1922; **34**: 289–96.

8   Jacobaeus HC. Die Thorakoskopie und ihre Praktische bedeutung. *Ergeb Ges Meb* (Berlin) 1925; **8**: 112–66.

9   Jacobaeus HC. The cauterization of adhesions in pneumothorax treatment of tuberculosis. *Surg Gynaecol Obstet* 1921; **32**: 493–500.

10 Jacobaeus HC. The cauterization of adhesions in artificial pneumothorax treatment of pulmonary tuberculosis under thoracoscopic control. *Proc R Soc Med* 1922–3; **16** (Parts 1&2, Section on Electrotherapeutics): 45–60.

11 Jacobaeus HC. The cauterization of adhesions in artifical pneumothorax treatment of pulmonary tuberculosis under thoracoscopic control. *Arch Radiol Electrotherapy* 1923; **28**: 97–146.

12 Davidson LR. A simple operating thoracoscope. *Am Rev Tuberc* 1929; **19**: 306–9.

13 Cutler JW. A technique and apparatus for intrapleural pneumonolysis. *Am Rev Tuberc* 1933; **28**: 528–36.

14 Friedel H. Importance of bronchological examination in cases of pleural disease. *Bronches* 1970; **20**: 77–82.

15 Day JC, Chapman PT, O'Brien EJ. Closed intrapleural pneumonolysis: an analysis of 1000 consecutive operations. *J Thorac Surg* 1948; **17**: 537–54.

16 Rogers BM, Moazam F, Talbert JL. Thoracoscopy. Early diagnosis of interstitial pneumonitis in the immunologically suppressed child. *Chest* 1979; **75**: 126–30.

17 Thomas P. Thoracoscopy: an old procedure revisited. In: Kittle CF, ed. *Current Controversies in Thoracic Surgery*. Philadelphia: Saunders, 1986: 101–6.

18 Page RD, Jeffrey RR, Donnelly RJ. Thoracoscopy: a review of 121 consecutive procedures. *Ann Thorac Surg* 1989; **48**: 66–8.

19 Hansen MK, Kruse-Andersen S, Watt-Boolsen S, Andersen K. Spontaneous pneumothorax and fibrin glue sealant during thoracoscopy. *Eur J Cardiothorac Surg* 1989; **3**: 512–14.

20 Wakabayashi A. Expanded applications of diagnostic and therapeutic thoracoscopy. *J Thorac Cardiovas Surg* 1991; **102**: 721–3.

21 Claes G, Drott C, Gothberg G. Thoracoscopy for autonomic disorders. *Ann Thorac Surg* 1993; **56**: 715–16.

22 Sang CTM, Braimbridge MV. Thoracoscopy simplified using the laparoscope. *Thoracic and Cardiovascular Surgery* 1982; **30**: 36.

23 Hutter JA, Harari D, Braimbridge MV. The management of empyema thoracis by thoracoscopy and irrigation. *Ann Thorac Surg* 1985; **39**: 517–20.

24 Ferguson MK. Thoracoscopy for empyema, bronchopleural fistula, and chylothorax. *Ann Thorac Surg* 1993; **56**: 644–5.

25 Coltharp WH, Arnold JH, Alford WC *et al*. Videothoracoscopy: improved technique and expanded indications. *Ann Thorac Surg* 1992; **53**: 776–9.

26 Donnelly RJ, Page RD, Cowen ME. Endoscopy assisted microthoracotomy: initial experience. *Thorax* 1992; **47**: 490–3.

27 Mack MJ, Aronoff RJ, Acuff TE *et al*. Present role of thoracoscopy in the diagnosis and treatment of diseases of the chest. *Ann Thorac Surg* 1992; **54**: 403–9.

28 Roviero GC, Rebuffat C, Varoli F *et al*. Videoendoscopic pulmonary lobectomy for cancer. *Surg Laparosc Endosc* 1992; **2**: 244–7.

Imaging equipment

P. Blenkinsopp

2

Introduction

The selection of imaging equipment for video-assisted thoracic surgery (VATS) can be very complex. Numerous aspects must be taken into consideration and many disciplines within the hospital will be involved in the decision-making process to make sure the equipment suppliers can meet the needs of the surgical team and the hospital.

A number of areas need to be carefully thought about, not only when purchasing the imaging equipment but also to enable its continued successful use:

- the technology involved
- theatre set-up
- ease of use and sterilisation
- care and maintenance
- service and back-up
- staff training.

This chapter considers the technical issues relating to imaging equipment for VATS procedures and identifies points of practical importance when selecting and using equipment.

Image technology
Video chips

First introduced in 1975, the charged coupled device (CCD) has developed into a rugged, lightweight, sensitive and high-quality imaging device. The CCD is an array of metal oxides which generates a charge proportional to the amount of light that hits the surface of the chip via light transmission from the endoscope. With the evolution of the Hyper Had CCD the chip is able to utilize the light via the endoscope to its full potential.

This is due to a film coating the chip which allows light to be focused in a more productive manner onto the pixels (electric wells), thus creating a far more light-sensitive CCD. The charge generated is then transferred for storage in pixels that are cut into the surface of the chip, which then transform the stored charge into a formulated analogue video signal. The information is transferred via electronics to a holding station on the chip where each piece of information is timed, then sent to the camera control unit for decoding and prepared for video output to the monitor, printer or video recorder.

Single-chip cameras

Because the individual pixels on the surface of the chip pick up photosensitive information only, a stripe filter which allows specific colour spectrums to pass through is placed over the surface of the CCD. This colour filter consists of four filter types: yellow, cyan, green and magenta. As the light enters the face of the camera, each filter allows only the specified spectrum of light to pass through. The camera creates shades of colour by combining the individual information from all the pixels into one image.

Since the single-chip camera must use four pixels to make up one piece of the image under the stripe filter, resolution and colour definition capabilities have been limited. However, the image quality of single-chip cameras has continued to improve with the use of better materials and miniaturisation which have increased the pixel density. Current camera heads are lightweight and, with the advent of the Hyper Had CCD, less powerful light sources are required. These factors have resulted in the production of high-quality, easy-to-use cameras, some with their own integral light source.

Three-chip cameras

Three-chip cameras address the problems of resolution and colour definition by incorporating three individual CCDs into one camera head. These CCDs represent each of the primary light colours: red, green and blue. The light enters the front of the camera housing from the endoscope then passes through a prism and is distributed evenly to the CCDs.

To contain the three 12 mm² CCDs and the prism, the camera head size for a three-chip camera has to be relatively large compared to many single-chip cameras (Fig. 2.1). This can be seen as a problem in some endoscopic procedures but, for laparoscopic and thoracoscopic surgery, the higher image quality gained from a three-chip camera is of greater importance.

This type of camera creates the image by passing the electronic information into the camera control unit and then onto the monitor and documentation devices via the red, green, blue signal process (Fig. 2.2a). Because the signals are separated throughout their route, 'noise' level (or image corruption) is at a minimum and colour fidelity is at a maximum, creating an extremely high-quality image for viewing during the operative procedure (Fig. 2.2b) and for producing documentation.

White set procedure

The electronic controls within the camera control unit must be correctly set for the camera to provide true colour reproduction. The primary colour spectrum is based on the

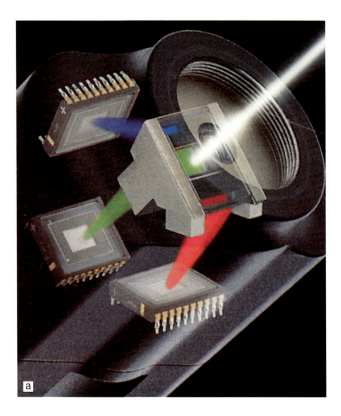

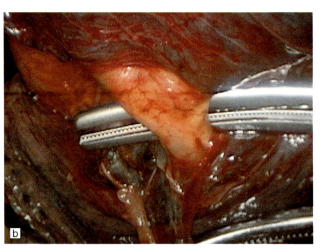

Figure 2.2 *(a) Diagrammatic representation of three-chip camera head demonstrating separation of light data into red, green and blue primary colours. (b) Example of a high quality image achieved during major pulmonary resection.*

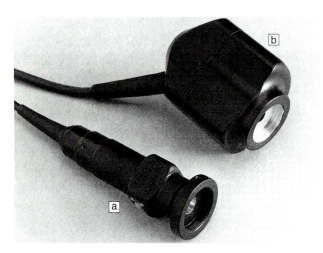

Figure 2.1 *Comparative sizes of single- (a) and three-chip (b) camera heads.*

colour white which represents the presence of all colours in proper balance. The white set procedure should therefore be carried out prior to the start of the surgical operation so as to re-establish the white balance parameters. The camera should also be reset if either an endoscope or light lead is changed during surgery as either of these items could affect the transfer of light to the camera head and CCD.

The following covers the white set procedure for many imaging systems:

- attach endoscope to camera head
- attach light lead to scope
- adjust light output from light source to achieve adequate image brightness on the monitor
- place into view a white gauze swab by aiming the scope at its centre, then focus scope
- depress white balance switch
- allow camera to complete the entire white set procedure before removing the swab from the aim of the scope.

Light level adjustment

Signal gain

It can be difficult to achieve adequate image brightness during thoracoscopic surgery. The dark hue of pigmented or collapsed lung and any free blood will 'absorb' light and therefore darken the picture. Some camera units have a facility called 'auto gain' which allows the image to be enhanced manually within the camera unit by increased signal amplification should very low light levels prevail. This is less likely to be required with the higher light sensitivity Hyper Had CCD but can still be a useful feature although at the expense of reduced image definition.

Automatic light level control

During surgical procedure, different levels of light are needed for close-up and panoramic views. When near tissue a reduced light level is required in order to eliminate glare from the tissue. There are two methods used to provide this adjustment:

- Light output control — a mechanical iris in the light source electrically controlled by the camera unit
- Light input control — an automatic shutter in the camera head.

The automatic shutter is faster and smoother in operation than the mechanical iris.

Video formats

There are several different systems for transmitting video signals. These formats vary in complexity and fidelity and are summarised below.

Composite format

A composite video signal carries video, synchronisation (sync) and colour signals together. Advantages of this system include the simplicity of a single coaxial cable, the ability to have long cable runs without significant loss of image, and compatibility with the video input of most domestic televisions. The system produces a relatively poor-quality image, however, as the available bandwidth allows a limited amount of information to be transmitted. Also, the effect of combining colour and brightness information in one signal is that intermodulation distortion and increased noise occur.

S-Video format (S-VHS, Y–C)

In this format, the brightness or luminance signal (Y) and the colour or chrominance signal (C) are transmitted separately using a multistranded shielded cable with mini-DIN plug connections. Separating the Y and C signals improves the signal-to-noise ratio and reduces cross interference between the two signals. The bandwidth is greater, allowing transmission of more information. A disadvantage of Y–C is that cable runs greater than about 4.5 m can be associated with signal loss.

Component format

A component output is split into three separate channels. A separate synchronisation signal is also usually required. There are two forms of component video:

1. RGB (Red, Green and Blue)

This is the purest form of video signal in which the three primary colours are output separately. As the three colour values and the synchronisation information each travel down separate cable elements, cross-signal interference is reduced to a minimum, resulting in excellent image clarity, colour definition and depth of field. This system is fully effective only when a three-chip camera is used with each CCD dedicated to a primary colour. If a single-chip camera unit has an RGB output the image quality can actually be degraded as the video signal from the CCD has to be processed electronically to derive an RGB output.

RGB is the optimum input to a monitor or video printer as the ultimate representation of the video image in these devices is via RGB processing and any other form of input has, therefore, to be converted back to RGB. A potential disadvantage of RGB is that colour reproduction which is a highly subjective judgement may not suit the user, and colour adjustment may not be possible in some monitors when using an RGB input.

2. YUV (Y, B–Y, R–Y)

This is a component signal in which the luminance information (Y) and two chroma channels (U and V) are presented separately. As with RGB, this format has the advantage of separation of the video signal elements so that interference and noise are minimized and excellent picture quality is obtained. The primary advantage of this form of signal, however, is that it is the format used for broadcast-quality videotape recording. YUV is used for this purpose rather than RGB as the YUV format equates to the way in which picture information is stored on the videotape.

A high quality camera unit should possess various video outputs all active in parallel. This allows the connection of monitors and image recording and archiving devices to the optimum type of video format for each. High quality video peripheral devices normally have a 'chaining' facility which allows a signal to be taken back out of the unit in the same format as the input. Where several devices require the same format, therefore, it is usually possible to connect these using interlinking cables. In this situation the one requiring the highest grade of signal should be placed first in the sequence. Also, the last may require a slider switch to be positioned so as to create a terminating resistance for the chain. Details regarding this form of interconnection are supplied by the equipment manufacturers.

Further aspects of video terminology are explained in Appendix 1.

Light sources

A high-powered light source is as important to a good image as the camera unit. If the camera has no auto-shutter facility, it must be able to control the light source iris in order to prevent white-out and glare.

The most commonly used types of light bulb are:

- metal halide
- halogen
- xenon.

The differences between the lamps are:

- light temperature (colour output of the lamp varying from a yellow white to the xenon bulb — a bluish white)
- lumen output (measured in watts)
- operational conditions
- cost (a xenon lamp > £1000, halogen and metal halide £40–500).

As with the camera control unit, the easier a lamp is to use the better; with less switches, buttons and sliders there is far less chance for user error. Likewise, it is important to consider how easy it is to change a lamp should one default during surgery (Fig. 2.3). There should be some form of bulb-life indicator, though lamps can blow at any time, so ideally a spare lamp should always be available; this is not so in many cases due to the cost.

Specific operation instructions for turning the light source on and off must be followed. The light should be placed on an imaging system trolley to allow for good air ventilation to cool the lamp. The light source will shut down if the theatre is abnormally warm; most have a thermostat to prevent overheating and will automatically turn off. Once back to a safe operational temperature they will function again.

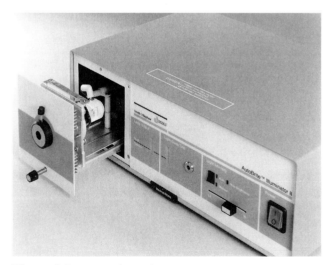

Figure 2.3 *Easy-to-change lamp operation.*

Video monitors

The third critical element to an excellent image is the monitor. As stated in the 'weak link theory' the image from a high resolution camera into a low resolution monitor is less than desired. Current monitors are now available with up to 750 lines of resolution; these come in 14 inch or 20 inch screens, with the 20 inch being the preferred size for thoracoscopy. The monitor should be of medical grade so as to ensure electronic safety.

Signal inputs and outputs on the back of the monitor should cover all three types of video format: composite, S-VHS and component.

Thoracoscopes

The thoracoscope (Fig. 2.4) has two functions once it has entered the thoracic cavity:

1. To transmit light into the cavity to enable the CCDs to function. This is accomplished by thousands of optic fibres positioned around the circumference of the thoracoscope carrying light from the light source via a light guide cable.
2. To present the image. This may be accomplished by a rod lens system taking the image to the CCD positioned in the back of the camera head or by locating the chip at the distal end of the thoracoscope. The distal and optical lenses of the laparoscope are best made from sapphire to prevent damage and therefore poor image quality. Some manufacturers will frost areas of the distal lens to help reduce glare.

There are currently many variables in the design of laparoscopes:

*   direction of view: 0, 30 and 45 degree
*   diameter: 2, 2.5, 5 and 10 mm
*   working length: 175 to 320 mm
*   autoclavable or non-autoclavable
*   direct view (eye piece) or video
*   end chip or telescope design.

The most commonly used scope is 10 mm in diameter with a view of 0° and a working length of 320 mm. Obviously there are variables, the major discussion being over the working length. At times, very little of the scope is actually in the thoracic cavity which may create difficulty for the camera person. Although a shorter scope would

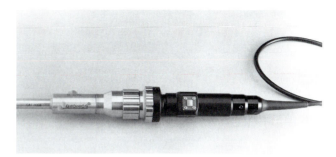

Figure 2.4 *Video laparoscope and camera head.*

reduce this problem, it is important to have a working length long enough to give a good view of the apex of the thoracic cavity. Therefore a compromise is made as few surgical departments can afford a range of scopes.

The decision to use autoclavable or non-autoclavable scopes depends on the hospital's sterilisation policy and facilities available. The key issue with autoclavable scopes is that both the distal and optical lenses are welded into their housings, as these joints would otherwise fail under the stress of autoclaving, allowing water ingress into the optics.

Contamination should not be removed by a moist swab as this will smear the distal lens so that image quality remains poor. An alcoholic preparation should be used to break down the grease film before an anti-fogging agent is applied.

It is possible to reduce the difficulties associated with changing video thoracoscopes, if this is part of the chosen operative technique, by utilising a camera unit which will accept more than one camera input. This enables both 0° and 30° scopes to be sterilised, mounted to their own camera heads, and connected to the camera unit so that both are available for use during the operative procedure.

Light guide cables

A light guide cable is interfaced between the light source and the light port on the scope, in order to transmit the light from the light source to the distal end of the scope. Light transmission is accomplished either by fibre optic bundles or a liquid medium.

Fibre optic cables can be sterilised by all methods available. They are flexible and therefore easy to handle. It is very important to do so with care in order to maintain their efficiency as damage to individual fibres will create inadequate light transmission.

Liquid light guides are capable of transmitting greater amounts of light and due to their construction they do not degrade as quickly as fibre optic guides, but it is not possible to autoclave liquid light guide cables and they can be difficult to handle as they are less flexible.

Coupling

A direct view scope (Fig. 2.5) will require a coupler to connect it to the camera head. Couplers vary in design, but they should be:

● easy to focus
● easy to attach securely to the scope
● lightweight
● vented to help reduce possible condensation.

To gain a full image on the monitor or documentation equipment a 30–35 mm coupler should be used.

Condensation can be a problem when using a coupler and direct view scope: both components must be thoroughly dried before the procedure commences, to prevent poor image quality. Image quality is improved also if the camera head and cable are sleeved and the scope autoclaved. The use of a coupler will make the change-over of scopes, from say a 0° to a 30° during surgery, a lot easier. Video laparoscopes screw directly into the camera head without the need for a coupler. The complete unit can then be soaked, reducing the risk of condensation which occurs with a soaking sterilization method. This reduces fogging but has a disadvantage when changing scopes as the connections are unsterile.

The best image is gained from the scope if the distal lens is kept free from condensation and contamination. Condensation is best avoided from the outset by warming the scope before it enters the thoracic cavity. Should condensation persist there are proprietary solutions on the market which are effective.

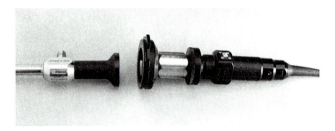

Figure 2.5 *A direct view scope with coupler and camera head.*

Documentation

Documentation varies from a still video print in a patient's records to full archiving or from simple video recordings to full edited presentations using picture in picture techniques.

Video recorders

These vary in quality from simple domestic VHS machines purchased from a local electrical store to broadcast-quality Betacam recorders. High end recording devices are obviously very expensive, but it is best to purchase the highest possible medical grade video recorder which can be afforded. S-VHS has now superseded the older U-Matic-type recorder; the image quality is similar and it is easier to review the tapes as U-Matic video units are now relatively uncommon. S-VHS units offer a good cost/quality ratio and probably represent the optimum compromise choice at present.

The entire procedure can be recorded and later edited, or a 'stop and start' type of editing can be performed during a procedure by using a foot pedal, a remote control or remote buttons which some camera manufacturers conveniently place on the camera head.

Recently digital tape machines have become available which offer exceptional picture quality with very low signal-to-noise ratios. These devices are currently significantly more expensive (two or three times more) than conventional analogue recorders and require a digital output from the camera unit via a 'firewire' connection. This technology is almost certain to become standard however, over the next three to five years. Digital tape media are also likely to dominate computer-based video editing, as relatively low data rates are needed for broadcast-quality results.

Video printing

A video printer freezes the signal from the video camera and converts it into a digital image which is then developed onto a special paper via thermal ink printing techniques. The printer can be activated either by a remote control pedal or by camera head buttons. Most printers allow single, quadruple or multiple images per print and have the capability to modify the image colour, contrast and brightness before printing. For optimum reproduction of the video image the printer input should receive at least S-VHS and preferably RGB signals.

Photography

For presentation purposes 35 mm photography produces the highest image quality. A still 35 mm film camera can be attached to a thoracoscope, but this is a cumbersome and tedious process. It is difficult to sterilise the camera, and the process requires disconnection of the video camera from the scope with consequent loss of the image from the monitor. Both sterility and picture composition are, therefore, compromised.

Digital imaging

The newer technology of digital imaging allows the camera signal to be processed via a computer which then digitises the image and transfers it to a mobile disk such as a standard floppy, optical floppy, a CD-ROM or the hard disk within the computer. Computer software is then used to enhance the picture by processing the image data to create a high resolution, nearly photographic-quality final image. The same process is used in the newer digital video camera systems now available; although the image is digitised, the signal output to the monitor or image capture device remains analogue.

Digital imaging is an excellent tool not only for patient archiving but due to its flexibility it can give high quality images for all types of presentation. The only drawback is cost.

Theatre set-up

Space and safety are the two critical areas when considering theatre set-up. Operating theatres are not designed to take the ever-growing array of equipment required in an environment of increasing technology, therefore space is at a premium. There will already be a large amount of equipment in the theatre suite — anaesthetic machines, diathermy and suction apparatus, trolleys for the instrumentation — and to this will be added a trolley for the imaging system and possibly another for an assistant's monitor (Fig. 2.6).

To make the set-up of the theatre easier, establish a routine for positioning the equipment, using imaging trolleys which are easy to manoeuvre and sturdy but not too obtrusive (Fig. 2.7). Use the minimum number of personnel in the theatre team to carry out this procedure safely.

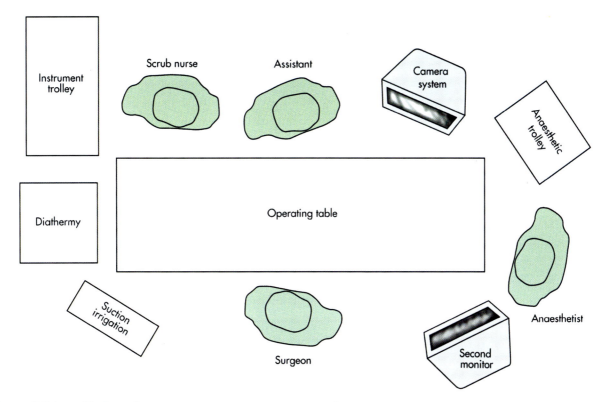

Figure 2.6 *A possible theatre layout incorporating an imaging system and monitor.*

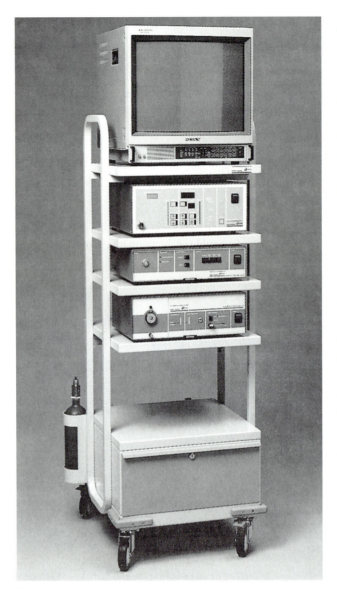

Figure 2.7 *Standard endoscopic trolley.*

Matters of safety also relate to the space available. There will be extra trailing leads; all cabling related to the imaging system should be wired through ducting incorporated in the trolley design.

Electronic safety checks will have been carried out on the imaging equipment by the hospital operating department assistant, although all the equipment should already have cleared the stringent regulatory testing required for protecting both the patient and the staff. Be sure that none of your existing electrical apparatus will interfere with or suffer interference from the new imaging equipment.

Sterilisation

Three sterilisation options exist: soaking, autoclaving and gas. Of these, soaking and autoclaving are compatible with rapid inter-case turn around.

Autoclaving is probably the simplest process, but not all theatre suites have their own autoclaves in which case equipment will have to be sent to a central sterilising unit and the potential advantage of rapid turn-round will be lost. It is imperative to ensure that the thoracoscope and light guide cable are designed for the autoclaving methods used. With this technique sterile sleeving will be required to enclose the camera head and cable, which are not usually autoclavable.

Soaking is a very easy and quick method for preparing equipment for surgery but can have significant drawbacks. Safety issues require that a ventilation cabinet must be used for glutaraldehyde sterilisation and the skin and eyes should be well protected. Peracetic acid is a safer method of soaking sterilisation although considered expensive. There are a number of new sterilisation fluids available which have yet to be extensively tested both by infection control departments and for compatibility with some of the materials used in the construction of camera heads, leads and light guide cables. At present, no soaking method can offer the absolute level of sterilisation provided by autoclaving. The distinct advantage of soaking, however, is that the thoracoscope, light guide, camera head and camera cable may be sterilised together.

Gas sterilisation with ethylene oxide has the advantage of causing least damage to endoscopic equipment but is generally impracticable due to the prolonged turnaround time inherent in this method (several days).

Where finance allows it is best to obtain as many scopes and light leads as you can in order to distribute the workload on these items so they not only last longer, but less time will be lost while sterilisation is performed; crucial should there be a number of thoracoscopic cases on the operating list.

Care and maintenance

A maintenance and service contract taken out with the system supplier will deal with equipment servicing and repairs. There are, however, aspects of equipment care which theatre staff can practise and which will help to retain the best possible image quality. All the items of video imaging equipment should be handled gently. Cables must not be coiled tightly and care should be taken not to damage them with towel clips. Cable connectors should be protected by placing any covers over the connector prior to immersion sterilisation.

A few minutes spent inspecting and testing equipment and, where necessary, substituting spares prior to using the video system can avoid many problems (Table 2.1).

The company supplying the equipment should provide comprehensive training for theatre staff on the use of the imaging system, together with details of service and warranty policies, the cost of service contracts and extended warranties. Service and warranty policies should be complied with so that should any piece of equipment fail that is under warranty then backup will be given within 24 hours. This will result in minimum down-time.

Troubleshooting is covered for the theatre staff during the commissioning of the imaging equipment, and is very dependent on the equipment purchased. The most common causes of equipment not performing to its optimum are: 'finger-tip problems' (e.g. wrongly-set switches), failure to white set, and faults in the light guide cables, camera lead, thoracoscope and coupler.

If a problem does occur, a set routine should be followed to try to identify the fault. It may be helpful for the routine to be written out by the supplier.

Signal cabling should not be tampered with. The risk of cable misconnections can be minimised by having a cable

Table 2.1

Theatre department equipment checks

System element	Comment	Action
Fibre optic light guide cable	This is the most vulnerable item in the imaging system. Degradation of the glass fibre light carriers will cause the image quality to deteriorate as insufficient light will be transmitted to allow the CCDs to function properly.	Visual inspection; light transmission test — replace if inadequate; ensure spare is available
Camera head cable	Damage to this will result in erratic picture transmission or complete system failure. The cable is frequently damaged at the junction with the head or at the cable connector which may also break.	Visual inspection; ensure spare field replaceable cable is available if applicable
Optical coupler	The coupler may suffer damage to the optical lenses or focusing ring or fluid may enter the coupler mechanism during sterilisation.	Inspect; replace with spare if malfunctioning
Thoracoscope	Poor light transmission results from damage to the fibre bundles. An image which cannot be focused is caused by the rod lens system becoming out of alignment. Damage to the distal and optical lenses and fogging result from fluid ingress.	Pre-use test; spare or disposable backup scope must be available

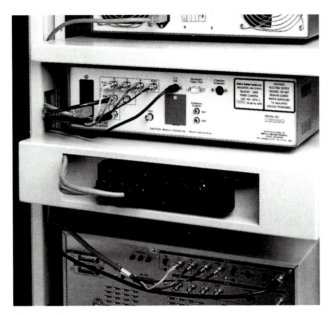

Figure 2.8 *Cable management system.*

management system (Fig. 2.8) on the image systems trolley, and the use of colour-coded labelling of cables and sockets.

The supplier's customer service or technical support telephone number must be readily available. As theatre personnel change, continuing education for theatre staff can prove very beneficial if offered by the supplier.

Technical advances

There have already been significant advances in minimal access surgery imaging technology with improved quality and sensitivity of CCD devices, automatic light level adjustment by auto shutters and image quality enhancement with high resolution cameras and digital processing. Development is currently underway in several fields which should yield considerable advantage in the future.

3-D imaging
3-D imaging requires either a double lens system within an endoscope feeding a twin camera head or twin end CCD

chips. Although such systems are under development at present, current designs tend to impose a size and/or weight premium. The viewing process utilises either a spectacle or helmet-and-visor approach or a special monitor system with rapidly alternating images: both are associated with user fatigue. Continued improvement in size, light quality, resolution, colour reproduction and user acceptability are required to make these systems practicable.

Electronic endoscopes
The primary advantage of the electronic end-chip endoscope is that light loss through the rod lens or fibre optic image transmission system of the endoscope is avoided. These devices offer the potential to reduce scope size below the current standard 10 mm with maintained image quality.

Reduction in CCD size
Reduction in CCD size is crucial to the successful development of both 3-D and electronic endoscope systems. It will also enable smaller and lighter-weight camera heads while retaining high quality and light sensitivity.

Autoclavable camera heads
Totally autoclavable electronic camera heads and cabling will soon be available which should improve turnaround time and obviate present problems with fluid-based disinfectant regimens.

High resolution systems
These will give pictures of greater clarity and definition and will be linked to high resolution television technology to yield image resolution of 1200 lines, i.e. 50% greater than any imaging system currently available.

Digital signal transmission
Use of digital video systems with digital 'firewire' interconnections between units will lead to the highest possible image quality.

Appendix 1: Video terminology

Video signals

These must convey information regarding the picture brightness (luminance), hue and colour (chrominance) and, also, vertical and horizontal synchronization information (sync).

Noise

Electrical noise can enter into the signal processing chain at various points and degrades image quality. The degree of noise is quantified on a logarithmic scale as the signal-to-noise (SN) ratio which is expressed in decibels (dB). The higher this value the lower the noise factor.

Bandwidth

This describes the frequency range over which frequency modulation can be used to transmit video signal information on a carrier frequency. Generally, the wider the available bandwidth the more video information that can be transferred and the better the resulting image.

Image resolution

The resolution of an imaging system describes the number of black lines which can be individually distinguished against a white background on the screen. Resolution is measured as both vertical and horizontal lines with the horizontal measurement generally being used for comparisons. The overall resolution of a system is the result of the additive interaction of all the elements in the signal chain but cannot exceed the level of the poorest component.

This is sometimes referred to as the 'weak link theory'. Typical line resolution values for system components are:

Medical grade monitor	750
3-chip camera	800
Domestic television	450
Betacam recorder	500
S-VHS recorder	400
Domestic VHS recorder	240

Camera resolution is determined by the quality of the CCD(s) used and is generally higher with three-chip cameras.

Television standards

There are three major television standards:

NTSC	(National Television Standards Committee)
PAL	(Phase Alternating Line)
SECAM	Sequentiel Couleur avec Mémoire

Video tapes made for presentation purposes must, therefore, be recorded in a format suitable for viewing in the intended country (see Appendix 2) or enquiries should be made to ascertain that appropriate display equipment is available.

Appendix 2: International video standards

PAL system

Australia, Austria, Belgium, China, Denmark, Finland, Germany, UK, Holland, Hong Kong, Italy, Kuwait, New Zealand, Norway, Portugal, Singapore, Spain, Switzerland, Thailand. Note variations:
PAL-M: Brazil; PAL-N: Argentina, Paraguay, Uruguay.

NTSC system

Bahama Islands, Bolivia, Canada, Chile, Colombia, Ecuador, Jamaica, Japan, Korea, Mexico, Peru, Taiwan, The Philippines, USA, Venezuela.

SECAM system

Bulgaria, France, Guiana, Hungary, Iran, Iraq, Monaco, Poland, Russia.

Planning and equipping a successful video-assisted thoracic surgery (VATS) procedure 3

W.S. Walker

Introduction

There is some debate as to what actually constitutes a video-assisted thoracic surgery (VATS) procedure.[1] At one extreme there are, for example, those operations which can be performed as entirely thoracoscopic procedures while at the other the procedure may be performed through a minithoracotomy with the use of rib retraction and predominant per incision visualisation. Somewhere in the middle lie those procedures which utilise videoendoscopic visualisation and endoscopic dissection but benefit from a small utility or access intercostal incision of 3–5 cm in length which is not spread but which does aid the insertion and use of bulky instruments and specimen delivery. In practical terms, whilst these differences will be strongly argued by proponents of the various techniques the important issue is that VATS is fundamentally simply a surgical technique which allows the operator to get at the operative field in a less destructive manner. The general principles of VATS surgery are, and must remain, identical to those of open thoracic surgery. This chapter considers the circumstances relevant to undertaking a successful VATS procedure: methods of access, optimising the operative conditions, instrumentation and safety.

Access
General considerations

In laparoscopic surgery instruments are inserted through gastight tubes or 'ports'. Whilst this approach may be used in VATS, it is often not necessary to use a tube as instruments may be inserted directly through the small intercostal stab incision.

In this discussion this will be referred to as a 'port' and where a physical tube device is intended this will be specified.

Simple biopsy procedures can be performed using two ports or even one if the thoracoscope incorporates a biopsy channel. Operative videothoracoscopic procedures, however, require at least three: one for the thoracoscope and two for instruments. The availability of two instrument ports is important as effective surgery requires the ability to manipulate and operate using a bimanual approach and this technique should, therefore, be acquired from the outset. Indeed, it could be argued that it is the bimanual operative capability that separates current video-endoscopic VATS procedures from conventional thoracoscopic procedures.

The first step in obtaining good access is to position the patient so as to open the interspaces on the operative side by arching the patient's thoracic cage as much as possible. Breaking the table centrally so as to drop the head and feet is of some value but is not nearly as effective as making extensive use of pillows, bags or, best of all, a mechanical bridge under the dependant chest (Fig. 3.1). Both positioning and draping must allow for rapid conversion to open thoracotomy.

Port placement
Triangulation

Three ports are best placed in a triangular configuration (Fig. 3.2).[2,3] This layout allows the optic to be inserted through any port according to the optimum view at any time. The optimum angle between the optic and any instrument is between 30 and 60° as the optic is then looking in the

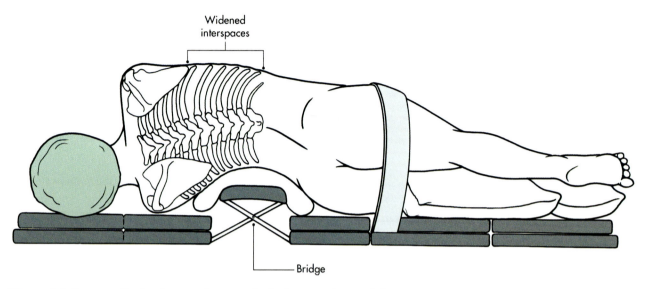

Figure 3.1 *Drawing of bridge elevating the operated side showing widening of the interspaces.*

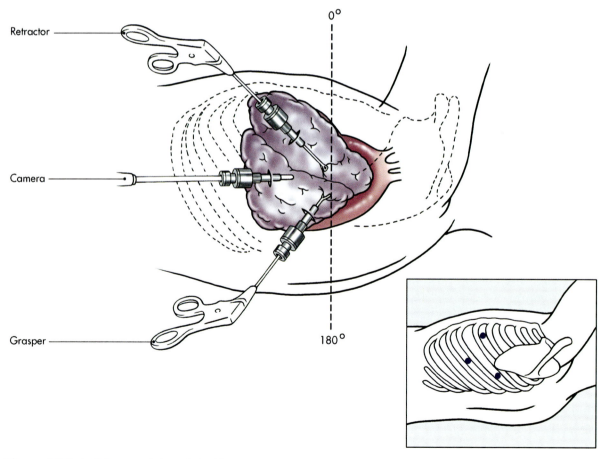

Figure 3.2 *Typical three-port 'triangulation' layout.*

general direction of the instrument. After 90° of angulation the instrument points back towards the viewer which reverses right and left and makes it very difficult to operate effectively. Below 30° the view obtained becomes parallel with the shaft of the instrument(s) with the result that depth perception is lost and it is difficult to determine the position of the end of the instrument. At either extreme it is easy to cross instruments which can then interfere or 'fence' (Fig. 3.3) with each other.

Many texts advise placing the optic centrally in the triangle but this involves the surgeon working around the camera person. In the author's opinion it is often better in thoracoscopic procedures to place the videothoracoscope at the posterior end of the port sequence. Although this

arrangement might appear to present a slightly 'side-on' view, it has several advantages. Manoeuvring is easier, the view provides a good appreciation of instrument depth (Fig. 3.4) and the posterior location of the videothoracoscope presents a view of the thoracic cavity which is similar to that obtained at a standard open posterolateral thoracotomy.

Location

In general, the exact location of the ports is determined by the intended procedure. One should, however, guard against the tendency to select completely different port positions for every procedure: it is often the case that only minor variations are needed between quite different operations, for example, simply moving the ports up or down the chest. This approach preserves broadly similar operative views and spatial relationships thereby facilitating understanding of a procedure for all the staff involved. On occasion, it may also be helpful to consider additional factors:

- An anteriorly placed port will be useful if very large instruments are to be inserted as the interspaces are wider anteriorly.
- A pleural drain will usually be left at the end of the procedure: one port should therefore be located in a comfortable drain position.
- A high anterior port will have a poor cosmetic result whereas an axillary, lateral mammary fold or submammary port will become invisible.

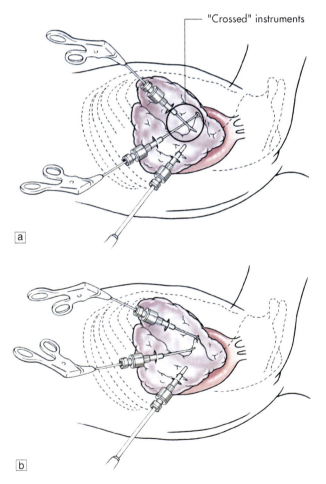

Figure 3.3 *A diagrammatic illustration of (a) incorrect instrument usage, showing 'crossing' and mutual interference of the dissecting instruments, and (b) correct bimanual use.*

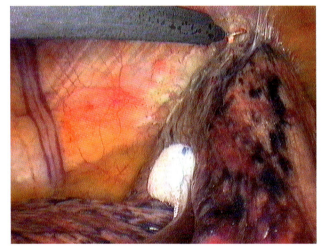

Figure 3.4 *Example of view at VATS during division of apical pleural adhesions using the posterior rather than the central port placement position for the videothoracoscope.*

- Previous drain sites are best avoided as the underlying lung is usually adherent to the chest wall.
- Small patients tend to have particularly narrow posterior interspaces and may experience less postoperative pain if the port sites are kept as far anteriorly as is consistent with safe and effective practice.

Surgical technique for port insertion

Each surgeon will evolve his or her own practice. A very common method is to make a stab incision through the skin and then push a forceps into the pleural cavity. The blades are then separated in order to enlarge the hole. In the author's view this is a crude and ineffective method for several reasons, principally: there is minimal haemostasis, the lung may be damaged (particularly if it is adherent to the parietal pleura) and the surgeon has no opportunity to ensure that the neurovascular bundle is avoided.

The following technique has been evolved on the basis of the author's personal experience and is offered in the belief that it may be of value to those with limited experience in this field of surgery.

Insertion

It is generally easier to create an anterior port first because the interspaces are wider and more superficial. Make a 2–2.5 cm cut through all dermal layers and spread the skin edges using a finger and thumb on either side of the incision. Use a cautery blade on low power to incise the subcutaneous fat taking care not to damage the skin edges. A pair of long forceps, e.g. Roberts, can then be inserted and the blades used to retract the wound edges. Divide or split the underlying muscle fibres until the chest wall is reached. Use the cautery to enter the chest along the top border of a rib under direct vision (Fig. 3.5). Careful haemostasis at all stages makes it easier to create the port safely and avoids the annoyance of port site oozing during the procedure, which can obscure the videoscope lens. Make a very small initial pleural incision. Air should hiss inwards when the first port is created. Gently use the obturator of a thoracoport or forceps to enlarge the pleural opening. Insert the port and withdraw the obturator. A thoracoscope can now be inserted and the interior of the thoracic cavity viewed. Further ports should be created using the same technique after determining the optimal

Figure 3.5 *Drawing of creation of a VATS port showing the use of long forceps blades as tissue retractors in order to expose the intercostal space.*

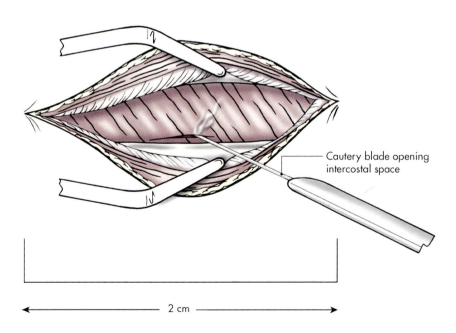

Cautery blade opening intercostal space

2 cm

sites based on the internal view and having excluded or mobilised adherent lung.

If lung is adherent beneath the initial port site try inserting a fingertip and sweeping it away. If this does not work easily, try making a new port in a different site. Fat patients are often best managed by making a deliberately large skin incision of 3–3.5 cm for the ports. This affords the surgeon a better view of the deeper tissues, allowing the remainder of the port to be created in the normal manner.

Closure

Use the thoracoscope to check for internal bleeding and to ensure that each port site is dry. If there is bleeding from a port site do not randomly cauterise the suspected area. This will likely result in a neuropraxic injury to the intercostal nerve and is frequently ineffective in controlling the bleeding. It is better to insert the corner of a swab using an artery forceps. This acts as a tampon and when it is removed after a few minutes the bleeding will frequently have stopped. If it has not, reinsert the swab and then slowly withdraw it until the bleeding point is exposed. Control this by accurate cautery or with deep sutures placed through the port site. In either case make sure that the intercostal nerve is not injured.

If a drain is to be inserted through the port site, a deep absorbable suture can be used to reduce the hole size and so improve the seal around the drain. Also the suture retaining the drain can be placed across the port wound so as to reduce the skin opening (Fig. 3.6). Otherwise, close the muscle and fat with several deep absorbable sutures and close the skin as preferred.

Gaining access through the port site

Decide whether to use a port or simply to pass instruments through the port site directly into the chest. A standard port (10 mm) must be used for the thoracoscope in order to keep it clean. A larger port (12 mm) may facilitate the passage of some instruments such as endoscopic staplers or clip appliers in fat people or through narrow posterior interspaces. Otherwise, it is often easier to operate without a port as curved and conventional instruments can be passed and a much wider range of movement is possible.

Regardless of whether or not a port is used, excessive leverage or torque at the port site should be avoided as this will injure the intercostal bundle and can result in

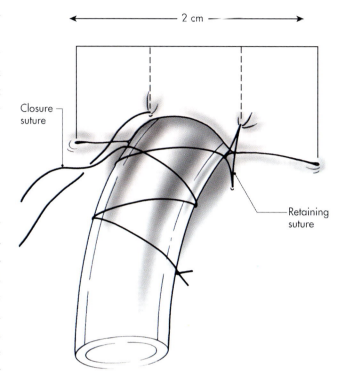

Figure 3.6 *Drawing of closed port site with drain.*

neuropraxic symptoms. This problem is less likely when a port is not used but the intercostal bundle can also be injured by direct trauma created during the passage of large instruments. The value of a minimal access approach is much reduced if the patient is left with persisting intercostal neuralgia.

Access — key points

- Position the patient so as to open the interspaces as much as possible
- Use a triangular port arrangement
- Avoid instrument 'fencing'
- Do not work towards yourself
- Use both hands
- Consider whether the port placement sites should be modified in view of the patient's circumstances
- Create the ports carefully and haemostatically under direct vision
- Consider whether it would be helpful to extend one port into a utility incision.

Optimising operating conditions

Ventilatory management

Room to operate within the chest is obtained in thoracoscopic surgery by a process which is the reverse of laparoscopic surgery. In abdominal procedures CO_2 is used to expand the abdominal cavity; in thoracic surgery space is obtained by reducing the volume of the ipsilateral lung. If this cannot be achieved — either because the pleural cavity is obliterated by adhesions or because the lung is hyperinflated — the procedure must be abandoned, as vision is impaired, there is no space within which to operate and safety is compromised. Pulmonary collapse can be achieved by:

- creation of a CO_2 pneumothorax
- reduced pulmonary ventilatory excursion
- selective lung ventilation.

Creation of a CO_2 pneumothorax requires a closed system so as to retain the CO_2 under pressure and gas-tight port tubes will, therefore, be necessary. It is best to insufflate CO_2 under direct vision through the side arm of a closed thoracoport containing the videothoracoscope. This allows the surgeon to visualise the lung and stop the gas flow when the degree of collapse achieved is adequate for the operative procedure intended. The intrapleural pressure should not exceed 10 mmHg (probably less in children) and the flow rate should be restricted to a maximum of 2 l/min in order to prevent rapid mediastinum movement.

CO_2 insufflation appears to be safe in clinical practice[4] although there is experimental evidence[5,6] to suggest that it can, potentially at least, have serious detrimental effects including mediastinal distortion, elevated central venous pressure and decreased cardiac output.

As with laparoscopic surgery, the requirement for a closed port system can be limiting as instruments are restricted to laparoscopic designs and mobility is reduced by the physical effects of the port. There are, however, potential advantages to this system. Oxygen is excluded from the thoracic cavity so that it should not be possible to initiate combustion by careless use of the electrocautery, single lumen endotracheal intubation can be used instead of double lumen intubation and the degree of insufflation/pulmonary compression can be varied by the surgeon as required.

Reduced ventilatory excursion may be achieved by high frequency jet ventilation. This technique can generate adequate operating conditions for a limited range of operative procedures such as pulmonary biopsy and wedge excisions or pneumothorax surgery. Lung motion is reduced but not eliminated and the volume is typically reduced only by 30–40%, so that access to the mediastinal and hilar regions and lung extremities remains poor. The primary advantage is continued ventilation, which may reduce the shunt effect inherent in one-lung anaesthesia and can prove valuable in managing elderly patients with poor lung function and in children who may be too small to allow double lumen endotracheal intubation. A closed system is not required and atmospheric pressure will aid pulmonary collapse.

Selective lung ventilation allows complete collapse of the ipsilateral lung which is motionless. This technique undoubtedly affords optimal operating conditions for any operative procedure, and is essential for major VATS procedures, particularly those involving dissection in or near the pulmonary hilum. Double lumen endobronchial intubation with selective lung ventilation is the preferred technique but different strategies may be required in children due to the size constraints imposed by current double lumen tube designs. Alternate techniques include the use of a bronchus blocker or deliberately advancing a conventional endotracheal tube into the contralateral main bronchus to exclude the ipsilateral lung. If selective lung ventilation is employed, open port tubes or simple port holes are used so that the lung will collapse on exposure to atmospheric pressure. It is important to allow adequate time for this process to occur and with emphysematous lungs 10 to 15 minutes may be necessary.

While a well placed double lumen tube provides excellent operating conditions, a misplaced tube is a disaster as it almost always results in air trapping and a hyperexpanded ipsilateral lung. Tube position should be checked bronchoscopically prior to proceeding with surgery as misplacement is common.[7] It is often possible to reposition a tube which has moved during surgery under bronchoscopic guidance[8] but if this cannot be rapidly achieved, this situation should be taken as an indication for conversion to an open procedure. The shunt through the collapsed lung may cause marked hypoxia. Continuous positive airway pressure has been advocated to improved this problem[9,10] but it may cause the lung to re-expand to a troublesome degree, and either intermittent insufflation of the operative lung with oxygen or delivery of continuous entrained oxygen to the lung may be useful alternative strategies. This problem is particularly noticeable in the initial phase of pulmonary collapse before hypoxic pulmonary vasoconstriction has occurred and, in our experience, oxygenation will usually improve as this process becomes established.

Adhesions

Adhesions are a significant problem. If they do not prevent adequate exposure for the intended procedure they may be ignored but it is generally safest to divide them under direct vision with a cautery. This allows the lung to collapse fully and makes it easier to manipulate or retract the lung, which may be necessary to correctly carry out a procedure or even to allow the pathology to be identified. The culprit apical bulla in a pneumothorax case may, for example, be surrounded by adhesions and if these are not divided the bulla can neither be identified nor controlled.

Theatre logistics

Video monitors should be positioned so as to provide a clear view for the surgeon, assistant(s) and scrub nurse. While this may seem self-evident, it is amazing how often the surgeon is forced into an awkward position simply because the monitors are not positioned intelligently. Positioning these at the top of the table is often recommended, but this is only suitable if the videothoracoscope is located centrally and inferiorly on the lateral chest and pointing towards the head. In general, the scope should point at the monitor so that the surgeon 'looks' in the same direction as the videothoracoscope. We have found that with a posterior scope placement site the monitors can be conveniently located opposite each other, providing excellent linkage between visualisation and functionality (Fig. 3.7).

The theatre lights should be dimmed and any windows covered if necessary to achieve low light levels. Trailing wires are dangerous and should at least be suspended above the table head. Cheap self-adhesive plastic cable conduit can easily be obtained from an electrical supplier and stuck to the theatre walls and ceiling where outlet sockets are on opposite walls, thereby removing the need for trailing wires completely. A major thoracic surgery instrument tray must be available beside the scrub nurse in case it is needed and the positioning of this should be taken into account when considering the theatre layout.

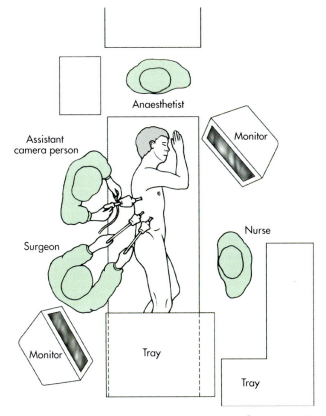

Figure 3.7 *Diagrammatic representation of one possible arrangement for the positions of the surgeon, assistant / camera person, nurse and monitors.*

Optimising operating conditions — key points

- Marked air trapping or dense pleural adhesions are indications for conversion to an open procedure
- CO_2 insufflation should be performed under videothoracoscopic control and requires a closed system with full endoscopic instrumentation
- Lung exclusion, ideally by double lumen endobronchial intubation, provides the optimal operating conditions — but pulmonary collapse may require 10–15 minutes to fully develop
- In general, all intrapleural adhesions should be divided before proceeding with a VATS procedure
- Monitors should be positioned in the same sense as the videothoracoscope and unnecessary wiring routed away from the operating table.

Instrumentation

Ports

As previously observed a physical port device is often not necessary. A variety of trochar and cannula devices are available (see Table 3.1 and Figs. 3.8–3.11) but for most purposes if a port is used a simple tube type is perfectly adequate. Reusable tube ports are available and should be preferred. Disposable types may be a better solution if CO_2 insufflation is used, however; in order to guarantee cleanliness, an integral valve mechanism is then required.

Telescopes

The technology underlying telescope design has been discussed in detail in Chapter 2. Currently, 10 mm videothoracoscopes predominate but the choice between an end-viewing 0 degree or angled (30°, 45°, 60° or greater) telescope is ultimately a matter for surgeon preference. A 0 degree instrument may offer the greatest versatility as it can be used for any procedure. It is certainly easier for the surgical team to follow the spatial relationships within an operative procedure if the viewing angle is constant rather than subject to variation (as is the case when the videothoracoscope is changed to one of a different angle during the procedure). Similarly, flexible thoracoscopes may add some confusion due to a constantly changing viewing angle, and optical transmission may be less efficient than with a rigid design. Angled or flexible 'scopes can, however, be of particular advantage in certain circumstances where it is difficult to visualise the operative field directly. They have, for example, been advocated for use in thoracoscopic take-down of the internal mammary artery during minimally invasive coronary artery bypass (MID CAB) procedures.

As optical transmission technology has developed the quality of the image provided by narrow calibre thoracoscopes has improved such that the view provided by a 5 mm instrument can be equivalent to that previously obtained with a 10 mm one. It would seem likely that the emphasis will shift towards narrower calibre instruments, particularly for small female patients, in order to reduce the risk of neuropraxic injury occurring at the videothoracoscope port site.

Operating instruments

Obtaining and handling specimens

Virtually any biopsy forceps can be put to good use within the chest including those used for rigid bronchoscopy. It is

Table 3.1

Port types available for VATS procedures

Port type	Characteristics
Rigid open tube cannula	Often has a spiral ridge winding along the cannula which serves to grip the chest wall tissue (Fig. 3.8)
Flexible open tube cannula	May exert less pressure on the intercostal bundle (Fig. 3.9)
Valved rigid cannula	Standard in laparoscopic practice and required for thoracoscopic procedures where CO_2 insufflation is used (Fig. 3.10)
Valved rigid cannula with cutting blade	Avoids the possibility of sharp trochar injury to tissues by using a direct vision device where the progress of the port through the chest wall can be directly monitored by the videothoracoscope (Fig. 3.11)

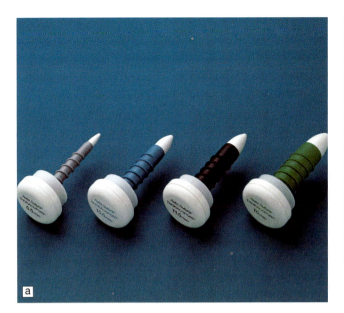

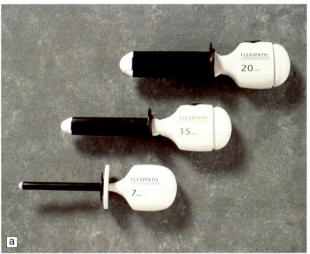

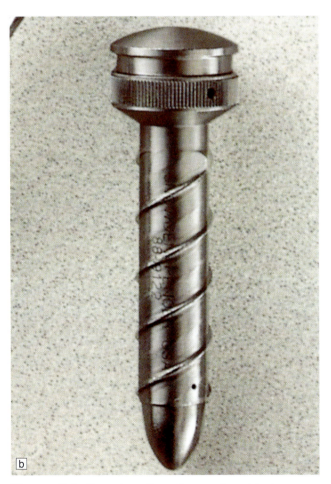

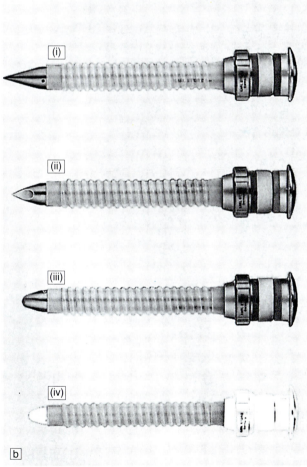

Figure 3.8 *Examples of rigid cannulae: (a) Autosuture (disposable) rigid cannulae, colour-coded according to size, and (b) Snowden-Pencer (reuseable) rigid cannula with obturator in situ.*

Figure 3.9 *Examples of flexible cannulae: (a) Ethicon (disposable) and (b) Storz (reusable) flexible cannulae, with (i) conical tip, (ii) pyramidal tip, and (iii) blunt tip trocars; (iv) Storz autoclavable flexible cannula.*

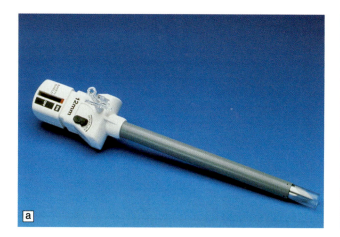

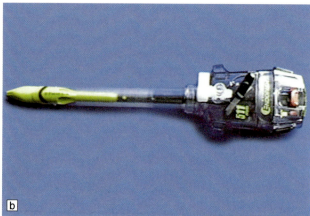

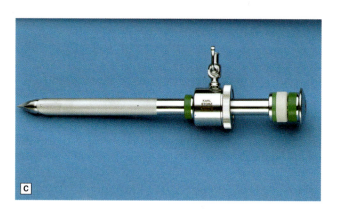

Figure 3.10 *Examples of valved rigid cannulae: (a) Autosuture (disposable) and (b) Ethicon standard (disposable) laparoscopic devices and (c) Storz (reusable) thoracoscopic device.*

helpful to use instruments with insulated shafts, e.g. many forms of mediastinoscopy biopsy forceps, as these can be used to cauterise the biopsy site. Soft tissue core biopsy needles work well for sampling pulmonary mass lesions. Biopsy and resection specimens can potentially seed tumour cell into the chest wall.[11] This can be prevented with small samples by inserting the biopsy instrument through a port tube so that chest wall tissue is shielded. Larger specimens will require to be placed inside a small polythene bag within the chest prior to extraction using either a purpose designed endoscopic bag (Fig. 3.12) or simply a sterile polythene bag used to package a sterile item.

Dissection

A large range of dissection instruments are available for thoracoscopic surgery and may be classified as:

1. conventional instruments
2. modified conventional instruments
3. endoscopic instruments (reusable and disposable).

(i) Standard conventional instruments

A Robert's forceps with a mounted peanut pledglet can serve as a palpation device while two can provide a bimanual capability. Light, long, straight and curved vascular clamps make very useful general instruments as they are hinged at about their mid points and can therefore, be opened widely through a small opening. They may be used as dissectors, clamps or pick-ups as required. Long scissors of the Nelson pattern are useful for division of broad areas of adhesion and for occasional use rather than opening a disposable item. In general, the larger instruments will work best when introduced through an anteriorly placed utility incision as the blades can then be opened most effectively.

Long Babcock forceps may be used to hold specimens but lung is best handled with broad-bladed ring pattern forceps. We have found that Rampley's sponge-holding forceps make effective lung forceps.

(ii) Modified conventional instruments

There are several eponymously named sets of thoracoscopic instruments on the market. Most of these contain some

28

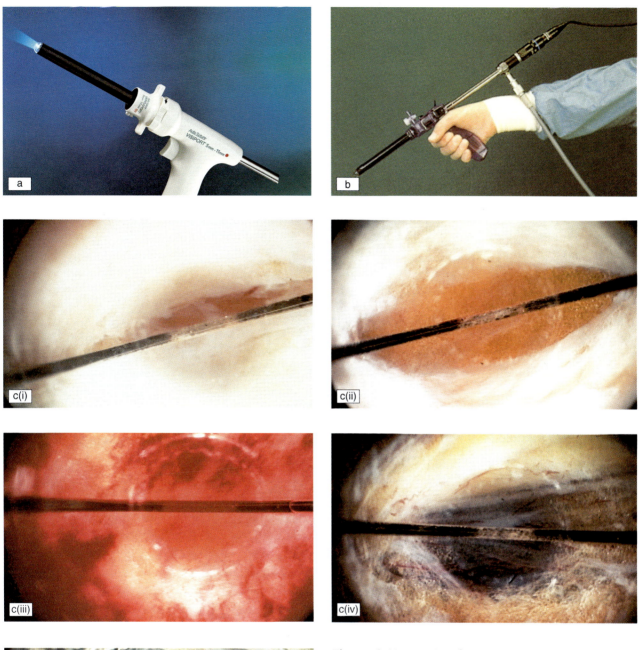

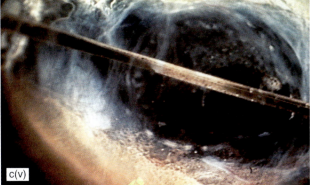

Figure 3.11 *Examples of disposable valved rigid cannula with cutting blade designs (a) and (b). These allow entry into the chest under direct vision as illustrated in images (c) (i)–(v) pictures obtained in the process of cutting through the tissue layers. This design allows the surgeon to see exactly when the thorax or abdomen is entered, thereby minimising the risk of inadvertent injury to the lung or abdominal viscera.*

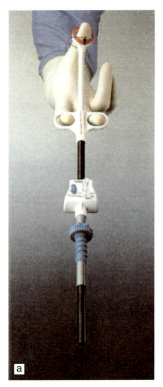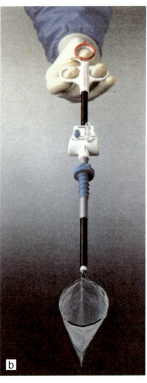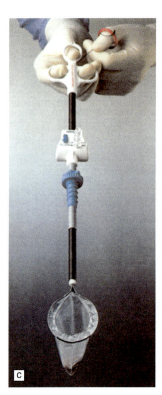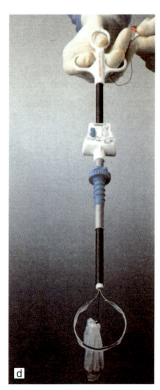

Figure 3.12 *Endoscopic specimen bag (Endobag™, Autosuture); four views showing Endocatch™ in action.*

useful instruments and others of somewhat limited value, as one surgeon clearly cannot have a sufficient range of experience to utilise or be able to endorse an entire range. Purpose-focused sets are of value e.g. Kaiser lung-holding ring forceps (Circom ACMI), while technique-orientated sets facilitate the performance of procedures in the manner of the associated surgeon. There are currently two such sets, both derived from modified conventional instruments, which deserve mention. These are:

● the Giudicelli instrument set (made by Stortz) designed primarily for Giudelli's 'minithoracotomy' lobectomy technique.
● the Lewis VATS instrument set (made by Thoramet) designed for general VATS pulmonary work but particularly suited to Lewis's 'simultaneously stapled' lobectomy technique.

These sets both move the hinge region of the instrument towards the middle, i.e. the portion of the instrument close to the port incision, in order to maximise opening. In addition the Giudicelli set employs an 'S' shaped bend (Fig. 3.21) in the instrument to enable the surgeon to operate through a minithoracotomy without obscuring his view

while the Lewis set utilizes offset 'switchback' blades (Fig. 3.22) to further increase jaw opening.

(iii) Endoscopic instruments
Endoscopic disposable scissors are cheap, light and very sharp; undoubtedly superior to reusable items, they should be used for preference. Disposable endoscopic dissectors — usually of the Maryland pattern — are also excellent, but satisfactory reusable items exist and may be preferred on economic grounds. Disposable endoscopic lung graspers are, in the author's opinion, of limited value and tend to slip easily but long, straight reusable endoscopic graspers are useful for manipulating the lung apex or as long peanut pledglet holders.

Suction is best performed using endoscopic devices. Reusable devices usually have a valve mechanism which can become sticky with repeated sterilisation; and disposable versions are available which also combine irrigation and cautery functions (Fig. 3.13). Suction should be performed beneath the surface of any fluid collection, and if smoke is being removed an open port should be available to allow through-flow of air, so as not to reduce the intrathoracic pressure which may encourage re-expansion of the lung.

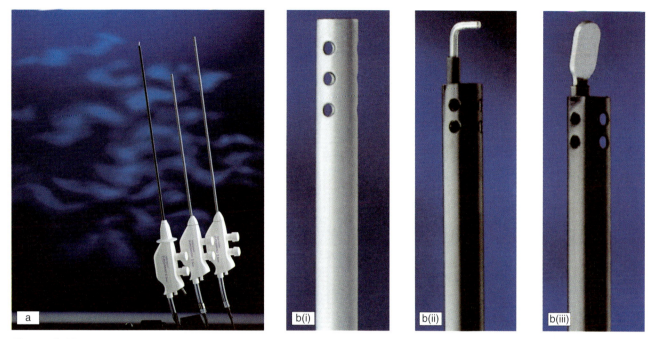

Figure 3.13 *(a) Combined sucker / diathermy / irrigation device (Autosuture) and (b) (i)–(iii) the different tips available.*

Design considerations

Unfortunately, many of the endoscopic instruments specifically designed for VATS appear to be derived from laparoscopic patterns and it is probably true to say that a great deal of development is still required. Some of the factors to take into account when selecting instruments are:

- *Jaw action*. Double action jaws (Fig. 3.14a) (i.e. those where each jaw moves equally) are almost invariably used in conventional instruments. These produce a smoother action than instruments with one moving jaw (Fig. 3.14b) which rock slightly from side to side when opened and closed (Fig. 3.14).
- *Jaw size*. Large curved jaws may facilitate dissection round relatively large structures in thoracic surgery. Laparoscopic instruments, however, must be inserted through a port and this consideration limits both the maximum possible deviation of the jaw from the axial line and the length of the blades. In thoracoscopic surgery it is common to insert instruments directly into the chest via a simple port incision so that the surgeon can insert instruments with large and angled or curved jaws as required.
- *Complexity*. Curved instruments (Fig. 3.15a) allow additional degrees of freedom of movement (Fig. 3.15b) and may be helpful for manoeuvring around structures. However, they do require additional expertise and may add unnecessary complexity for most practical purposes.

- *Grip*. Conventional instruments usually employ a scissors grip whereas many endoscopic instruments utilise a pistol grip. Both are perfectly satisfactory, but the scissors grip may feel more natural. It lends itself more easily to fingertip use for delicate manoeuvres.
- *Cost*. Endoscopic instruments are expensive and less robust than conventional ones. Is an endoscopic pattern needed? Disposable instruments are a very expensive solution — will a reusable item suffice? Is a specific instrument required at all?

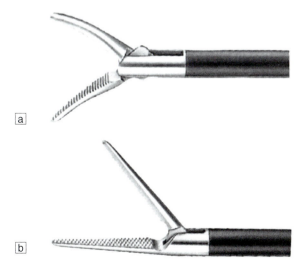

Figure 3.14 *Photograph comparing (a) double moving and (b) single moving blades.*

Staplers

Endoscopic linear staplers are available with 30, 35, 45 or 60 mm jaw lengths (Fig. 3.16) and are now also available with 45 degree bilateral anvil articulation (Fig. 3.17). Different staple leg length sizes are denoted by colour-coded cartridges which should be selected using a purpose-designed tissue thickness gauge according to the thickness of the tissue to be divided. However, few surgeons bother to do this as the correct loads have become well established (Table 3.2).

The 30 and 45 mm staplers can be introduced through a 12 mm port tube or directly through a port site but the 60 mm staplers are very wide (>15 mm) and should be inserted through an anterior port site or access incision.

The structures of the pulmonary hilum tend to radiate centrifugally. Conversely, instruments inserted through ports or port sites pass in a centripetal manner towards

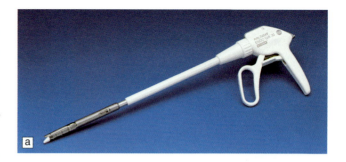

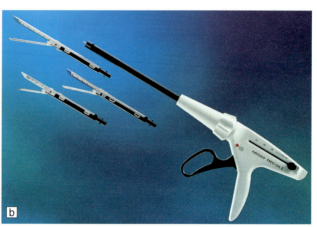

Figure 3.16 (a) Standard Autosuture EndoGIA 30, Stapler and (b) EndoGia II multiple cartridge stapler.

the hilum and, therefore, are orientated in a largely parallel direction to the hilar structures. The use of stapling devices, on the other hand, requires that structures to be divided should be at right angles to the stapler. This incongruity can only be resolved by angling the stapler (which is helped by the new roticulating 45 mm devices) and by orientating the hilar structures using slings. Slings also allow the surgeon to elevate structures, facilitating dissection and the passage of larger instruments.

Other instruments and devices

A variety of other instruments and techniques — some novel and others applications of established practice — have been described in the relevant literature.

Oesophageal identification is facilitated by the use of an illuminated bougie (Fig. 3.18) which may obviate the use of an endoscope during oesophageal myotomy procedures. One of the potential advantages of VATS is rapid patient mobilisation and discharge, but this is not

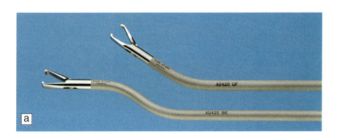

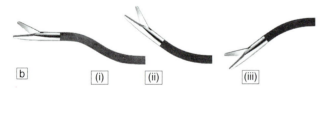

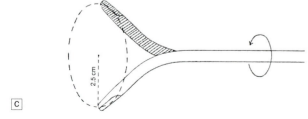

Figure 3.15 (a) Storz Cuschieri pattern instruments and (b) the different tips to fit them: (i) bayonet shaped, (ii) coaxial curved up and (iii) coaxial curved down. (c) Sketch to show how coaxial instruments allow dissection behind anatomical structures by rotating the outer tube, so that the risk of tissue ruptures is decreased.

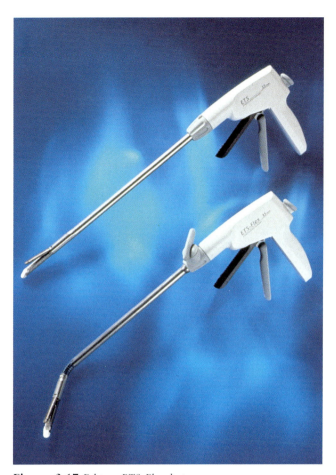

Figure 3.17 *Ethicon ETS-Flex device.*

Table 3.2

Endoscopic stapler colour-codes and usage

Cartridge colour	Staple size (mm)	Use
Grey	2.0	Thin walled blood vessels
White	2.5	Other blood vessels, thin bullae
Blue	3.5	Most lung tissue, normal oesophagus
Green	4.8	Bronchus, very dense lung tissue, thick oesophagus

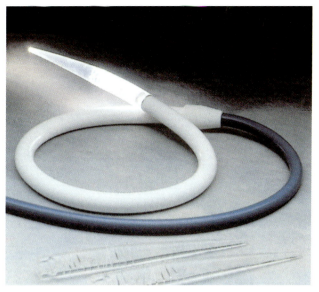

Figure 3.18 *Illuminated oesophageal bougie (Endolumina: BioEnterics).*

possible in the presence of continuing air leakage from lung closure sites. Attempts to deal with this problem have included the application of fibrin-based tissue glue to the staple lines and, more recently, the use of pericardial (Figs. 3.19a–c)[12] and Goretex[13] strips to buttress staple lines. Figures 3.19 (d)–(g) show the Ethicon stapleline sealant system. Although these measures have been of some help, the recent development of a polyethylene glycol-based gel polymer specifically designed as a biological sealant offers the exciting prospect of near zero post-operative air leakage.[14] If this goal can be achieved, early discharge may become a much more easily achieved objective, and the advantages of the VATS approach more clearly identifiable.

Attempts to utilise lasers for shrinkage of bullae and pulmonary parenchymal excision have not proved advantageous due to prolonged air leak, and standard unipolar and bipolar electrocautery remain the mainstay of small vessel haemostasis in VATS. These can usefully be augmented by Helium and Argon ion beams for coagulation of oozing areas. The ultrasonic harmonic scalpel (Fig. 3.20) can be used to coagulate small vessels and appears to work well in laparoscopic surgery.[15] It may offer advantages in a VATS context by reducing smoke production and collateral tissue damage and by avoiding electrical hazards.

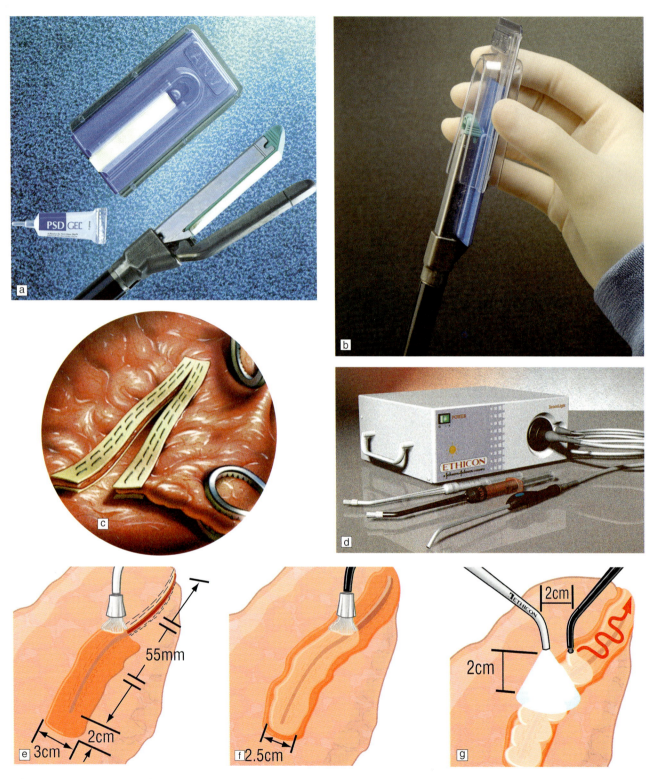

Figure 3.19 *Two strategies for sealing pulmonary staple lanes. (a) Peristrips system (from Somatech Medical Ltd); (b) Peristrips on stapler blades; and (c) Peristrips Dry buttress staple lines during lung resection procedure. (d) Ethicon Advaseal® sealant system, light generator, seal and brush applicators and light wand; (e) application of Advaseal® primer to pulmonary staple line; (f) application of Advaseal® sealant within boundaries of primed tissue and (g) activating light beam. Note: beam should follow sealant application closely.*

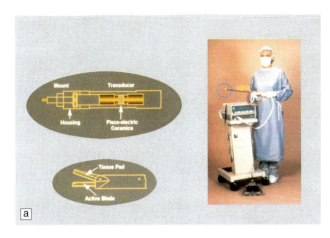

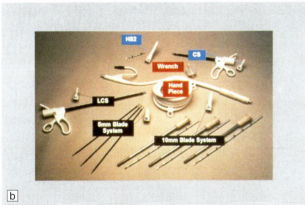

Figure 3.20 *(a) UltraCision machine and (b) various blades for the device.*

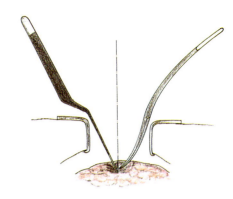

Figure 3.21 *Sketch showing side view of 'S'-shaped dissecting forceps (left) and scissors from the Giudicelli VATS instrument set. The curve allows manoeuvrability without compromising the surgeon's view, when operating under direct vision through a mini thoracotomy.*

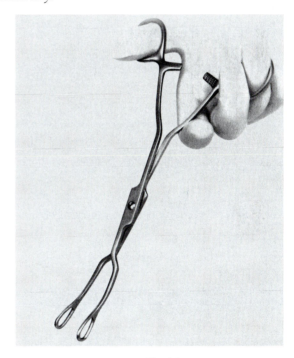

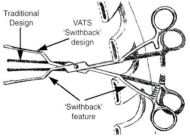

Figure 3.22 *Sketch illustrating the 'switchback' design of forceps from the Lewis VATS instrument set. This offers a usefully wide jaw opening within a narrow operating space.*

Instrumentation — key points

- Instrument selection for VATS should be purpose-orientated and based on surgeon preference
- Conventional long forceps, scissors and vascular clamps are particularly useful
- Select a few VATS instruments rather than purchase a complete set
- Novel instrument shapes may add to rather than reduce procedure complexity
- Few disposable dissection instruments are necessary but endoscopic scissors and Maryland dissectors are economic and probably superior to reuseable versions
- Staplers and cartridges must be selected according to the type and thickness of tissue to be divided
- Measures to reduce postoperative pulmonary air leakage may increase the potential benefits of a VATS procedure.

35

Safety

Diathermy

(i) Use of metallic ports

The high frequencies and voltages inherent in monopolar diathermy equipment can cause inadvertent charging of metal instruments and telescopes during endoscopic use, due either to direct contact or to capacitive coupling.[16] The charge can then discharge on to the viscera and cause burn injuries. This problem is particularly likely when the thoracoscope and any metallic instruments have been inserted through plastic ports, as these act as insulators, preventing the charged instrument from discharging into the body via the insertion site. A metal port will earth any conductive instrument passed through it and should, therefore, always be used for the thoracoscope, at least, as this is the largest metal object in the chest.

(ii) Monopolar versus bipolar

Bipolar diathermy provides a limited current path with minimal collateral current spread. It does, however, require the use of a specific bipolar instrument and, although these come in thoracoscopic versions, monopolar diathermy is generally more convenient, as it can be applied through most of the current endoscopic instruments. Subject to the considerations discussed in (i) above, monopolar diathermy is generally entirely safe for thoracoscopic use but:

- lower power settings should be employed than with open surgery;
- bipolar diathermy should be used when working near:
  - the heart (risk of dysrhythmias)
  - vertebral foramina (risk of spinal cord injury)
  - oesophageal mucosa (risk of perforation).

(iii) Air leakage

Major air leaks flood the thoracic cavity with oxygen-rich gas. In this situation sparks from the diathermy may cause an intrathoracic fire. If the cautery is to be used in this situation it is safer to flush the thoracic cavity with CO_2 in order to reduce the explosion risk.

(iv) Precautions against ventricular fibrillation

In any situation where diathermy is used near the heart it is sensible to have remote defibrillation pads applied to the patient prior to surgery so that ventricular fibrillation can be easily corrected.

The most obvious procedures where this might apply are formation of a pericardial window and endoscopic dissection of the internal mammary artery.

Use of instruments

(i) General handling

Instruments should be inserted and advanced only when the surgeon can see the direction the instrument follows. Advancing the instrument unsighted increases the risk of inadvertently puncturing structures; the tips of any instrument, particularly scissors, must be visible at all times. When scissors are to be used or a clamp or stapler applied, the surgeon must check that the blades or jaws of the instrument do not include or jeopardise other structures.

(ii) Stapler technique

Endoscopic staplers have proved to be extremely safe in clinical practice but if misfired or misused they can result in a potentially serious intraoperative situation. Correct usage requires that the surgeon ensures that:

- the tip of the device can be seen
- only the intended structure will be divided
- the tissue for division is of uniform and appropriate thickness
- it lies within the 'cut' markers on the device
- the correct staple leg length has been chosen
- the cartridge is correctly loaded.

It is important to remove any loose staples from the jaws of the instrument and to make sure that tissue does not encroach on the hinge area of the stapler jaws as either may jam the instrument. It can be helpful to apply sterile lubricating jelly to the jaws of the instrument; this eases the passage of the instrument between structures and prevents loose staples being shed into the operative field as these stick to the jelly. If a large vessel is to be divided, a centrally-placed clamp is a wise precaution.[17]

Coping with haemorrhage

Occasionally it is necessary to convert to open thoracotomy in an emergency manner because of calamitous bleeding occurring at the time of a major intrathoracic procedure. This situation is best dealt with by forward planning. This includes several key elements: the patient should be positioned and draped so that conversion to an immediate major thoracotomy is feasible; every member of the surgical team must be well trained in general open thoracic surgery[18] and the necessary equipment and trays must be immediately to hand beside the patient. We believe it is sensible for all major VATS cases to have arterial pressure monitoring, a large calibre i.v. line *in situ* and blood readily available within the operating theatre area.

Although the instinctive reaction to haemorrhage is to attempt to control the bleeding by placing a vascular clamp, this is a dangerous policy as the videothoracoscopic view is usually lost within seconds and it is very difficult to clamp safely within that time frame. It is better to use those few seconds of vision to insert a swab mounted on a stick through the utility incision and get the assistant to press on the bleeding area. This manoeuvre reduces the chance of creating further damage, and controls blood loss whilst the surgeon opens the chest.

Safety — key points

- Use a metal port for the videothoracoscope
- Use bipolar cautery near the heart, oesophagus and spine
- Ensure that remote difibrillator pads are in place when using cautery near the heart
- Always make sure that a cutting instrument or stapler is properly positioned and fully in view before dividing tissue
- Consider placing a vascular clamp centrally when a significant blood vessel is to be stapled
- Always ensure that the appropriate skilled staff and equipment are available for immediate conversion to open thoracotomy in the event of intraoperative haemorrhage
- Do not grab for a major bleeder with a vascular clamp; use a swab stick to control blood loss by direct pressure whilst the chest is opened.

References

1 Lewis RJ. VATS is not thoracoscopy [letter]. *Ann Thorac Surg* 1996; **62**: 631–2.

2 Landreneau RJ, Mack MJ, Hazelrigg SR *et al*. Video-assisted thoracic surgery: basic technical concepts and intercostal approach strategies. *Ann Thorac Surg* 1992; **54**: 800–7.

3 Landreneau RJ, Mack MJ, Keenan RJ *et al*. Strategic planning for video-assisted thoracic surgery. *Ann Thorac Surg* 1993; **56**: 615–9s.

4 Wolfer R, Krasna M, Hasnain JU, McLaughlin JS. Hemodynamic effects of carbon dioxide insufflation during thoracoscopy. *Ann Thorac Surg* 1994; **58**: 404–8.

5 Jones DR, Graeber GM, Tanguilig GS, Hobbs G, Murray GF. Effects of insufflation on haemodynamics during thoracoscopic procedures. *Ann Thorac Surg* 1993; **55**: 1379–82.

6 Hill RC, Jones DR, Vance RA, Kalantarian MD. Selective lung ventilation during thoracoscopy: effects of insufflation on haemodynamics. *Ann Thorac Surg* 1996; **61**: 945–8.

7 Smith G, Hirsch N, Ehrenwerth J. Placement of double lumen endobronchial tubes. Correlation between clinical impression and bronchoscopic findings. *Br J Anaesthesia* 1986; **58**: 1317–20.

8 Benumof J, Partridge B, Salvatierra C, Keating J. Margin of safety in positioning modern double-lumen endotracheal tubes. *Anaesthesiol* 1987; **67**: 729–38.

9 Caplan L, Turndorf H, Patel C *et al*. Optimization of arterial oxygenation during one lung anaesthesia. *Anesthes Analg* 1980; **59**: 847–51.

10 Horswell JL. Anaesthetic techniques for thoracoscopy. *Ann Thorac Surg* 1993; **56**: 624–9.

11 Downey RJ, McCormack P, LoCicero J. Dissemination of malignant tumours after video-assisted thoracic surgery: a report of 21 cases. *J Thorac Cardiovasc Surg* 1996; **111**: 954–60.

12 Cooper JD. Technique to reduce air leaks after resection of emphysematous lung. *Ann Thorac Surg* 1994; **57**: 1038–9.

13 Vaughn CC, Wolner E, Dahan M *et al*. Prevention of air leaks after pulmonary wedge resection. *Ann Thorac Surg* 1997; **63**: 864–6.

14 Data presented by Ethicon. *European Association for Cardiothoracic Surgery*, Copenhagen, Denmark, September 1997.

15 Swanstrom L, Pennings J. Laparoscopic control of short gastric vessels. *J Am Coll Surg* 1995; **181**: 347–51.

16 Voyles CR, Tucker RD. Education and engineering solutions for potential problems with laparoscopic monopolar electrosurgery. *Am J Surg* 1992; **164**: 57–62.

17 Craig SR, Walker WS. Potential complications of vascular stapling in thoracoscopic pulmonary resection. *Ann Thorac Surg* 1995; **59**: 736–8.

18 Statement of the AATS/STS Joint Committee on thoracoscopy and video-assisted thoracic surgery. *J Thorac Cardiovasc Surg* 1992; **104**:

Thoracic sympathectomy and splanchnicectomy

4

J.G. Geoghegan and P.J. Broe

Introduction

Surgical interruption of intrathoracic autonomic neural pathways has a number of useful clinical applications, particularly upper thoracic sympathectomy for upper limb hyperhydrosis and splanchnicectomy for relief of pancreatic pain. Prior to the development of thoracoscopic techniques, surgical access to both of these autonomic pathways was demanding and was associated with significant morbidity and patient discomfort. Recent advances in endoscopic technology have led to the almost universal adoption of the endoscopic transthoracic route as the preferred technique for upper limb sympathectomy and have also rekindled interest in thoracic splanchnicectomy as a treatment for pancreatic pain.

Anatomical and functional considerations

Topographical anatomy of the thoracic sympathetic chain

The sympathetic chain enters the thorax over the neck of the first rib and continues in a plane beneath the parietal pleura and superficial to the intercostal vessels (Fig. 4.1). It lies on the necks of the ribs in the upper third of the thorax but as the thoracic spine increases in size, the chain comes to lie over the costovertebral joints in the mid thorax and then on the sides of the vertebral bodies in the lower third before passing under the medial arcuate ligament to become continuous with the lumbar chain.

There are usually 10 or 11 ganglia along the chain which may be duplex in places. The first thoracic ganglion and the inferior cervical ganglion usually fuse to form the Stellate ganglion which is located on the neck of the first rib. Additional and highly variable interganglionic connections run parallel to the main trunk and fibres may pass directly from the sympathetic chain (commonly at the level of the second ganglion) to the brachial plexus. This connection is referred to as the nerve of Kuntz and is present in about 10% of individuals (Fig. 4.2).

Preganglionic sympathetic nerve fibres arise from the spinal segments as myelinated fibres and leave the spinal cord in the corresponding spinal nerves. They join the sympathetic ganglia as white rami communicantes and synapse within in the ganglia but may run up or down the sympathetic chain before doing so. Unmyelinated postganglionic fibres leave the sympathetic chain as grey rami communicantes and rejoin the corresponding spinal nerve (Fig. 4.3).

Sympathetic spinal level relationships

Preganglionic fibres for the head and neck emerge from the spinal medulla at the T1 and T2 level. Preganglionic fibres destined for the heart leave from T1-4 and ascend to the cervical ganglia, from which they exit as cardiac nerves. Branches also pass direct from the thoracic sympathetic trunk at T2-4 to the cardiac and pulmonary plexuses. Cardiac visceral sensory fibres pass along the direct branches from the cardiac plexus and up the inferior and middle cardiac nerves to ultimately enter the cord via spinal nerves T1-5. Preganglionic fibres for upper limbs emerge from spinal nerves T2-7 and reach the arm via the ipselateral brachial plexus while those passing to the abdominal structures exit from spinal levels T6-12.

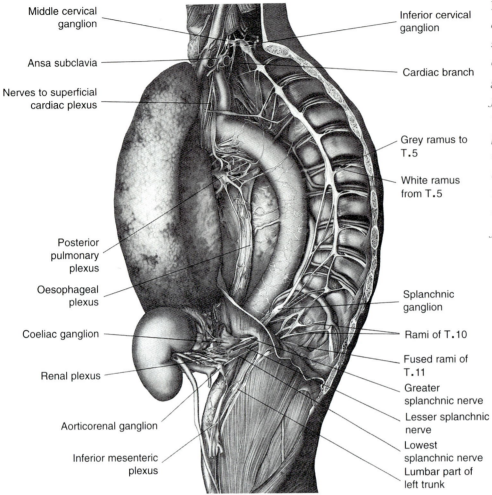

Middle cervical ganglion

Ansa subclavia

Nerves to superficial cardiac plexus

Posterior pulmonary plexus

Oesophageal plexus

Coeliac ganglion

Renal plexus

Aorticorenal ganglion

Inferior mesenteric plexus

Inferior cervical ganglion

Cardiac branch

Grey ramus to T.5

White ramus from T.5

Splanchnic ganglion

Rami of T.10

Fused rami of T.11

Greater splanchnic nerve

Lesser splanchnic nerve

Lowest splanchnic nerve

Lumbar part of left trunk

Figure 4.1 *An anatomical dissection of the left thoracic sympathetic chain. The inferior cervical and first thoracic ganglia are usually fused to form the stellate ganglion, which is often covered by a fat pad and is not therefore seen thoracoscopically. The splanchnic branches are seen arising from the lower sympathetic ganglia. (Reproduced with permission from Gray's Anatomy, 37th ed. Edinburgh: Churchill Livingstone, 1987: 1162.)*

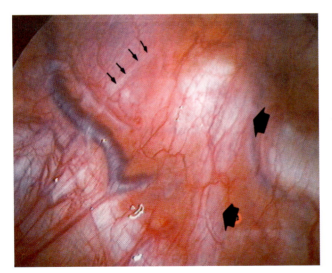

Figure 4.2 *Close-up view of the sympathetic chain (marked by large arrows) with an accessory fibre clearly seen running parallel (marked by small arrows). (Courtesy of Dr. D. Gossot.)*

The stellate ganglion is of particular surgical importance as damage to this structure may interrupt the sympathetic innervation to the eye resulting in Horner's Syndrome (ipselateral meiosis, ptosis, anhidrosis and enophthalmos).

The splanchnic nerves

These are the largest branches of the thoracic sympathetic trunk and arise from the 5th and subsequent ganglia (Fig. 4.1). They pass anteriorly, medially and inferiorly on the bodies of the thoracic vertebrae and contain pre- and post-ganglionic and visceral sensory fibres. There are three nerves. The greater splanchnic nerve which is the largest and most proximal arises by branches from 5th to 9th thoracic ganglia and pierces the crus of the diaphragm to enter the coeliac ganglion. The lesser splanchnic nerve is formed from branches arising from the sympathetic chain in the region of the 9th and 10th ganglia and descends between the chain and

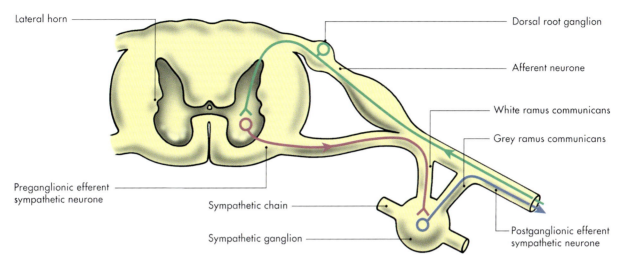

Figure 4.3 *Schematic representation of the interconnections between the sympathetic ganglion and the spinal nerve.*

the greater splanchnic nerve to pierce the diaphragm close to the greater nerve before it too enters the coeliac ganglion. The lowest splanchnic nerve is difficult to visualise surgically as it emerges from the last thoracic ganglion, pierces the diaphragm and enters the renal plexus.

Levels of surgical significance

The functional relationships of each spinal level of the sympathetic chain are variable and interpretations differ between authors in this regard. However, from a surgical perspective where ablation of the sympathetic innervation to a structure is under consideration, the appropriate levels may be summarised as in Table 4.1.

Table 4.1

A working guide to the approximate relationships of function to spinal levels of the sympathetic chain (See Figure 4.1)

Target area	Interruption level
Hand	T2 and T3
Axilla	T4 and T5
Heart	T1 to T4
Coeliac ganglion	Greater and lesser splanchnic nerves

Thoracoscopic sympathectomy

Ablation of the sympathetic outflow to the upper limb has been recognised for many years as an effective treatment for a variety of vasospastic and vascular disorders. A variety of surgical approaches to the upper thoracic sympathetic chain have been used, both cervical (supraclavicular) and transthoracic. The transthoracic endoscopic method was first described by Hughes in 1942,[1] but it is only with recent improvements in endoscopic and video technology that it has gained wider acceptance and superseded other surgical approaches. Compared to the supraclavicular approach, endoscopic transthoracic sympathectomy gives better visualisation of the sympathetic chain, quicker postoperative recovery, a lower complication rate, and a superior cosmetic result. The supraclavicular approach is technically difficult, resulting in a higher risk of pneumothorax and an incidence of Horner's Syndrome in up to 10% of cases.[2] Brachial plexus injury is reported in most series of sympathectomy by the supraclavicular route but has not been reported following thoracoscopic sympathectomy.

Indications

The most common indication for upper thoracic sympathectomy is palmar hyperhydrosis. The value of sympathectomy for this condition was first reported in 1920 by Kotzareff[3] and numerous reports in the scientific literature attest to its effectiveness. Hyperhydrosis is a distressing and socially disabling condition which affects predominantly the palms, axillae and feet. Conservative treatment with aluminium chloride or iontophoresis may be tried but the benefits are usually short-lived. Before advising operation, causes of secondary hyperhydrosis should be excluded, in particular thyrotoxicosis and phaeochromocytoma. Anxiety states may also be associated with hyperhydrosis; psychological assessment may be appropriate in some patients before proceeding with sympathectomy.[3]

Other clear indications for sympathectomy include reflex sympathetic dystrophy and frostbite. Sympathectomy is highly effective in reversing the syndrome of reflex sympathetic dystrophy (causalgia, Sudek's atrophy).[5,6] This is characterised by burning pain, cyanosis, and sweating of a limb following major nerve or bony injury. The patient is typically very protective of the limb and, with prolonged immobilisation, oedema and stiffness result. Over time, progressive atrophic changes occur with the development of fibrosis and joint contracture. Sympathectomy produces excellent results in 80–90% of patients if performed early in the evolution of the syndrome; however the late changes are irreversible and sympathectomy is ineffective if delayed until joint contracture has occurred. Sympathectomy is also effective in ameliorating the effects of frostbite injury, especially if performed within 36–72 hours of cold exposure.[7,8]

Sympathectomy has also been suggested as a treatment for Raynaud's phenomenon: however, in general the results have been disappointing.[9,10] Extensive experience has shown that patients with mild Raynaud's disease usually have a good early response but nearly all eventually relapse, whereas patients with severe Raynaud's syndrome with trophic changes and ulceration rarely achieve even a temporary response. Most surgeons have therefore abandoned sympathectomy for Raynaud's disease. Acrocyanosis is occasionally severe enough to warrant surgical treatment and sympathectomy usually produces a good and sustained response.

Sympathectomy is occasionally tried for digital ischaemia secondary to microembolism, digital atherosclerosis, or Buerger's disease. In the absence of any proximal reconstructible lesion there are limited therapeutic alternatives and sympathectomy may be worth trying since occasionally a gratifying result is obtained.

Experience with thoracoscopic sympathectomy for relief of refractory angina pectoris is largely anecdotal but occasional instances of good symptomatic outcome have been reported. Based on electrocardiographic studies, it has been suggested[11] that the underlying mechanism for any beneficial effect of sympathectomy in this condition may be the shift in balance between sympathetic and vagal tone towards the latter.

Operative technique

A preoperative chest X-ray should be performed to exclude any undetected pulmonary disease which might preclude one-lung anaesthesia or prevent adequate access to the upper thoracic sympathetic chain. Endoscopic transthoracic sympathectomy is performed under general anaesthesia using a double-lumen endotracheal tube. The patient may be placed supine (Fig. 4.4a) or in the lateral position (Fig. 4.4b), and access is improved by placing a sandbag under the shoulder as this improves access to the axilla. The supine position allows bilateral sympathectomies to be performed. Recently, Cuschieri has advocated the use of a semi-prone position on the basis that the lung will naturally fall downwards and away from the posterior chest wall, thereby improving access to the sympathetic chain. In the authors' unit, however, we recommend that one side is done first to allow assessment of the patient's response to the procedure before proceeding with the other side.

A 1 cm skin incision is made in the mid-axillary line over the fourth intercostal space. The underlying lung is disconnected from the ventilator allowing the lung to collapse. The pleural space is entered by blunt dissection with an artery forceps, a 10 mm port inserted and the thoracoscope introduced. Carbon dioxide is not routinely

Table 4.2

Summary of indications for sympathectomy

Established indications	Controversial indications
Hyperhydrosis	Raynaud's disease
Reflex sympathetic dystrophy	Digital ischaemia
Frostbite	Angina pectoris

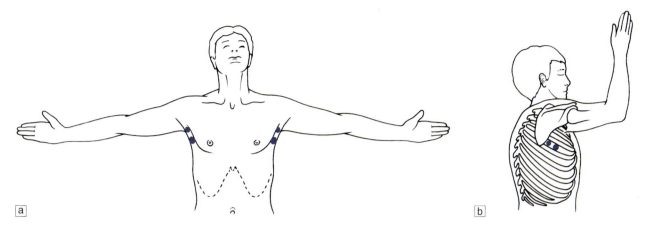

Figure 4.4 *Supine (a) and lateral (b) positions for VATS / thoracoscopic sympathectomy. Note that insertion of cannulae into the axillary and mammary fold areas produces a better cosmetic result.*

insufflated into the pleural cavity although this is occasionally necessary to further collapse the lung, in which case the line pressure should be maintained <10 mmHg. A second (5 mm) port is inserted under endoscopic control in the third or fourth intercostal space adjacent to the 10 mm port. Some surgeons prefer to insert this port in the mid-clavicular line to avoid interference between the camera and the diathermy probe; however, this does diminish the cosmetic result of the operation. Any adhesions tethering the apex of the lung are divided with diathermy. Careful

attention to haemostasis is vital, particularly when the lateral position is used as blood pooling in the paravertebral gutter may obscure the sympathetic chain.

The upper thoracic sympathetic chain is identified beneath the parietal pleura, running over the necks of the ribs (Figs. 4.5, 4.6 and 4.7). The stellate ganglion is usually not visible as it lies beneath a characteristic fat pad on the neck of the first rib (Fig. 4.8). The position of the chain can be confirmed by running a probe along the neck of the rib and feeling the solid trunk of the sympathetic chain rolling underneath it.

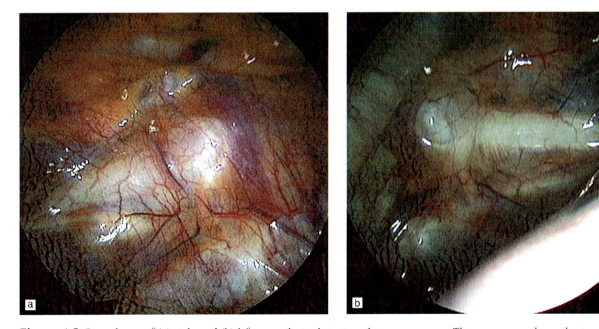

Figure 4.5 *General view of (a) right and (b) left sympathetic chain in a thin young woman. The structure can be easily visualised.*

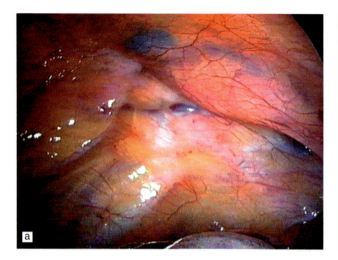

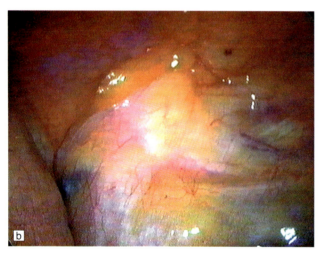

Figure 4.6 *General view of (a) right and (b) left sympathetic chain in an obese middle-aged male. The structure is much harder to visualise through the thicker pleura and extrapleural fat layer.*

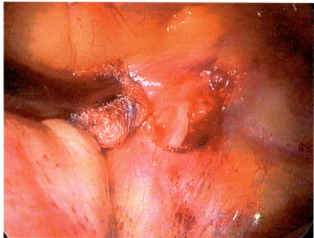

Figure 4.7 *The pleura has been opened in the same patient as seen in Fig. 4.6(b), giving a clear view of the left sympathetic chain.*

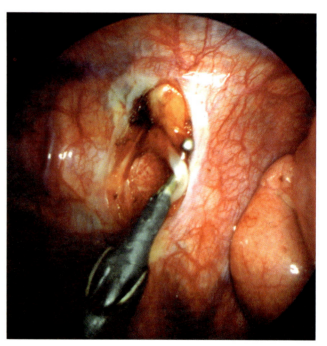

Figure 4.8 *The fat pad over the stellate ganglion is clearly seen in this view of the proximal part of the dissection of the right sympathetic chain. (Courtesy of Dr. D. Gossot).*

The sympathetic chain is then interrupted in the preferred manner. There are basically three technical approaches to thoracoscopic sympathectomy which may be summarised as:

- cautery ablation of the chain at several ganglia
- excision of a segment of the sympathetic chain
- division of the rami communicantes to a segment of the chain with preservation of the main trunk.

Of these, cautery interruption of the chain is the simplest and most common approach (Fig. 4.9). Some surgeons divide the chain with scissors above the second thoracic ganglion (Fig. 4.10) to avoid transmission of

diathermy current to the stellate ganglion and so reduce the likelihood of causing a Horner's syndrome. This is generally not considered necessary. Excision of a segment of the chain is comparable to open surgical practice but apart from offering the opportunity to confirm removal of sympathetic nervous tissue on pathological analysis, it does

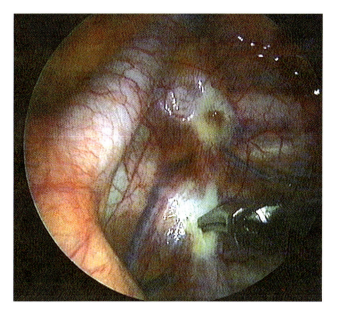

Figure 4.9 *Simple cautery interruption of the left sympathetic chain.*

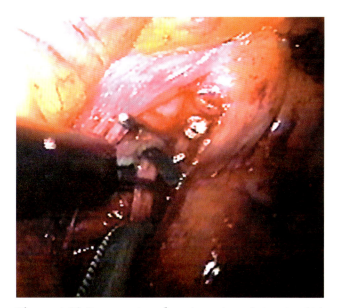

Figure 4.10 *Demonstration of an alternative technique in which the chain (left again) is clipped and divided prior to cautery interruption.*

not seem to confer any specific advantages and does involve a more extensive dissection with increased risk of troublesome bleeding from posterior thoracic wall veins. Careful and meticulous diversion of the rami communicantes whilst preserving the main sympathetic trunk is a novel approach suggested by Wittmoser[12] with a view to reducing

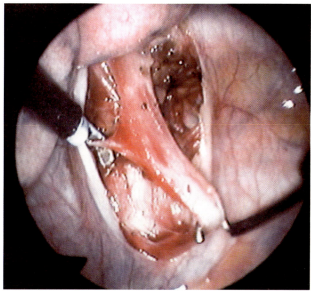

Figure 4.11 *The Wittmoser technique: the sympathetic trunk has been elevated and the rami are being divided. (Courtesy of Dr. D. Gossot).*

the adverse effects of sympathectomy, notably compensatory hyperhidrosis. This technique requires elevation of the sympathetic chain (Fig. 4.11). The authors use unipolar diathermy at the level of the second and third ribs.

The extent of sympathectomy that should be performed has been the subject of some debate. Interruption of the chain at the level of the second and third ribs adequately sympathectomises the hand and this has been the authors' practice. Extending the sympathectomy to the level of the fourth and fifth ganglia has been recommended by some authors for axillary hyperhidrosis, but there is some evidence that this results in a higher incidence of compensatory hyperhidrosis. Extended upper thoracic sympathectomy has a failure rate as high as 40% in the management of axillary hyperhydrosis and axillary skin excision may be considered a better alternative for this condition.[3]

On completion of the sympathectomy, the lung is reinflated under direct vision. If carbon dioxide insufflation has been used, the second port is opened to the outside prior to removal to allow the gas to escape. The muscle layer at the 10 mm port site is sutured with a 2/0 absorbable suture and the skin incisions closed with a subcuticular absorbable suture. A chest drain is not routinely inserted and a chest X-ray is taken in the recovery room.

Postoperative care

The effect of the sympathectomy is usually apparent immediately with the hand feeling warm and dry. Occasionally, the patient may experience a transient return of sweating on the first or second postoperative day. This resolves within 24 hours and reassurance is all that is required. Postoperative pain is usually controlled with oral analgesics. The patient may be discharged the following day and can usually return to work within a week. In some units, this procedure is performed as a day case, although there is a small risk of pneumothorax occurring as a delayed event after the postoperative chest X-ray and, for this reason, the authors prefer to observe the patient overnight.

Complications

Pneumothorax

The reported incidence of pneumothorax in recent series of endoscopic transthoracic sympathectomy is approximately 1%.[13–16] Reinflation of the lung under direct vision and suture of the muscle layer of the chest wall at the 10 mm port site should reduce the incidence of pneumothorax. A significant pneumothorax can usually be aspirated and insertion of a chest drain is rarely necessary.

Horner's syndrome

Horner's syndrome may occur because of injury to the stellate ganglion by direct or transmitted electrocautery. The reported incidence is 2–5%.[10–13] Prevention is by accurate identification of the anatomy, with care being taken to avoid diathermy to the sympathetic chain above the level of the second rib. The use of bipolar diathermy may also help reduce the incidence of this complication. In most cases, Horner's syndrome following thoracoscopic sympathectomy proves to be transient and resolves within 6 weeks.

Postoperative chest or arm pain and paraesthesia

Injury to the intercostal or intercostobrachial nerves may cause unpleasant pain or paraesthesia in their distribution. The sympathetic chain should be cauterised over the neck of the rib and not over the intercostal space to avoid this complication.

Compensatory hyperhidrosis

This condition is characterised by an increase in sweating in other areas of the body, especially the trunk, following thoracic sympathectomy. It has been well documented by various authors reporting large series (Table 4.3).

These data suggest that it is a common symptom (average incidence: 58.4%) but only rarely of disabling severity (average

Table 4.3

Incidence of compensatory hyperhidrosis following thoracoscopic sympathectomy

Author	Yr	Patients	Any compensatory sweating	Disabling compensatory sweating
Sachor[17]	1994	150	50	Not stated
Herbst[18]	1994	323	67.4	Not stated
Drott[19]	1995	850	55	2
Rennie[20]	1996	235	60	1
Gossot[21]	1997	124	65.3	1.6

(Adapted from: Gossot D, Toledo L, Fritsch S, Celerier M. Thoracoscopic sympathectomy for upper limb hyperhidrosis: looking for the right operation. *Ann Thorac Surg* 1997; **64**: 975–8.)

incidence: 1.76%) and one which appears to be independent of the sympathectomy technique used. This phenomenon probably represents a physiological thermoregulatory response as it has been estimated that up to 40% of sweat gland function is lost after extensive bilateral upper thoracic sympathectomy.[22] One theoretical strategy for reducing the incidence of this problem would be to restrict the degree of sympathectomy performed. This approach has been advocated by O'Riordan[23] and Bonjer[24] who have suggested single level sympathetic chain interruption at the second and third ganglia, respectively, and by Rennie[20] and Lemens[25] who have advocated restricting the interruption to the second and third ganglia. Gossot[21] investigated the effect of division of the rami only leaving the chain itself intact — the Wittmoser technique. He compared the results obtained in 54 hyperhidrotic patients undergoing conventional sympathectomy, with 62 undergoing division of the rami communicantes alone. No recurrence was experienced in the conventional group but there was a 5% risk of recurrence in the rami communicantes group (p<0.05). The incidence of compensatory hyperhidrosis was the same in both groups at about 70% but embarrassing (as opposed to disabling) symptoms were greater in the conventional group (50%) in comparison with the rami group (21%) (p<0.001). Compensatory hyperhidrosis is, therefore, so common as to merit detailed pre-operative explanation to the patient regarding this side effect. The incidence is diminished with a selective Wittmoser technique but at the expense of an increased risk of recurrence.

Gustatory sweating, conversely, occurs rarely (<5%) and may be due to aberrant regeneration of the sympathetic fibres.[26] Kux[13] has reported successful correction of this problem by excision of the lower third of the stellate ganglion.

Long-term results

Success rates of approximately 95% with low long-term recurrence rates have been reported from several centres (Table 4.4). Palmar hyperhidrosis is a benign condition and its treatment should combine low morbidity and no mortality, with a good cosmetic result and patient satisfaction. Endoscopic transthoracic sympathectomy fulfils all of these criteria and has deservedly become the preferred method of performing upper thoracic sympathectomy.

Thoracoscopic splanchnicectomy

A number of strategies are available for the management of pain due to unresectable or recurrent pancreatic cancer and chronic pancreatitis. Neurolytic methods can provide excellent pain relief, reducing or removing the patient's requirement for narcotic analgesics. A variety of techniques for pancreatic denervation has been described of which percutaneous coeliac plexus block is the most widely practised.[27] Pain eventually recurs in the majority of patients following coeliac plexus block and, although the procedure may be repeated, the duration of effective pain relief shortens with subsequent blocks.

Table 4.4

Success rates with sympathectomy

Author	Year	Surgical approach	Number of patients	Success rate (%)
Kux[13]	1978	Endoscopic	63	93
Conlon[26]	1987	Supraclavicular	75	95
Byrne[14]	1990	Endoscopic	86	85
Edmondson[15]	1992	Endoscopic	25	92
O'Riordan[23]	1993	Supraclavicular	86	100
Claes[16]	1993	Endoscopic	450	99

In addition, a number of serious complications have been reported following percutaneous coeliac plexus block including paraplegia, monoparesis with loss of bladder and anal sphincter function, and sexual dysfunction.[27,28] Thus while it may prove useful as a temporising procedure, coeliac plexus block has not generally been effective as definitive therapy for chronic pancreatitis. Good results for coeliac ganglionectomy have been reported by Mallet-Guy in Lyons but a number of other authors have failed to reproduce equivalent success rates.[29] Operative exposure of the coeliac axis area in the patient with chronic pancreatitis, who may have had a previous resection, is a difficult undertaking which does not appear to be justifiable in the light of published reports of its effectiveness.

Transthoracic division of the splanchnic nerves with vagotomy for the treatment of chronic pancreatitis was first reported in 1947 by Rienhoff and colleagues.[30] Since then, a number of reports of transthoracic splanchnicectomy have demonstrated sustained relief from pain in approximately two-thirds of patients with chronic pancreatic pain.[31-3] The transthoracic approach avoids dissection in an operative field scarred by inflammation, previous surgery or percutaneous neurolytic block. However, the need for thoracotomy to achieve these results has prevented wider adoption of this procedure.

Thoracoscopic splanchnicectomy is a recently described approach that combines the benefits of a visually controlled division of the splanchnic nerves with the low morbidity and reduced patient discomfort associated with minimal access techniques.[34,35] There has been some controversy as to how extensive a neurectomy is required for adequate pain relief. Some authors recommend bilateral splanchnicectomy, although most reports suggest that left splanchnicectomy can produce equally effective pain relief. Right splanchnicectomy alone has not been shown to produce favourable results. One report[36] suggested that bilateral truncal vagotomy reduced recurrent episodes of pain in alcoholic pancreatitis by reducing acid stimulation of pancreatic secretion, and some authors perform bilateral vagotomy at the same time as left splanchnicectomy. There is insufficient data available to evaluate the role of vagotomy in this context, and its addition to the procedure should be considered empirical. The authors do not routinely include bilateral vagotomy as part of this procedure because of lack of evidence of benefit and concerns over its effects on gastric emptying.

Indications

Thoracoscopic splanchnicectomy is indicated for pain control in patients with unresectable or recurrent pancreatic cancer or for patients with chronic pancreatitis in whom the only alternative surgical option is pancreatic resection.

Operative technique

Thoracoscopic splanchnicectomy is performed under general anaesthesia with the patient in the right lateral position using a double-lumen endotracheal tube to allow single lung ventilation. A pre-operative chest X-ray should be performed to exclude any pre-existing pulmonary disease that might preclude single lung ventilation or cause pleural adhesions. Usually, four ports are required. The thoracoscope is introduced through a 10mm port which is inserted in the sixth intercostal space in the mid-axillary line and the remaining ports are inserted under thoracoscopic control. A second 10 mm port is inserted in the eighth intercostal space in the anterior axillary line, through which a fan retractor is inserted to retract the lower lobe of the lung and the diaphragm. The last two ports, through which the operating instruments are passed, as placed in the ninth intercostal space, mid-axillary line (5 mm port) and the seventh intercostal space, posterior axillary line (10 mm port) (Fig. 4.12).

The sympathetic chain is readily identified running along the necks of the ribs, lateral to the aorta. Through the pleura, the greater and lesser splanchnic nerves can be seen coursing anteriorly and medially as they pass down towards the diaphragm (Fig. 4.13). The parietal pleura is incised over the sympathetic chain and lifted anteriorly, exposing the splanchnic branches. The greater splanchnic nerve usually receives branches from the fifth to the tenth sympathetic ganglia, while the lesser splanchnic nerve receives branches from the ninth to the eleventh ganglia. Each of these splanchnic branches is electrocoagulated and, optionally, clipped, leaving the main sympathetic chain intact (Fig. 4.14).

The authors do not routinely perform vagotomy as part of this procedure because of concerns about its effect on gastric emptying and lack of clear evidence that it is of benefit. However, if desired, the anterior and posterior vagi may be identified and divided on the anterior and posterior aspects of the oesophagus as it passes through the diaphragm.

The lung is reinflated under vision as the ports are removed. A single 28 Fr chest tube is inserted and removed on the second postoperative day. The wounds are closed with absorbable sutures; 2/0 to the muscle layer and subcuticular 4/0 to the skin.

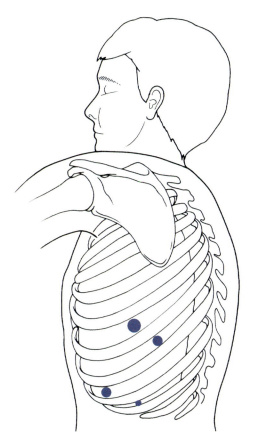

Figure 4.12 *Operative positioning and port sites for VATS splanchnicectomy.*

Complications

None of the reported cases of thoracoscopic splanchnicectomy have recorded any complications.[34,35,37,38] However, the total number of cases is very small and with increasing experience complications specific to the procedure may emerge. Delayed gastric emptying occurs commonly if bilateral truncal vagotomy is added to the procedure. In one series of open splanchnicectomies in which vagotomy was routinely performed, delayed gastric emptying occurred in 11 of 14 patients, although only one required a drainage procedure.[31]

Long-term results

Onset of pain relief occurs very rapidly in almost all patients. In the few reported cases of thoracoscopic splanchnicectomy, good control of pain was achieved in all patients. Cuschieri and colleagues[35] reported that pain was controlled until death by this procedure in three patients

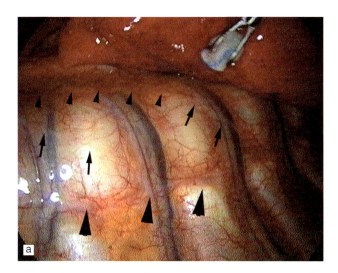

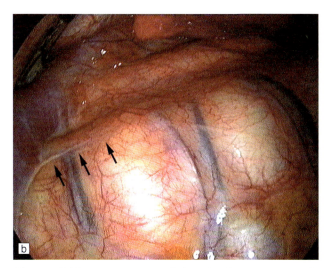

Figure 4.13 *Operative views of the splanchnic nerves: (a) the proximal portion of the greater splanchnic nerve (indicated by short arrowheads), the sympathetic chain (indicated by large arrowheads) and two branches passing from the sympathetic chain to the greater splanchnic nerve (indicated by arrows). In (b) the distal portion of the greater splanchnic nerve (indicated by arrows) is shown as it pierces the diaphragm.*

with pancreatic cancer. In five patients with chronic pancreatitis the pain recurred at variable intervals depending on the severity of the disease. Le Pimpec Barthes[37] recently reported results obtained in 20 patients undergoing splanchnicectomy for pancreatic carcinoma. All were opiate-dependent and 16 experienced complete relief of pain post-operatively. Interestingly, whereas 12 of 16 patients undergoing a unilateral splanchnicectomy procedure were

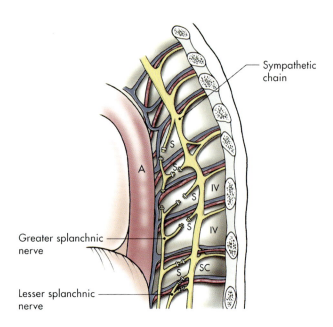

Figure 4.14 *Diagram of the splanchnic nerve branches divided during left thoracoscopic splanchnicectomy. S, splanchnic nerves; A, aorta; IV, intercostal vessels; SC, sympathetic chain.*

rendered pain free this was achieved in all four of those undergoing a bilateral approach. The authors suggested that a bilateral approach was not generally necessary, however, as an initial left procedure it is usually effective. A subsequent right-sided procedure could be a second-line option for those with persisting symptoms. Similar results have been described by Noppen[38] in a smaller series of seven patients with chronic pancreatitis, five of whom obtained "excellent" pain control with thoracoscopic splanchnicectomy.

Results obtained from series of open splanchnicectomies suggest that two-thirds of patients with chronic pancreatitis achieve permanent pain relief following left splanchnicectomy. For recurrent or persistent pain, right splanchnicectomy may offer further improvement, although the numbers of patients who have undergone this are too small to quantify the benefit accurately.

The adoption of thoracoscopic techniques should allow splanchnicectomy to become a more widely used procedure in the management of pain due to pancreatic cancer and chronic pancreatitis. With increasing experience, this procedure should become established in the repertoire of the thoracic surgeon.

References

1   Hughes J. Endothoracic sympathectomy. *Proc R Soc Med* 1942; **35**: 585–6.
2   Adar R, Kurchin A, Zweig A, Mozes M. Palmar hyperhidrosis and its surgical treatment: a report of 100 cases. *Ann Surg* 1977; **186**: 34–41.
3   Kotzareff A. Resection partielle de trone sympathetique cervical droit pour hyperhidrose unilaterale. *Rev Med Suisse Romande* 1920; **40**: 111–13.
4   Moran KT, Brady MP. Surgical management of primary hyperhydrosis. *Br J Surg* 1991; **78**: 279–83.
5   Schumaker HBJ, Abramson DI. Post traumatic vasomotor disorders. *Surg Gynaecol Obstet* 1949; **88**: 417.
6   Kirklin JW, Chenoweth AE, Murphey F. Causalgia: a review of its characteristics, diagnosis, and treatment. *Surgery* 1947; **21**: 321.
7   Schumaker HBJ, Kilmen JW. Sympathectomy in the treatment of frostbite. *Arch Surg* 1964; **89**: 575.
8   Golding MR, Martinez A *et al*. The role of sympathectomy in frostbite, with a review of 68 cases. *Surgery* 1965; **57**: 774.
9   DeTakats G, Fowler EP. The neurogenic factor in Raynaud's phenomenon. *Surgery* 1962; **51**: 9.
10 Johnson ENM, Summerly R, Birnotingl M. Prognosis in Raynaud's phenomenon after sympathectomy. *Br Med J* 1965; **1**: 962–4.
11 Tygesea H, Claes G, Drott C *et al*. Effect of endoscopic transthoracic sympathicotomy on heart rate variability in severe angina pectoris. *Am J Cardiol* 1997; **79**: 1447–52.
12 Wittmoser R. Thoracoscopic sympathectomy and vagotomy. In: Cuschieri A, Buess G, Perissat J, eds. *Operative manual of endoscopic surgery*. New York: Springer, 1992: 110–33.
13 Kux M. Thoracic endoscopic sympathectomy in palmar and axillary hyperhydrosis. *Arch Surg* 1978; **113**: 264–6.
14 Byrne J, Walsh TN, Hederman WP. Endoscopic transthoracic electrocautery of the sympathetic chain for palmar and axillary hyperhydrosis. *Br J Surg* 1990; **77**: 1046–9.
15 Edmondson RA, Banerjee AK, Rennie JA. Endoscopic transthoracic sympathectomy in the treatment of hyperhydrosis. *Ann Surg* 1992; **215**: 289–93.
16 Claes G, Götheberg G, Drott C. Endoscopic electrocautery of the thoracic sympathetic chain — a minimal invasive method to treat palmar hyperhydrosis. *Scand J Plast Reconstr Hand Surg* 1993; **27**: 29–33.
17 Sachor D, Jedeikin R, Olsfanger D *et al*. Endoscopic transthoracic sympathectomy in the treatment of primary hyperhidrosis. *Arch Surg* 1994; **129**: 241–4.
18 Herbst F, Plas EG, Fugger R, Fritsch A. Endoscopic thoracic sympathectomy for primary hyperhidrosis of the upper limbs: a critical analysis and long term results of 480 operations. *Ann Surg* 1994; **220**: 86–90.
19 Drott C, Guthberg G, Claes G. Endoscopic transthoracic sympathectomy: an efficient and safe method for the treatment of hyperhidrosis. *J Am Acad Dermatol* 1995; **33**: 78–81.
20 Rennie JA. Compensatory sweating: an avoidable complication of thoracoscopic sympathectomy? *Minimally Invasive Therapy and Allied Technology* 1996; **5**: 101 [Abstract].
21 Gossot D, Toledo L, Fritsch S, Celerier M. Thoracoscopic sympathectomy for upper limb hyperhidrosis: looking for the right operation. *Ann Thorac Surg* 1997; **64**: 975–8.
22 Shelley WB, Florence R. Compensatory hyperhydrosis after sympathectomy. *N Engl J Med* 1960; **263**: 1056–8.
23 O'Riordain DS, Maher M, Waldron DJ, O'Donovan B, Brady MP. Limiting the anatomic extent of upper thoracic sympathectomy for primary palmar hyperhidrosis. *Surg Gynaecol Obstet* 1993; **176**: 151–4.
24 Bonjer HJ, Hamming JF, duBois NAJJ, van Urk H. Advantages of limited thoracoscopic sympathectomy. *Surg Endosc* 1996; **10**: 721–3.
25 Lemmens HJ. Importance of the second thoracic segment for the sympathetic denervation of the hand. *Vasc Surg* 1982; **16**: 23–6.

26 Conlon KC, Keaveny TV. Upper dorsal sympathectomy for palmar hyperhydrosis. *Br J Surg* 1987; **74**: 651.

27 Leung JWC, Bowen-Wright M, Aveling W, Shorvon PJ, Cotton PB. Coeliac plexus block for pain in pancreatic cancer and chronic pancreatitis. *Br J Surg* 1983; **70**: 730–2.

28 De Conno F, Caraceni A, Aldrighetti L *et al*. Paraplegia following coeliac plexus block. *Pain* 1993; **55**: 383–5.

29 Mallet-Guy PA. Late and very late results of resections of the nervous system in the treatment of chronic relapsing pancreatitis. *Am J Surg* 1983; **145**: 234–8.

30 Rienhoff WF, Baxter BM. Pancreolithiasis and chronic pancreatitis: preliminary report of a case of apparently successful treatment by transthoracic sympathectomy and vagotomy. *JAMA* 1947; **134**: 20–1.

31 Harlan Stone H, Chauvin EJ. Pancreatic denervation for pain relief in chronic alcohol pancreatitis. *Br J Surg* 1990; **77**: 303–5.

32 Hurwitz A, Gurwitz J. Relief of pain in chronic relapsing pancreatitis by unilateral sympathectomy. *Arch Surg* 1950; **61**: 372–8.

33 Connolly FE, Richards V. Bilateral splanchnicectomy and lumbodorsal sympathectomy for chronic relapsing pancreatitis. *Ann Surg* 1950; **131**: 58–63.

34 Worsey J, Ferson PF, Keenan RJ, Julian TB, Landreneau RJ. Thoracoscopic pancreatic denervation for pain control in irresectable pancreatic cancer. *Br J Surg* 1993; **80**: 1051–2.

35 Cuschieri A, Shimi SM, Crosthwaite G, Joypaul V. Bilateral endoscopic splanchnicectomy through a posterior thoracoscopic approach. *J Roy Coll Surg Edinb* 1994; **39**: 44–7.

36 Stone HH, Mullins RJ, Scovill WA. Vagotomy plus Bilroth II gastrectomy for the prevention of recurrent alcohol-induced pancreatitis. *Ann Surg* 1985; **201**: 684–9.

37 Le Pimpec Barthes F, Chapuis O *et al*. Thoracoscopic splanchnicectomy for control of intractable pain in pancreatic cancer. *Ann Thor Surg* 1998; **65**: 810–3.

38 Noppen M, Meysman M, D'Haese J, Vincken W. Thoracoscopic splanchnicectomy for relief of chronic pancreatic pain: experience of a group of pneumonologists. *Chest* 1998; **113**: 528–31.

5

Pleural diseases and aspects of trauma

R.G.C. Inderbitzi

Pleural diseases

Inspection of the pleural cavity and biopsy of abnormal tissue is one of the oldest applications of thoracoscopy. Although transthoracic needle biopsy is still widely practised for pleural-based disease, this approach permits only random sampling and is limited by small specimen sizes (1–2 mm diameter). An endoscopic approach allows samples to be taken under direct vision and, with the introduction of video imaging technology, magnification is available to aid interpretation of appearances. The combination of this development with the evolution of minimal access instrumentation and video-assisted thoracic surgical techniques allows larger and more accurately identified samples to be taken and facilitates progression to definitive surgical intervention.

Diagnostic effectiveness of thoracoscopy

Interpretation of the appearance of the pleural cavity in the context of suspected disease is complicated by the frequency of pleural abnormalities. Residues from previous, mainly inflammatory, pleural processes are found to a greater or lesser extent in 80% of postmortems performed on adults[1] and hyaline plaques on the parietal pleura and fibrosis of the visceral pleura (Fig. 5.1) are examples of past inflammatory changes which are often encountered during thoracoscopy.[6] Sampling under direct vision, particularly with the ability to dissect and therefore select target areas, when combined with clinical information provides a reliable morphological diagnosis in 90–97% of cases.[1] Diagnostic sensitivity is reported at 95% for malignancy and 100% for benign disease.[2,3] As an investigation for pleural effusion, thoracoscopy has a sensitivity of 92–97% with a specificity of 99%.[3]

Anatomical and physiological considerations

Visceral pleura

Microscopically, the visceral pleura is composed of multiple layers. The outer surface layer is formed by mesothelial cells which are bound together by desmosomes. Beneath this are three sparsely cellular sublayers of fibrous connective tissue which are bounded by the outer elastic lamella. The inner lamella borders on the alveolar walls and is continuous with the interstitial connective tissue of the lung in the region of the interlobular septa. The connective tissue layers closest to the lung contain a plexus of lymph vessels which may be identified clinically as the chessboard pattern created by carbon pigment accumulation. Communicating lymph vessels run between this plexus and the lymph plexus of the bronchial tree at the level of the smallest bronchioles so that the lymph drainage of the visceral pleura tends to follow that of the underlying portion of lung. The blood supply to the costal and diaphragmatic regions of the visceral pleura is derived from the pulmonary arteries while the other areas are supplied by the bronchial arteries with anastomoses to the pulmonary arteries.

Parietal pleura

The parietal pleura lines the thoracic cavity and is attached to the endothoracic fascia. It is conventionally described as consisting of costal, cervical, mediastinal and diaphragmatic portions and has a similar structure to the visceral pleura but with variable thickness. The diaphragmatic and mediastinal pleurae can be relatively insubstantial but fatty tissue

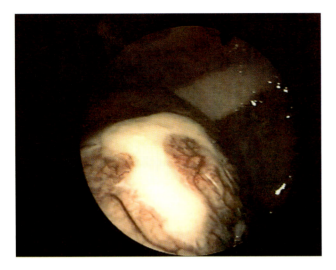

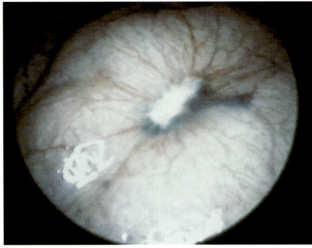

Figure 5.1 *Hyaline plaques of diverse aetiology on the parietal and visceral pleura.*

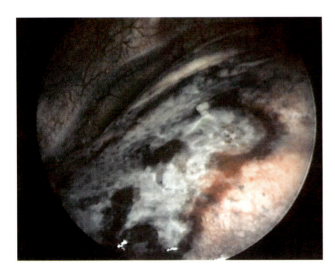

running parallel to the ribs is embedded in the costal pleural stroma while the interpleural layer is more dense over the ribs than over the muscular intercostal area. The lymphatics in the parietal pleura are particularly important. There is a rich plexus of vessels which communicate directly with the pleural cavity through stomas situated between the mesothelial cells allowing fluid, fibrin and corpuscular substances to be transported away.[1] This drainage passes from the costal pleura mainly to the intercostal and parasternal nodes though some upper spaces drain to the axillary nodes. The pleura over the first intercostal space and the cervical pleura drain to the deep cervical nodes. The mediastinal pleura drains to the tracheobronchial and mediastinal nodes. The diaphragmatic pleura drains to the parasternal, middle phrenic and posterior mediastinal nodes but also communicates with a plexus on the abdominal surface of the diaphragm thereby accounting for trans-diaphragmatic spread of pleural tumours. The blood supply is derived from the underlying somatic arteries.

Pleural fluid

The pleural space contains about 3 ml of fluid but there is continuous passage of fluid through the space. Fluid, as a low protein filtrate (<1.4 g/dl), enters and is reabsorbed through both the parietal and visceral pleurae but, as the pulmonary capillary pressure is less than that in the systemic circulation, there is greater reabsorption through the visceral pleura leading to a net flow from parietal to visceral pleura. Greatly accelerated fluid generation or impaired removal will result in an effusion which is classically designated on the basis of protein content as an exudate (>3 g/dl) or as a transudate (<3 g/dl). Transudates

Transudative (<3 g/dl)	Exudative (>3 g/dl)
Congestive heart failure	Infections
Constrictive pericarditis	Malignancy
Nephrotic syndrome	Immunological diseases
Cirrhosis	Inflammatory diseases
Peritoneal dialysis	Lymphatic abnormalities
Hypoalbuminaemia	Fluid movement from abdomen
Malignancy	Iatrogenic
Atelectasis	
Urinothorax	

Table 5.1

Usual causes of transudative (low protein) and exudative (high protein) pleural effusions

General diagnostic technique — keypoints

Successful diagnostic thoracoscopy is more likely if the following principles are observed:

1. The entire pleural cavity should be available for inspection. Adhesions (Fig. 5.2) must, therefore, be divided.
2. Fibrin and adhesions are often located precisely where the biopsy should be taken (Fig. 5.3).
3. Multiple and wide-ranging specimens should be taken from all areas where changes are apparent and should include bacteriological samples as it is not possible to determine the nature of abnormalities by inspection alone.
4. The specimens should be as deep and as large as possible. A layer of fibrin is frequently present over abnormal tissues so that a deep biopsy is necessary in order to reach beneath this layer (Fig. 5.3). A deep bite helps the histopathologist to comment on zonation and maturation. Also, additional analyses may be necessary and these are easier to obtain from larger specimens.
5. A full range of samples must be taken: fibrin, adhesions, parietal pleura with underlying thoracic wall and visceral pleura with subjacent lung.
6. It is sensible to site the thoracoscope on the opposite side of the chest from a localized abnormality in order to present the best possible view of the target area or lesion.
7. Specimens should be placed in a bag within the pleural cavity prior to extraction in order to minimise the risk of tumour cell implantation in the port sites.

are usually the result of increased hydrostatic pressure or reduced colloid osmotic pressure in the vascular system whereas exudates tend to develop as a result of inflammatory and neoplastic diseases causing increased capillary permeability (Table 5.1). Diagnostic accuracy is improved by including the pleural fluid:serum lactic dehydrogenase (LDH) ratio (>0.6 in an exudate).

Pleural tumours

Benign tumours

A pleural lipoma develops in the fat layer outside the parietal pleura and is usually discovered as an incidental finding on a standard chest X-ray, CT scan or MRI scan (Fig. 5.4). If the tumour appears to be growing it can be

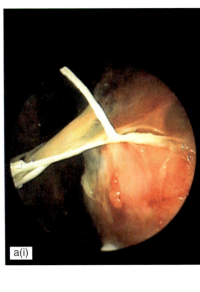
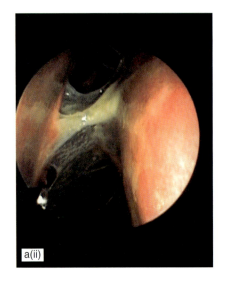
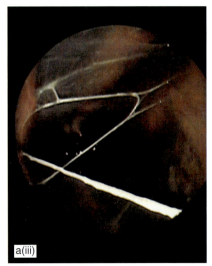

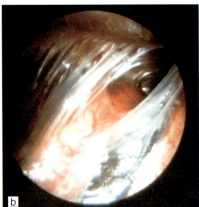
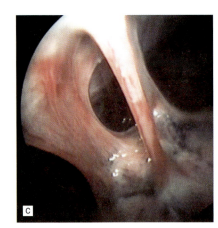

Figure 5.2 *Various types of intrapleural adhesions: (a) fine, (b) medium and avascular and (c) dense and vascular. It is essential that specimens from these are sent for bacteriological and histological analysis.*

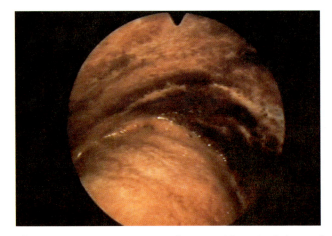

Figure 5.3 *The pleural sheet is often covered by multiple layers of fibrin. To obtain a useful histological specimen, deep biopsies are mandatory. The picture shows the parietal pleura in the region of the costophrenic recess in a patient with malignant effusions due to metastatic breast cancer.*

removed easily by thoracoscopic techniques using a retrieval bag.[5]

Benign local pleural fibromas are often asymptomatic, chance radiographic findings. They originate in the visceral pleura in 80% of cases and can range in size from 2 to 30 cm in diameter.[1] This tumour is a good example of the difficulties which may be caused by small biopsy samples as it may then be difficult to exclude the possibility of a sarcomatous mesothelioma.

Primary malignant pleural tumours

Localized malignant mesothelioma is generally a firm encapsulated tumour. In contrast to pleural fibromas, clinical symptoms are not uncommon and take the form of chest pain, coughing, dyspnoea and fever. Histological diagnosis based on a thoracoscopic biopsy sample is straight-forward.[7,12]

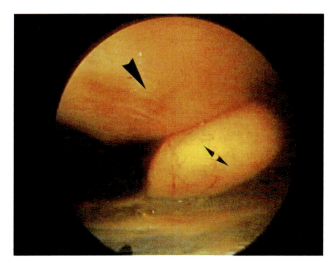

Figure 5.4 *Lipoma of the parietal pleura.*

Diffuse malignant pleural mesothelioma originates from any portion of the parietal, visceral or mediastinal pleura and grows selectively along the pleural surfaces (Fig. 5.5). Diffuse mesotheliomas tend to arise in the lower part of the pleural cavity but, as the disease progresses, the ipselateral lung may become completely encased and the surface invaded. Hilar lymph node involvement is seen in the later stages. Clinically, the first sign is frequently recurring pleural effusion and even at more advanced stages there are almost always remnants of encapsulated effusion present in the basal and dorsal thoracic regions between tumour masses.

Thoracoscopy is an effective procedure in the diagnosis of this disease. Tumour implantation at thoracotomy sites is well described with mesothelioma. The use of an extraction bag is therefore essential[8] and port sites should be placed so as to co-incide with a thoracotomy wound in the event that a pleuro-pneumonectomy is planned.

Thoracoscopic features of malignant mesothelioma include:

- effusion — often turbid or bloodstained
- multiple small pleural nodules
- tumour plates several centimetres thick
- 'knot-like' structures
- pulmonary encasement and fissural spread.

Multiple biopsies should be taken. Spindle, epithelial and mixed patterns of cell morphology are commonly recognised. Immunohistochemistry is required for firm diagnosis with the presence of cytokeratin expression aiding differentiation of a spindle cell mesothelioma from fibroblasts in a florid inflammatory situation and the absence of carcinoembryonic antigen (CEA) differentiating an epithelial mesothelioma from adenocarcinoma.

Secondary pleural tumours

Pleural metastases (Figs. 5.6 and 5.7) are at least twenty times more common than primary pleural tumours and may occur early in the course of disseminated malignant disease

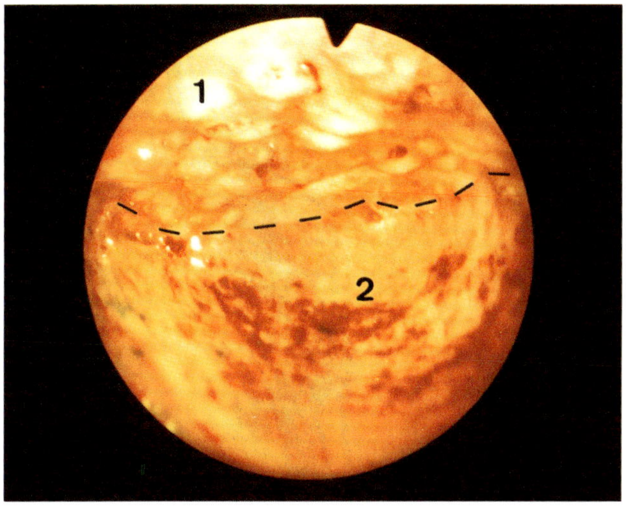

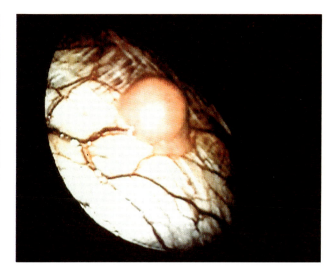

Figure 5.5 *Diffuse malignant mesothelioma: tumorous nodes on the parietal pleura (1). Thickened pleura in the area of the diaphragma (2).*

Figure 5.6 *Metastasis of a malignant thymoma on the diaphragma.*

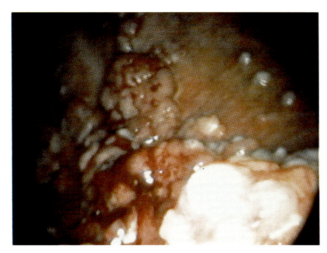

Figure 5.7 *Diffuse pleural metastasis and malignant effusion in a patient with cancer of the colon.*

due to the rich concentration of pleural lymphatic and blood vessels. It can be difficult to distinguish large and broad-based metastases from diffuse malignant mesothelioma on visual inspection so that generous sampling is required to provide adequate tissue for analysis.

Malignant pleural effusion

Malignant pleural effusions are common and in over 80% of cases occur bilaterally. The incidence increases with age such that more than 50% of exudative effusions in patients over 60 years old are due to malignant disease. The probability of pleural involvement varies with different malignancies but malignant pleural effusions can be expected to occur with a frequency of 26–49% for carcinoma of the breast, 10–24% for bronchogenic carcinoma, 16–17% for ovarian carcinoma and 7–15% for malignant lymphoma.[10,11] In such cases, the pleural cavity is almost always infiltrated by tumour cells and the diagnosis can be confirmed in more than half the cases by cytological examination of aspirated fluid. The effusion results either from increased capillary permeability owing to distended or destroyed capillary endothelium or from tumorous lymphatic drainage.[11] However, it is not rare for hypoalbuminaemia to cause or contribute to pleural effusions in cachectic patients.

Clinical features include shortness of breath, coughing and chest pain. Fluid can be detected on X-rays in the posteroanterior (PA) view when there is more than 175 cm³ or in the lateral view with as little as 100 cm³.[12] The symptoms arising from a malignant effusion are often the

first indications of disease. They are then the dominant cause of the patient feeling ill and further restrict the quality of life when prognosis is already extremely poor. The survival time after diagnosis of malignant effusion is usually less than one year.[10]

After excluding the possibility of successful systemic oncological therapy, the aim of any treatment must be fast, effective and lasting alleviation of the respiratory symptoms. This is usually achieved by draining the effusion and effecting a pleurodesis, often simply by injecting a sclerosent directly into the drainage tube. Obliteration of the pleural cavity with chemical pleurodesis by local instillation of sclerosing substances is the most common method, but is associated with recurrence rates of up to 30%.[13] Thoracoscopic pleurodesis was first proposed by Béthune in France in 1935.[14] Guérin and Boniface reported a series of 792 cases, 630 malignant and 162 non-neoplastic effusions, with no recurrences in 90% of cases.[15] Boutin, in Marseilles, reported equally impressive results in his personal experience of 300 cases of malignant effusion with a success rate of over 90% after talc pleurodesis.[7] He also reviewed the literature covering a total of 1244 patients treated with talc pleurodesis and found an average success rate of 87%. Hartmann and Gaither in a randomised study of 124 patients with malignant effusions[16] compared pleurodesis using bleomycin or tetracycline with thoracoscopic talc poudrage and discovered that the latter produced significantly better results at 30 and 90 days in the surviving patients. The various thoracoscopic pleurodesis techniques have been compared in animal experiments.[17] This comparison of pleurodesis using tetracycline, talc, mechanical abrasion, Nd:YAG laser scarification of the pleura, photocoagulation and the argon beam coagulator showed that only talc poudrage was able to match the effectiveness of mechanical abrasion.

The success of pleurodesis depends primarily on careful evaluation of the patient as not all malignant effusions can be managed by thoracoscopic pleurodesis. The following conditions must be met:

- the compressed lung must be shown clinically and radiologically to be fully expanded following drainage of the effusion
- evacuation of the pleural cavity and decompression of the lung must lead to significant alleviation of the respiratory symptoms.

Technique of talc (kaolin) insufflation

We use video thoracoscopy for this intervention. Two ports are normally sufficient. A lateral decubitus position is preferable but the respiratory status of the patient must be taken into consideration. If there is dyspnoea or orthopnoea, pleurodesis can be performed in the semi-sitting position. If the operator has enough experience, local anaesthesia combined with sedation is almost always adequate. Although the pleura is thickened and has correspondingly reduced sensitivity in cases of chronic effusion, pleural pain caused by the strongly hyperosmotic talc particles can be severe and will require effective analgesia. Sterile kaolin powder (up to 50 g) is sprayed with an atomiser and distributed on the parietal and visceral pleura under vision as homogeneously as possible. A multi-holed thoracic drain is required to empty the entire thoracic cavity from the base to the apex and so ensure adhesion of the pleural membranes. The author believes that the drain should remain in position for at least 72 hours and be on suction at about 4 cm H_2O.

The possible complications of thoracoscopic talc pleurodesis are those inherent in thoracoscopy and are not generally dangerous. They include:

- surface lung injuries
- thoracic wall bleeding
- local infection
- local tumour implantation in the port sites.

Thoracoscopically guided talc pleurodesis represents an effective first treatment for malignant effusion and can be performed as a minimally invasive intervention involving few complications in patients in poor general condition. It is not in the patient's interest to delay pleurodesis once the diagnosis has been made and the chance of curative therapy has been excluded. Quality and duration of life are impaired and loss of protein caused by the effusion increases the catabolic metabolic state. Also, the chance of successful pleural adhesion decreases with growth of the tumour, formation of loculations and thickening of the visceral pleura.

Pleurisy

Inflammatory changes of the pleura are primarily the result of pathological processes in adjacent organs, particularly the lungs but systemic diseases are frequently associated with non-specific pleural inflammation and often with effusions (Fig. 5.8).[1,6,18]

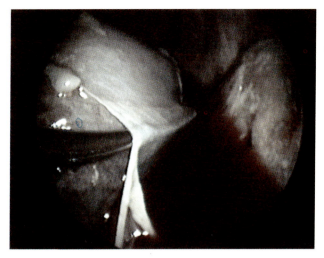

Figure 5.8 *Non-specific pleurisy with a layer of fibrin on the surface of the lung in a patient six weeks after thoracoscopic parietal pleurectomy. The figure shows decortication of the lung by an endoscopic dissector.*

Acute, non-specific pleurisy usually occurs as a reaction to diseases of the lungs, pneumonia, tumours and infarction. After initial oedema of the pleura, the second phase involves serofibrinous fluid passing into the pleural cavity. Depending on the cause, the effusion takes the form of either a transudate or an exudate and is haemorrhagic or purulent. Fibrin deposits form a web pattern on the pleura. Purulent

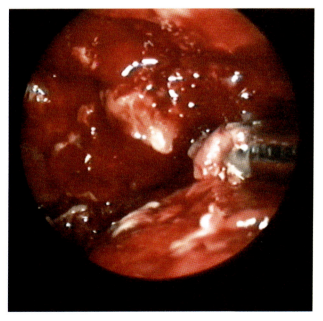

Figure 5.9 *Empyema in a patient with tuberculosis.*

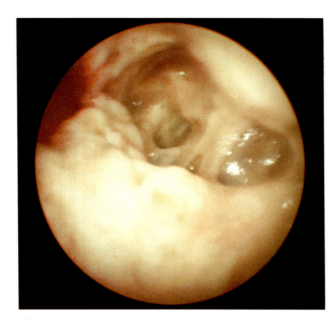

Figure 5.10 *Empyema with granulation tissue in the sinus phrenico-costalis. Decortication is being performed by a specially designed shaver.*

pleurisy is caused by an infection and is the basis for a later empyema. After several days or weeks the advance of the disease is marked by the development of granulation tissue (Fig. 5.9). Pleurisy finally leaves broad-area and band-like fibroses with whitish-grey thickening of the pleura and adhesions between the pleural membranes. There is extensive vascular proliferation in the area of the interpleural adhesions.

It is not possible to reliably distinguish thoracoscopically between a tumour and acute or subacute pleurisy. Even cytological assessment may be difficult due to reactive changes in the mesothelial cells. It is essential, therefore, to collect an adequate number of representative specimens of a suitable size and depth to allow conclusive histological diagnosis.

Granulomatous pleurisy
This group includes:

- tuberculosis
- sarcoidosis
- anthracosilicosis
- pleural involvement in rheumatic diseases
- iatrogenic, foreign body reactions.

Pleural tuberculosis is of particular interest to the thoracoscopist[7] as this disease is on the increase worldwide, and thoracoscopy is a highly effective method of obtaining the diagnosis. Miliary granulomas which are usually intrapulmonary and close to the pleura can be seen endoscopically, and granulomas are also found in thin webs of fibrin. Fresh, fibrinous adhesions provide excellent samples for cell culture in suspected tuberculosis cases. With an aggressive policy towards thoracoscopic diagnosis, caseogenic forms of tuberculosis, tuberculous pleural empyema (Fig. 5.10) and calcified post-tuberculous pleural deposits should seldom be encountered.

Chylothorax

Chylothorax, the accumulation of lymph in the pleural space, is a potentially serious condition and remains a challenging clinical problem. There are a variety of causes (Table 5.2) and therapy is to some extent determined by the aetiology of the chylothorax.

Conservative management combines pleural drainage with fluid and electrolyte replacement and parenteral feeding. Despite apparently adequate replacement therapy there is a net loss of protein, fat soluble vitamins, electrolytes and lymphocytes and post surgical patients may have difficulty tolerating the high volumes of intravenous fluids required to replace drain loss and maintain hydration. Spontaneous remission may often occur after a variable time interval but approximately 50% of cases will ultimately go on to require surgical intervention.[19,20]

Ligation of the thoracic duct was first proposed by Lampson in 1948[21] and remains the procedure of choice in patients with post traumatic or post surgical chylous fistula as there is usually a discrete duct laceration. However, this

Table 5.2
Causes of chylothorax

Neoplasms	c50%
Surgical injury or trauma to the thoracic duct	25%
Thrombosis of jugular or subclavian veins	25%
Postactinic damage and other causes	2%

procedure is complicated by the highly variable thoracic duct anatomy (Fig. 5.11) which has an atypical course in 40–60% of cases and even ligation of a successfully identified duct may fail due to the presence of lymphatic collaterals and numerous lymphovenous anastomoses.[26] It is essential to localize the point of duct leakage in order to either directly control the leak or to be sure of occluding the duct below that level. Bipedal lymphangiography allows accurate preoperative localisation[22,25] and intraoperative visualisation is possible if the patient is given a drink containing 50 ml of full fat cream prior to surgery as the chyle will become pure white.

The introduction of videothoracoscopic techniques has made an increasing variety of surgical strategies possible.[22–4] Direct measures include: placing a clip or ligature on the proximal duct, suture of the thickened pleura around the leaking point and application of fibrin sealant to the leaking point. Where the leakage is over a wide area due perhaps to increased lymphatic pressure or disruption from neoplastic obstruction or inflammatory disease so that a direct duct procedure is inappropriate, videothoracoscopic intervention may serve two useful functions. It allows a thorough diagnostic examination of the pleural cavity and pleurodesis may be carried out using various techniques including: pleurectomy, talc insufflation, fibrin glue or tetracycline.[27]

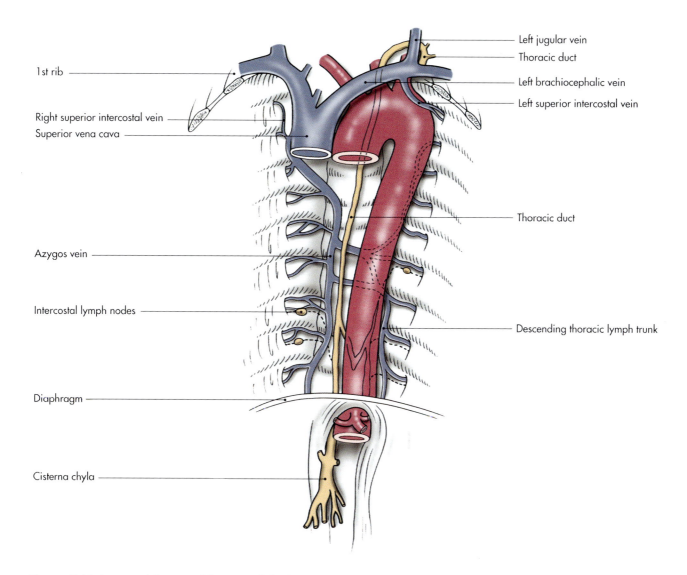

Figure 5.11 *Anatomical drawing of the course of the thoracic duct.*

Surgical technique (see also Chapter 6)

The patient is placed in the lateral decubitus position and the procedure performed under general anaesthesia with double-lumen intubation. Port site placement is based on the preoperative findings regarding location of the leak, adhesions, loculated fluid collections and any tumour masses. Generally, three ports are required. Intrathoracic adhesions should be divided and fluid completely aspirated. Following either direct management of a leaking point or duct occlusion or pleurodesis a single drain is inserted.

Despite reduction in mortality from 45% to 2% with surgical as opposed to conservative management, enthusiasm for early surgical intervention has been tempered by the morbidity of a thoracotomy. Thoracoscopic management represents a much less invasive procedure and should be considered immediately after the diagnosis has been proved. At this stage adhesions are either absent or flimsy and easy to divide.

Empyema

In pleural empyema, fibrin exudates are deposited in the thoracic cavity. Shallow breathing resulting from pleuritic pain promotes rapid organisation of these deposits by fibrocytes with accompanying destruction of the mesothelium and adhesion of both pleural membranes. The end result is marked restriction and even total loss of pulmonary mobility with a corresponding decrease in vital capacity. This sequence of events is most noticeable when there is bacterial infection. Not every contaminated pleural effusion develops into an empyema, although if bacterial infection is present, the probability is high.[28–31]

By definition, empyema is characterised by a collection of pus in the pleural cavity. The pathological development can be divided into three stages:

1. exudative
2. fibrinopurulent, and
3. fibrosing/organising.

These stages are however not clearly demarcated and often overlap and coexist in different regions of the thoracic cavity, resulting in loculations and basal recesses.

When bacterial pleurisy with the possible danger of empyema is suspected, evaluation of the effusion is important in determining subsequent actions. If the effusion is no longer serosanguineous but viscous or if it clots quickly after being drawn off owing to a high protein content, adequate aspiration by thoracocentesis is not possible and surgical intervention is necessary. When this stage is reached, cell counts and glucose and lactate dehydrogenase levels are of less prognostic importance.[28–30,32]

With the onset of the fibrinopurulent phase, sail-like adhesions form, the pleural membranes become adherent and loculations are created. The process progresses to fixation and reduced pulmonary expansion. With the invasion of fibroblasts, the visceral pleura finally loses its elasticity and a 'pulmonary cortex' results.

In the exudative to early fibrinopurulent phase of empyema, thoracoscopic intervention can prevent the advance of the disease. Loculations can be opened and aspirated under vision and adhesions divided. In contrast to Braimbridge's study group,[33–5] the authors are convinced that not one but three portals are necessary to be able to work under endoscopic vision and with the aid of an assistant. Thoracoscopic surgical intervention at this stage allows the pleural cavity to be returned to a single chamber cavity by lavage and instituting drainage at the lowest point.[36,37]

In the late fibrinopurulent phase, scarring in the recesses can be evacuated with a shaver and fresh deposits on both pleural membranes removed with a dissector. If the latter proves impossible, the authors' experience indicates that despite a free pleural cavity an early open decortication should be performed. Even if the pleural cavity is sterile, the trapped lung can no longer expand and decortication is therefore required. Immediate progress in the endoscopic treatment of this serious disease could be made if patients were referred for thoracoscopy at an earlier stage than usually occurs as organised pleural structures can often be found within only two weeks of the first symptoms.[38]

Surgical technique

The operation is performed in the lateral position under general anaesthesia with double-lumen intubation. The positions of the three ports are selected on the basis of the CT scan but are typically located between the fourth and eighth intercostal spaces. In the exudative to early fibrinopurulent phase, the aim of the intervention is to free and examine the whole thoracic cavity including the fissures. Any fluid that is present is carefully aspirated through the first port and the telescope is then introduced. The second port is then established based on the endoscopic findings. Using the dissector, palpator and suction tube, adhesions are divided step by step and fluid, fibrin bands and pus are evacuated by alternate irrigation and aspiration. When the space is sufficiently large to introduce the third trocar, the suction–irrigation tube is used parallel to the palpator/dissector to make dissection easier. Fresh adhesions between the two pleural membranes are carefully broken through with the palpator or dissector and sail-like adhesions are divided. Once the whole pleural cavity is free including the various recesses and the interlobar fissures, lavage is started alternately irrigating and aspirating warm Ringer's lactate in 500 ml aliquots until between four and five litres have been used. An apical drain is then placed through the fourth intercostal space and a dorsobasal drain is inserted through an additional incision and positioned under video-thoracoscopic vision at the deepest point in the pleural cavity.

Even at the early fibrinopurulent stage, the recesses are usually covered by thick fibrin deposits. They must be examined, unequivocally identified, exposed with the dissector and removed with the shaver. The shaver must only be used with the blade pointing towards the thoracoscope.

After freeing the whole pleural cavity and removing the fibrin deposits from both pleural membranes, the lung is cautiously ventilated. It must be seen to expand completely, i.e. up to the thoracic wall. If this is the case, drainage is established as described above and the intervention is completed. If, however, there is still a dead space between the lung and the evacuated pleural cavity and if the lung cannot be freed thoracoscopically, open decortication must be performed.

Results

Several groups[39,40,41] have now reported on significant series of patients undergoing VATS management of empyema (Table 5.3). Taken collectively these would suggest that an immediate conversion rate to open thoracotomy is required in approximately 17% of cases due to more advanced than anticipated pathology while a further 5–10% will require late thoracotomy due to recurrence of empyema or poor initial result. There is some limited evidence to suggest that discharge is more rapid and pulmonary function well preserved after a VATS procedure.[39,41]

Aspects of trauma

Videothoracoscopy is, necessarily, an elective intervention in the care of patients with thoracic trauma which must follow assessment, resuscitation and the immediate management of life-threatening conditions. Experience with the application of videothoracoscopy in trauma is limited and a proper understanding of its role and potential is still evolving. In suitable cases, however, it offers a number of diagnostic and therapeutic possibilities.

Indications

The patient must be in a stable, controlled condition and able to withstand both the physiological effect of one lung

Table 5.3

Results of VATS management of empyema

Report	No. of patients	Conversion rate: Immediate	Late	Post-op stay (days)	Mortality
Angelillo-Mackinlay[38] 1996	31	10%	0	6.8	3.2%
Lawrence[39] 1997	44	4.8%	24%	5.3	–
Striffler[40] 1998	67	28%	4%	12.3	4%

ventilation and the time delay inherent in performing the procedure. It is not suitable for patients with severe hypovolaemia, active major blood loss, respiratory or cardiac insufficiency or multiple thoracic wall injuries.

Currently, videothoracoscopic intervention in the context of trauma has been described[18,42–48] in the management of various situations (Table 5.4), including:

- pulmonary injury
- haemothorax
- empyema
- thoracic duct injury
- diaphragm injury
- retrieval of foreign bodies.

Of these, evacuation of haemothorax is probably the single most common use of VATS techniques in trauma and is described in further detail below. Many of these applications are not new and have been undertaken using simple monocular thoracoscopy for some years but infrequently and in selected cases. Videothoracoscopy or VATS provides a detailed view of the hemithorax with the opportunity to inspect any suspect area closely and with

magnification affording the surgeon greater diagnostic confidence and facilitating endoscopic intervention. Consequently VATS assessment of thoracic trauma cases has proved to be of significant value in avoiding unnecessary thoracotomy, with Liu and colleagues[49] reporting that 12 patients out of 50 (24%) undergoing VATS assessment where thoracotomy would otherwise have been indicated were spared this outcome.

Haemothorax

Thoracoscopic treatment of haemothorax has been performed for many years. Various authors have described the possibilities of thoracoscopic haemostasis using a flexible endoscope.[50,51] Kaiser describes the evacuation of a haematoma using a mediastinoscope.[52] He and Jones[53], who performed thoracoscopy to localise and evacuate bleeding as an urgent measure in 32 patients with traumatic haemothorax, both point out the advantages of an early endoscopic intervention: the haematoma is not yet organised and, with few fibrin deposits, complete evacuation and effective drainage of the thoracic cavity is possible.

Diagnosis	Intervention
Isolated persistent pneumothorax	Wedge resection ± pleurectomy
Persistent haemothorax (>1500 mm/24h)	1. Evacuated
	2. Haemostasis
Clotted haemothorax	Lavage, evacuation
Possible diaphragmatic rupture (Fig. 5.12)	Repositioning of intra-abdominal organs
	Reconstruction
	1. Confirm diagnosis
Pericardial effusion	Pericardial window formation
Persistent atelectasis	Diagnostic
	Controlled reinflation of the lung
Injuries to the thoracic duct	Leak closure ± pleurodesis
Pneumatocele due to lung lacerations	1. Exposure
	2. Drain placement
Signs of intrathoracic infection	1. Adhesiolysis
	2. Lavage
	3. Drainage

Table 5.4

Indications for video thoracoscopy in trauma patients with stable vital functions

In cases of haemothorax, the therapeutic procedure depends primarily on the cause and extent of the source of bleeding. If the intrathoracic haemorrhage is accumulating slowly and is not causing cardiovascular instability, a drain is normally placed both for therapy and to assess the rate of blood loss. Explorative thoracotomy is indicated if there is persistent blood loss greater than 500 ml/h for more than three hours or 150 ml/h for six hours through the chest tube. If a haemothorax cannot be evacuated by drainage within a few days, operative evacuation is also necessary. The same guidelines apply to video thoracoscopic interventions.

Surgical technique

The thoracoscopic intervention is performed under general anaesthesia with double-lumen intubation with the patient in the lateral position. The three incisions are planned based on PA and lateral view thoracic X-rays according to the position and extent of the haematoma. Initially, approximately 300 ml of CO_2 are carefully insufflated through a Verres needle. If the insufflation pressure is above 10 mmHg and/or gas flow is slow, blind gas insufflation is stopped since the tip of the cannula may be located in clotted blood. Instead, an incision is made with the scissors and a trocar inserted to allow viewing with the 0° scope. If the light is absorbed by the haematoma, this can be partly evacuated by alternate irrigation and suction which quickly improves the lighting conditions. The next step is to define the anatomic structures and the boundaries of the haematoma so as to avoid further damage to lacerated lung parenchyma. Older haematomas often have membranes with a matt sheen resembling the visceral pleura of atelectatic regions of the lung. If a source of bleeding is found (intercostal vessel, small vein) it is closed, if possible, with fibrin glue, a suture or a clip. The pulmonary fissures and recesses must be exposed and examined as these often harbour encapsulated remnants of the haematoma. The operator should also be on the lookout for other pathological findings such as atelectatic lung tissue or lacerations of the lung parenchyma. Mistaking the adherent parietal pleura of an atelectatic pulmonary lobe for the capsule of the haematoma can lead to accidental injury to the lung when the 'haematoma' is opened.

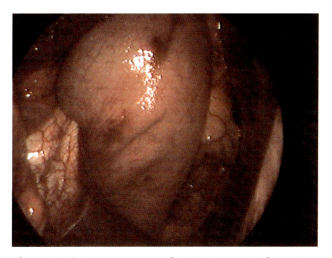

Figure 5.12 *Traumatic rupture of the diaphragm. The figure shows the herniation of the stomach into the thoracic cavity.*

Diaphragmatic injury

In a stable patient with radiographic features suggestive of possible diaphragmatic injury, VATS exploration of the thoracic cavity may be a useful diagnostic tool. This technique allows the surgeon to differentiate diaphragmatic eventration/paralysis from acute diaphragmatic rupture (Figure 5.12) in a much less invasive manner than an explorative thoracotomy.

Future development

As with many areas of videothoracoscopic surgery, further developments in instrumentation and alternate methods of tissue sealing and repair will expand the range of possible interventions in traumatic cases. It is also probable that developing experience in thoracoscopic techniques in general may be transferred to the management of traumatic cases. For example, the experience gained with the use of laser devices, tissue glues and sealants to achieve accurate haemostasis and aerostasis during surgery on the pulmonary parenchyma[47] is potentially applicable to the management of traumatic pulmonary parenchymal lacerations. The assessment and management of major intrathoracic injuries is a particularly exciting area of development where the use of a videothoracoscopic approach offers the opportunity to avoid further compounding the primary injury by performing a major thoracotomy. Current experience is largely anecdotal but already includes repair of oesophageal tears[47,48] and management of diaphragmatic injuries.

References

1   Müller KM. Erkrankungen der Pleura — pathologische Anatomie. In: Nakhosteen JA, Inderbitzi R (eds) *Atlas und Lehrbuch der thorakalen Endoskopie*. Berlin: Springer Verlag, 1994; 325–40.

2   Harris RJ, Kavuru MS, Mehta AC *et al*. The impact of thoracoscopy on the management of pleural disease. *Chest* 1995; **107**: 845–52.

3   Boutin C, Loddenkemper R, Astoul P. Diagnostic and therapeutic thoracoscopy: techniques and indications in pulmonary medicine. *Tuber Lung Dis* 1993; **74**: 225–39.

4   Fry WA, Siddiqui A, Pensler JM, Mostafavi H. Thoracoscopic implantation of cancer with a fatal outcome. *Ann Thorac Surg* 1995; **59**: 42–5.

5   Furrer M, Inderbitzi R. Fallbericht: Endoskopisch Resektion eines 5 cm grossen ntrathorakalen Lipoms. *Pneumologie* 1992; **46**: 334–5.

6   Brandt HJ, Loddenkemper R, Mai J (eds). *Atlas of diagnostic thoracoscopy*. 1985; Stuttgart: Thieme.

7   Boutin C, Viallat JR, Aelony Y. *Practical Thoracoscopy* 1991b. Berlin: Springer Verlag.

8   Canto A, Blasco E, Casillas M *et al*. Thoracoscopy in the diagnosis of pleural effusion. *Thorax* 1977; **32**: 550–4.

9   Moore DWO. Malignant pleural effusion. *Sem Oncol* 1991; **18**: 59–61.

10 Chernow B, Sahn SA. Carcinomatous involvement of the pleura. *Am J Med* 1977; **63**: 695–702.

10 Stenzl W, Rigler B, Tscheliessnigg HK, Beitzke A, Metgler H. Treatment of postsurgical chylothorax with fibrin glue. *J Thorac Cardiovasc Surg* 1983; **31**: 35–36.

11 Hausheer FH, Yabro JW. Diagnosis and treatment of malignant pleural effusion. *Sem Oncol* 1985; **12**: 54–75.

12 Woodring JH. Recognition of pleural effusion on supine radiographs: how much fluid is required? *Am J Roentgenol* 1984; **142**: 59–64.

13 Furrer M, Inderbitzi R. Pleurodeseverfahren beim malignen Pleuraerguss. *Schweiz Med Wschr* 1992; **122**: 181–183.

14 Béthune N. Pleural poudrage. A new technique for the deliberate production of pleural adhesions as a preliminary to lobectomy. *J Thorac Cardiovasc Surg* 1935; **4**: 251–61.

15 Boniface E, Guerin JC. Intérêt du talcage par thoracoscopie dans les traitement symptomatique des pleurésies récidivantes. A propos de 302 cas. *Rev Mal Resp* 1989; **6**: 133–9.

16 Hartman DL, Gaither JM, Kesler KA *et al*. Comparison of insufflated talc under thoracoscopic guidance with standard tetracycline and bleomycin pleurodesis for control of malignant pleural effusions. *J Thorac Cardiovasc Surg* 1993; **105**: 743–8.

17 Bresticker MA, Oba J, LoCicero III J, Greene R. Optimal pleurodesis: a comparison study. *Ann Thorac Surg* 1993; **55**: 364–7.

18 Inderbitzi R. *Surgical thoracoscopy*. Berlin: Springer Verlag, 1993.

19 Ferguson MK, Little AG, Skinner DB. Current concepts in the management of postoperative chylothorax. *Ann Thorac Surg* 1985; **40**: 542–5.

20 Milson JW, Kron IL, Rheuban KS, Rodgers BM. Chylothorax: an assessment of current surgical management. *J Thorac Cardiovasc Surg* 1985; **89**: 221–7.

21 Lampson RS. Traumatic chylothorax. A review of the literature and report of a case treated by mediastinal ligation of the thoracic duct. *J Thorac Surg* 1948; **17**: 778–91.

22 Inderbitzi RGC, Krebs T, Stirnemann P, Althaus U. Treatment of postoperative chylothorax by fibrin glue application under thoracoscopic view with use of local anaesthesia. *J Thorac Cardiovasc Surg* 1992; **104**: 209–10.

23 Kent RB, Pinson TW. Thoracoscopic ligation of the thoracic duct. *Surg Endosc* 1993; **7**: 52–3.

24 Shirai T, Amano J, Takabe K. Thoracoscopic diagnosis and treatment of chylothorax after pneumonectomy. *Ann Thorac Surg* 1991; **52**: 306–7.

25 Sachs PB, Zelch MG, Rice TW *et al*. Diagnosis and localization of laceration of the thoracic duct: usefulness of lymphangiography and CT. *AJR* 1991; **157**: 703–5.

26 Zerkowski HR, Hakim K, Rüter F, Roth G, Reidemeister JC. Application of fibrin glue in the operative treatment of chylothorax. In: *Fibrin sealing in surgical and nonsurgical fields: cardiovascular surgery, thoracic surgery*. Berlin: Springer Verlag, 1994, Vol 6; 148–54.

27 Adler RH, Levinsky L. Persistent chylothorax. *J Thorac Cardiovasc Surg* 1978; **76**: 859–64.

28 Good JT, Taryle DA, Maulitz RM, Kaplan RL, Sahn SA. The diagnostic value of pleural fluid pH. *Chest* 1980; **78**: 55–9.

29 Houston MC. Pleural fluid pH: diagnostic, therapeutic, and prognostic value. *Am J Surg* 1987; **154**: 333–7.

30 Light RW, Girard WM, Jenkinson SG, George RB. Parapneumonic effusions. *Am J Med* 1980; **69**: 507–12.

31 Potts DE, Taryle DA, Sahn SA. The glucose-pH relationship in parapneumonic effusions. *Arch Intern Med* 1978; **138**: 1378–80.

32 Orringer MB. Thoracic empyema — back to basics. *Chest* 1988; 901–2.

33 Hutter JA, Harari D, Braimbridge MV. The management of empyema thoracis by thoracoscopy and irrigation. *Ann Thorac Surg* 1985; **39**: 517–20.

34 Ridley PD, Braimbridge MV. Thoracoscopic debridement and pleural irrigation in the management of empyeam thoracis. *Ann Thorac Surg* 1991; **51**: 461–4.

35 Rosenfeldt FL, McGibney D, Braimbridge MN, Watson DA. Comparison between irrigation and conventional treatment for empyema and pneumonectomy space infection. *Thorax* 1981; **36**: 272–7.

36 Oakes DD, Sherck JP, Brodsky JB, Mark JB. Therapeutic thoracoscopy. *J Thorac Cardiovasc Surg* 1984; **87**: 269–73.

37 Weissberg D, Kaufmann M, Schwecher I. Pleuroscopy in clinical evaluation and staging of lung cancer. *Poumon-Coeur* 1981; **37**: 241–3.

38 Silen ML, Naunheim KS. Thoracoscopic approach to the management of empyema thoracis. Indications and results. *Surg Clin North Am* 1996; **6**(3): 491–9.

39 Angelillo Mackinlay TA, Lyons GA, Chimondeguy DJ *et al*. VATS debridement versus thoracotomy in the treatment of loculated postpneumonia empyema. *Ann Thorac Surg* 1996; **61**: 1626–30.

40 Lawrence DR, Ohri SK, Moxon RE, Townsend ER, Fountain SW. Thoracoscopic debridement of empyema thoracis. *Ann Thorac Surg* 1997; **64**: 1448–50.

41 Striffler H, Gugger M, Im Hof V *et al*. Video-assisted thoracoscopic surgery for fibrinopurulent pleural empyema in 67 patients. *Ann Thorac Surg* 1998; **65**: 319–23.

42 Sosa JL, Puente I, Lemasters L *et al*. Videothoracoscopy in trauma: early experience. *J Laparoendosc Surg* 1994; **4**: 295–300.

43 Uribe RA, Pachon CE, Frame SB *et al*. A prospective evaluation in thoracoscopy for the diagnosis of penetrating thoracoabdominal trauma. *J Trauma* 1994; **37**: 650–4.

44 Koehler RH, Smith RS. Thoracoscopic repair of missed diaphragmatic injury in penetrating trauma: case report. *J Trauma* 1994; **37**: 515.

45 Nel JH, Warren BL. Thoracoscopic evaluation of the diaphragm in patients with knife wound of the left lower chest. *Br J Surg* 1994; **84**: 713–14.

46 Bartek JP, Grasch A, Hazelrigg SR. Thoracoscopic retrieval of foreign bodies after penetrating chest trauma. *Ann Thorac Surg* 1997; **63**: 1783–5.

47 Wong MS, Tsoi EK, Henderson VJ *et al*. Videothoracoscopy: an effective method for evaluating and managing thoracic trauma patients. *Surg Endosc* 1996; **10**(2): 118–21.

48 Lang-Lazdunski L, Mouroux J, Pons F *et al*. Role of videothoracoscopy in chest trauma. *Ann Thorac Surg* 1997; **63**(2): 327–33.

49 Liu DW, Liu HP, Lin PJ, Chang CH. Video-assisted thoracic treatment of chest trauma. *J Trauma* 1997; **42**(4) 670–4.

50 Dimitri WR. Massive idiopathic spontaneous haemothorax — case report and literature review. *Eur J Cardiothorac Surg* 1987; **1**: 55–8.

51 Ratliff JL, Johnson N, Clever JA. Pluroscopy and cautery control of intrathoracic haemorrhage with a flexible fiberoptic bronchoscope. *Chest* 1977; **71**: 216–17.

52 Kaiser D. Thoracoskopische Hämatomausräumung beim unvollständig entleerten Hämatothorax. *Hefte zur Unfallheilkunde* 1987; **189**: 328–32.

53 Jones JW, Kitahama A, Webb WR, McSwain N. Emergency thoracoscopy. A logical approach to chest trauma management. *J Trauma* 1981; **21**: 280–4.

54 Mancini M, Smith LM, Nein A, Buechter KJ. Early evacuation of clotted blood in hemothorax using thoracoscopy: case reports. *J Trauma* 1993; **34**: 144–7.

Diagnosis and treatment of mediastinal lesions

6

M. Boaron, S. Artuso, N. Santelmo, G. Corneli and N. Lacava

Introduction

The management of mediastinal lesions is an excellent application of video-assisted thoracic surgery (VATS) techniques. Other minimally invasive surgical biopsy techniques, such as mediastinoscopy and mediastinotomy, although useful in specific indications, can be limited by restricted vision and access. With a VATS approach, however, a magnified view is obtained which provides detailed visualisation and facilitates delicate surgery. This may be useful in many surgical procedures within the mediastinum, notably the removal of masses close to the intervertebral foramina or in the upper thoracic inlet. It is also possible to inspect the whole hemithorax so that related or synchronous abnormalities can be identified.

Dissection is relatively bloodless as the mediastinal structures are surrounded by poorly vascularised fatty tissues and deep-seated abnormalities can, therefore, be biopsied or removed with equal precision and safety to that provided by surgical dissection via an open thoracotomy. The addition of a 5 cm unspread utility thoracotomy allows mini-invasive video-assisted mediastinal procedures to be undertaken using conventional instruments. This may be useful when dealing with lesions where a purely thoracoscopic approach would be hazardous, or as a means of providing added safety for surgeons with less experience in thoracoscopic surgical techniques.

As with all minimally invasive procedures, postoperative pain and disability are generally reduced. Overall operative time is usually comparable with an open procedure and may be shorter in some cases as there is no major thoracotomy wound to close.

Surgical anatomy of the mediastinum: distribution of mediastinal mass lesions

The mediastinum may be divided into three compartments for classification of mass lesions: anterior, visceral and paravertebral (Fig. 6.1). The anterior compartment lies between the sternum and the anterior surfaces of the pericardium and the great vessels. These surfaces constitute the anterior border of the visceral compartment which contains the intrathoracic organs and therefore extends posteriorly to the vertebral column. The paravertebral compartment comprises the paravertebral spaces. Within this classification, the commoner mediastinal lesions are distributed as shown in Table 6.1.

The older classification of superior, anterior, middle and posterior mediastinum (Fig. 6.2) can be confusing as it utilizes arbitrary boundaries between these areas. The superior mediastinum, in particular, lies above a line drawn from T4 to the manubrial–sternal junction and therefore includes elements of the three compartments described above. Similarly, the posterior mediastinum includes both the paravertebral compartment and that portion of the visceral compartment which lies behind the trachea and heart. Consequently, compartmental position is of less value in inferring the diagnosis of a mediastinal abnormality in this classification system.

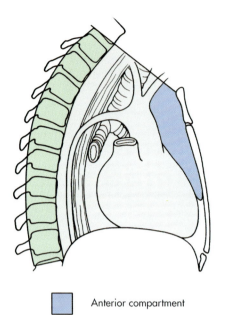
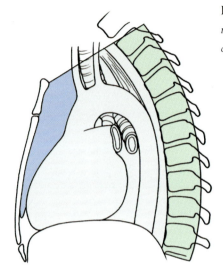

Figure 6.1 *Topography of the mediastinum showing anterior, visceral and paravertebral compartments.*

■ Anterior compartment

□ Visceral compartment

■ Paravertebral compartment

Table 6.1

Distribution of the commoner mediastinal lesions

Compartment	Pathology
Anterior	Lymphoma, thymoma, thymic hyperplasia, germ cell tumours (teratomas, dermoid cysts, malignant germ cell tumours)
Visceral	Secondary mediastinal tumour, lymphoma, retrosternal thyroid, aortic aneurysm, hiatus hernia, lymphadenopathy, enterogenous cyst, bronchogenic cyst, pleuropericardial cyst, ganglionoma
Posterior	Neurogenic tumour, lymphoma, haemangioma meningocele, vertebral abscess

Alternative invasive mediastinal diagnostic techniques

Modern CT and MRI imaging techniques can usually suggest the diagnosis of a mediastinal abnormality depending on the location and physical characteristics of the lesion (Fig. 6.3). Other clinical inputs may contribute to the diagnostic process such as the history and examination (thymoma with myasthenia), biochemical analyses (alpha fetoprotein and beta human chorionic gonadotrophin [HCG] in germ cell lesions) and isotope scans (ectopic parathyroid). It is often the case, however, that noninvasive methods cannot provide adequate certainty for long-term management so that a biopsy is required. A VATS procedure, on the other hand, is a sophisticated, expensive and potentially time-consuming technique and may not be appropriate for some biopsy procedures if other simpler, cheaper and equally effective minimal access surgical options are available. The choice includes:

● fine-needle aspiration biopsy
● needle core biopsy
● mediastinoscopy
● anterior mediastinotomy.

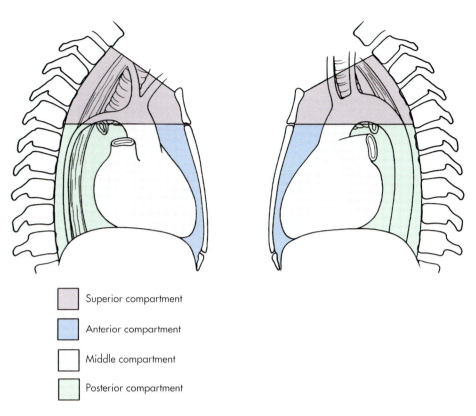

Figure 6.2 *Topography of the mediastinum (previous classification).*

Superior compartment

Anterior compartment

Middle compartment

Posterior compartment

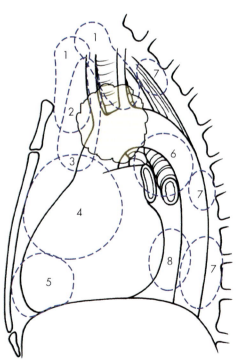

Figure 6.3 *Topography of mediastinal lesions. (1) Goitre, (2) lymph node tumours, primary and metastases, (3) thymoma, (4) dermoid/teratoma, (5) pleuro-pericardial cyst, (6) bronchogenic cyst, (7) neurogenic tumour, (8) enterogenous cyst.*

Fine-needle aspiration biopsy can provide a rapid and reliable diagnosis with minimal trauma and at low cost in suitable cases.[1] A needle core biopsy should be the procedure of first choice for a large mediastinal mass, particularly when lymphoma is suspected, as the larger tissue sample is associated with high (>90%) diagnostic accuracy.[2–3] Pretracheal and paratracheal masses may be sampled by transbronchial needle biopsy[4] and if this is unhelpful mediastinoscopy should be undertaken. Pathological subaortic or preaortic lymph nodes or a large anterior mediastinal mass placed immediately behind the costal cartilages are easily accessible through an anterior mediastinotomy (Chamberlain procedure). Both mediastinoscopy and mediastinotomy are effective and highly accurate techniques but are limited in anatomical range and in the size of specimen which can reasonably be managed. Visualisation may also be relatively impaired although the view at mediastinoscopy can now be greatly improved by the use of instruments with videoimaging optics.[≠] The specific advantage of mediastinoscopy over a VATS approach for

≠ Karl Storz GmBH & Co., Tuttlingen, Germany

mediastinal node biopsy is the opportunity to sample both paratracheal zones whereas sampling by bilateral VATS would be time-consuming and impractical.

In some cases, access to the mediastinum may not be required at all. The commonest causes of a mediastinal mass are metastatic carcinoma or lymphoma both of which may often be diagnosed on biopsy of more accessible deposits elsewhere. Approximately half of the patients with a mediastinal lymphomatous mass will, for example, have nodes palpable in the neck and excisional biopsy of one of these would be the least invasive method of getting a tissue sample.

VATS in the diagnosis and management of mediastinal lesions

General indications

A VATS approach is complementary to other minimal access techniques and is, consequently, most appropriately used where it may contribute additional or better information or where more than a simple biopsy procedure is required. It is, therefore, indicated in the diagnosis, staging and treatment of mediastinal masses or lymphadenopathy in the following circumstances:

- other techniques (needle biopsy, mediastinoscopy or mediastinotomy) have failed, are contraindicated or are inappropriate to the location of the lesion
- concurrent assessment or treatment of pulmonary, pleural or pericardial involvement is required
- excision of a cyst or encapsulated tumour is anticipated
- mediastinal pathology occurring in paediatric patients who are too small to undergo mediastinoscopy.

Aspects of general technique

Anaesthesia

The authors routinely employ a double lumen tube but a Univent* tube can be helpful in patients with small calibre airways. For operations close to the diaphragm, particularly in patients with poor respiratory reserve, selective block of the inferior lobar bronchus can be obtained by the use of a Fogarty-type catheter positioned under fibre optic bronchoscopic guidance.

Instruments

Trocars. Wide and flexible trocars (15–20 mm Flexipath†) allow bent endoscopic instruments and conventional tools to

be introduced. In thin patients however, the trocars for operative endoscopic instruments can be removed and instruments inserted directly through the ports. This approach also makes it easier to use conventional instruments.

Optic. The procedure routinely starts with a 0° optic for exploration of the pleural cavity and in most instances this is adequate for the whole operation. When it is necessary to view a lesion from various angles, a 30° optic is more helpful and may facilitate delicate dissection in a narrow field.

Endoscopic instruments. Routine disposable equipment may be sufficient for simple biopsy procedures but bent or rotating instruments are often helpful. Endoscopic clip appliers (Endo-clip‡, Ligaclip ERCA†) are indispensable for haemostasis. Endo-loops† are seldom used for the purpose, but can be used to lift and pull a lesion after binding its base. Endo-staplers (Endo-Gia‡, Linear Cutter Endopath†) must be available for all major procedures.

As blunt dissection is most commonly employed in mediastinal surgery, endoscopic blunt dissectors are very useful and safe (Endopath Endoscopic Dissector†, Endoscopic Kittner#).

The authors make extensive use of bipolar coagulation forceps during mediastinal dissection as only the tissue grasped between the instrument's prongs is coagulated. This avoids inadvertent electrical damage or thermal injury to nearby structures, which can be a significant risk in VATS procedures due to the lack of stereoscopic vision. Bipolar forceps are very helpful for dissecting soft tissues using a process of alternately coagulating and then tearing them little by little. This intermittent action minimises the amount of smoke in the field and although apparently slow, it is safe and actually relatively fast as no time is lost due to blood oozing or in removing excessive smoke.

It is essential to extract any specimens in endoscopic bags (Endo Catch#, Endopouch†) in order to avoid tumour seeding.

* Fuji Systems Corporation, Tokyo, Japan
† Ethicon Endo-Surgery
‡ United States Surgical Corporation, Norwalk, Conn., USA
# O.R. Concepts, Inc. Roanoke, Tex. USA

Conventional instruments

It is quite common to employ conventional instruments such as scissors, ring forceps, right angled clamps and vascular clamps and a conventional round-end sucker with the end bent by about 60° can also be useful for suction, dissection, displacement and traction (Fig. 6.13).

A small paediatric Finocchietto retractor should be available in case it is necessary to open the utility thoracotomy.

Swabs can be used as in open chest surgery but the authors pass a suture through the swab to avoid the risk of leaving one inside the chest. As with all major VATS procedures, a complete set of instruments for emergency thoracotomy must always be available.

Patient positions

Routine. The routine position is a lateral one with the arm raised for procedures on the upper mediastinum (Fig. 6.4) and with the arm forward for procedures on the lower mediastinum (Fig. 6.5).

Abduction of the arm limits the space for ports, but trocars can be inserted where the chest walls are thinner, and one can be located in the axilla. In this position, if necessary, a lateral emergency thoracotomy can be performed in a few seconds.

The classical position for posterolateral thoracotomy with the upper arm forward is more versatile as regards trocar placement, and as the arm is displaced anteriorly, facilitates handling the instruments. In either case, the table is broken to aid lung and diaphragm displacement and to minimise the need for endoscopic retractors.

Anterior mediastinal lesions. For operations on the anterior mediastinum the patient is placed supine but with the hemithorax elevated by 20–45°, in order to displace the lung laterally, without retractors. With the patient in this position and the arm raised, an axillary trocar can be inserted in the third space and at the same time a cervicotomy or mediastinoscopy can be carried out. This approach is particularly useful for thymic surgery (Fig. 6.6). If a cervicotomy plus bilateral thoracoscopic approach is employed the patient is supine with a support under his back and a lifter in traction behind the manubrium (Figs. 6.7–6.8).

Costovertebral sulcus lesions. For lesions of the costovertebral sulcus, the patient is positioned rolled prone by 120° in order to displace the lung anteriorly (Fig. 6.9).

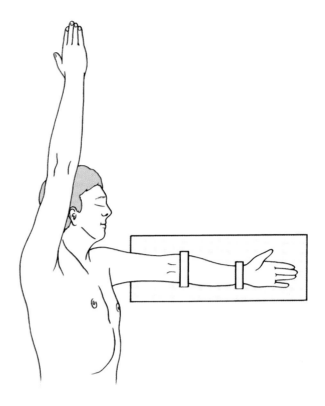

Figure 6.4 *Routine lateral position for VATS on the upper mediastinum.*

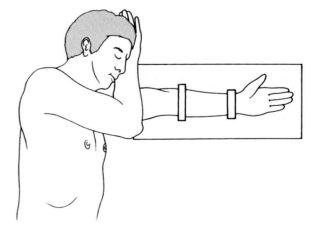

Figure 6.5 *Routine lateral position for VATS on the lower mediastinum.*

Whichever position is to be used, the patient must be secured so as to allow the full movement of the operating table in any direction.

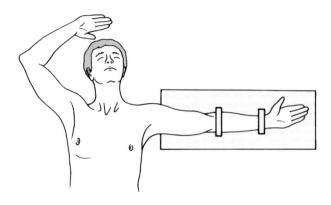

Figure 6.6 *The position for breast surgery allows a good approach to the anterior mediastinum and simultaneous cervicotomy or mediastinoscopy.*

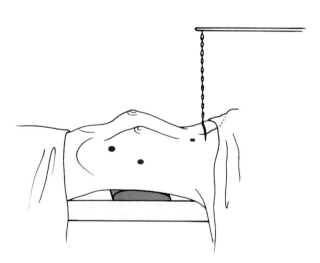

Figure 6.7 *The position of patient and ports for VATS extended thymectomy through a cervicotomy plus bilateral thoracoscopy.*

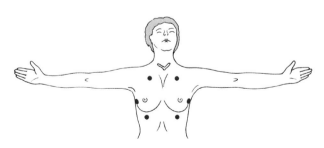

Figure 6.8 *The position of trocars for VATS extended thymectomy through a cervicotomy plus bilateral thoracoscopy.*

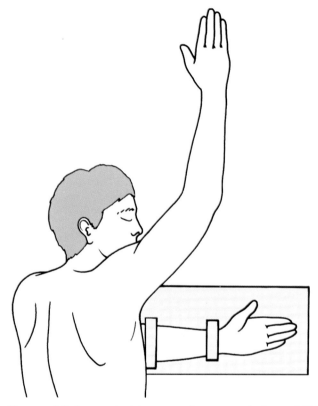

Figure 6.9 *Paravertebral lesions are best approached in a 120° position, to displace the lung anteriorly.*

Position of the surgeons

The positioning of the operating team is shown in Figure 6.10 but the location of the monitors will vary according to the site of lesion. The use of two monitors allows the whole surgical team to follow the procedure and ensures that both the surgeon and the assistant are not forced into uncomfortable positions (Figs. 6.10–6.11).

Trocar positions. In general, the use of a classical diamond arrangement avoids crossing instruments within the chest cavity. After introducing the optic and having explored the pleural cavity and mediastinum, the operative instrument trocars can be safely inserted under direct vision. Choice of the correct position may be helped by transillumination or by insertion of a long fine needle through the proposed port site.

Drains. One or two drains are usually placed at the end of the procedure as for any open chest operation. If the procedure has not involved the lung or drainage of a pleural effusion the necessity of leaving drains is a matter for debate.[6]

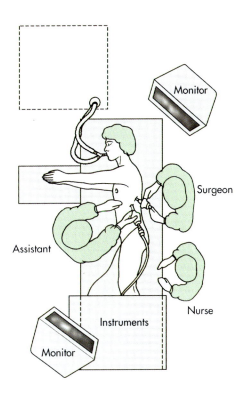

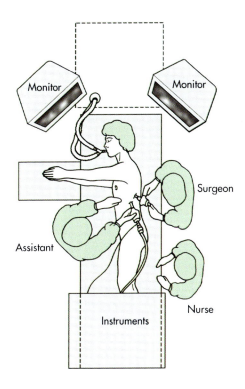

Figure 6.10 *With two monitors available, surgeons are not compelled to work in uncomfortable positions.*

Figure 6.11 *Another possible two-monitor layout for the VATS operating theatre.*

Specific applications of VATS in mediastinal disease

Biopsy of the indeterminate mediastinal mass

As previously discussed, a VATS approach is a highly effective biopsy technique which enables the surgeon to take a large sample under direct vision. The proximity of other anatomical structures can be readily appreciated and an opinion formed as to likely operability if this issue is in question. There is also the opportunity to assess and if necessary biopsy or manage concurrent intrathoracic disease processes.

Technique

Positioning and port positions will vary according to the location of the mass. The mediastinal pleura is often thickened over a mass and should be incised over a mass so that the biopsy obtains a good sample of abnormal tissue. It is prudent to aspirate with a fine gauge needle prior to sampling. Highly vascular tumour may be best managed by a needle core biopsy taken under direct vision so that pressure can then be placed on the puncture site with a pledget afterwards.

Lymph node biopsy and staging in bronchogenic carcinoma

It is frequently necessary to biopsy mediastinal lymph nodes either to obtain a diagnosis in cases of unexplained lymphadenopathy, e.g. sarcoid or lymphoma, or in the assessment of bronchogenic carcinoma. The value of excluding all but very limited N2 disease prior to undertaking pulmonary resection for bronchogenic carcinoma has been well established and accurate post resectional staging is also of increasing importance in defining patients with unsuspected N2 disease many of whom are now managed under neo-adjuvant therapy protocols.

Mediastinoscopy should remain the method of choice for biopsy of unexplained lymphadenopathy and for primary pre-resectional surgical assessment of the mediastinum. This technique is validated by the ability to sample pretracheal and both contralateral and ipselateral paratracheal nodes, the proven value of a positive finding in the context of bronchogenic carcinoma and the minimal access nature of the procedure. Anterior mediastinotomy is of proven value for the assessment of Station 5 lymph nodes but is probably less effective than a VATS procedure because of the limited surgical field obtained.

Neither mediastinoscopy nor mediastinotomy allow sampling of paraoesophageal and pulmonary ligament nodes and access to the subcarinal region is greatly restricted. These regions are therefore conventionally sampled or cleared at open surgery whereas a VATS exploration provides a minimally invasive method of accessing lymph nodes in these regions. Also, in bronchogenic carcinoma cases, the opportunity exists to exclude unsuspected inoperability and to take a concurrent needle biopsy of the primary pulmonary mass if histology is unknown.

Surgical technique

The patient is positioned in the routine position for access to the upper mediastinum and the operating table is foot tilted downwards. Trocars are placed in the midaxillary line on the seventh space (optic) and in the fourth and sixth intercostal space in the anterior and posterior axillary line, respectively (Fig. 6.12).

Biopsy

If the mediastinal pleura is not involved, it is opened after gentle coagulation to avoid oozing. Pathological nodes are usually easy to recognise and occasionally 'pop' out through the pleural dissection. If stone-like mediastinal infiltration is encountered, a 1.8 mm Menghini needle can be inserted through the chest wall to take core biopsies under direct vision. Generally, this is sufficient to provide satisfactory specimens, but, depending on the amount of bleeding the needle biopsy provokes, it is easy to decide if a surgical biopsy can be taken safely.[5]

Mediastinal lymph node dissection

Complete lymph node sampling may be performed either for staging, or to achieve a radical lymph node dissection prior to undertaking lung resection for cancer. The trocars should be inserted one space lower so that the pulmonary ligament can be divided easily to allow access to Station 9 nodes. The lung is then displaced anteriorly and the

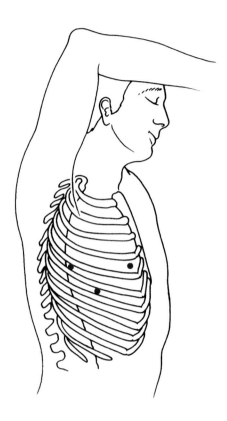

Figure 6.12 *Position of ports for biopsies of the upper mediastinum.*

mediastinal pleura is opened at the posterior hilar reflection. Blunt dissection with pledgets and the bipolar coagulator is used to remove the paraoesophageal (Station 8) and subcarinal (Station 7) nodes. This procedure is relatively easy on the right side but more difficult on the left, particularly for the Station 7 nodes. In the right chest, it mediastinoscopy has not been performed, the mediastinal pleura is then incised from the azygos vein to the thoracic inlet following the course of the vagus nerve. The azygos is lifted and displaced to display group 4 and 2 (right paratracheal) nodes (Fig. 6.13) which can be sampled or excised. The use of gentle blunt dissection and bipolar coagulation or endoscopic clips avoids bleeding. In the authors' experience an angulated metal sucker is extremely useful when dissecting soft tissues as it can be used both to keep the field dry and to displace anatomical structures (Fig. 6.13).

On the left side the subaortic (Station 5) and preaortic (Station 6) nodes are easily recognised and removed although care must be taken to avoid damaging the recurrent (Fig. 6.14) and phrenic nerves. Using this

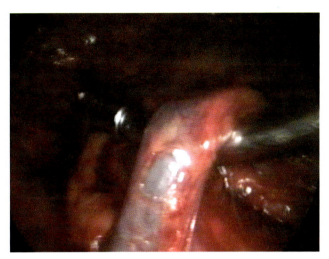

Figure 6.13 *Right paratracheal lymphadenectomy. The azygos vein is lifted by a bent metal sucker, allowing the surgeon to reach right paratracheal lymph nodes.*

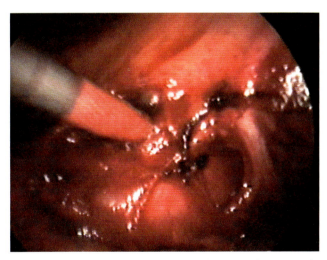

Figure 6.14 *Subaortic lymph nodes biopsy. Subaortic nodes (Group 5) have been removed and vagus and recurrent nerves are clearly visible.*

approach any growth or lymph node group in the mediastinum can be reached and biopsied safely and with limited dissection providing that pathological adhesions do not conceal the anatomical structure and make the approach inadvisable.[5–18]

In order to reduce the open and shut thoracotomy rate due to either local inaccessibility or advanced nodal disease it has now become quite common to perform a thoracoscopic evaluation, immediately prior to thoracotomy, both for advanced pulmonary and mediastinal neoplasms.[5–10]

Management of discrete mediastinal pathologies

A VATS approach is now the procedure of choice for the removal of cysts and a variety of small encapsulated tumours from the mediastinum. Should the dissection become hazardous, conversion to open thoracotomy is required. Even if it is necessary to convert to an open technique, however, the preceding videothoracoscopic procedure is often so advanced that a targeted unspreaded mini-thoracotomy rather than a full open thoracotomy is adequate to complete the operation safely. The approach is still, therefore, less invasive than with a standard thoracotomy.

Mediastinal cysts

The most common cysts are pleuropericardial, thymic, bronchogenic, and enteric.

Pleuropericardial cysts

Pleuropericardial cysts do not usually require surgical management as they can be reviewed at serial follow-up or aspirated. Removal may be indicated if they become large, or aspiration proves to be inadequate or the patient becomes psychologically stressed by the presence of a known lesion.

Technique

As for any thoracoscopic operation close to the diaphragm the patient is positioned at about 90°, with the arm forward (Fig. 6.5), and the bed tilted to displace the diaphragm or the inferior lobe downwards. The optic is positioned in the anterior–mid-axillary line in the 4th space, and trocars for operative instruments in the 6th space.

Removal of these lesions is usually simple, as there is almost always a good plane of dissection around the cyst. Caution is required to avoid severing or coagulating the phrenic nerve or breaking the pericardium and injuring the heart or initiating a dysrhythmia. Initially, the cyst can be partially detached by a combination of sharp and blunt dissection, without having to grasp it. It is both difficult and unnecessary to attempt to remove it intact so, after freeing as much of the cyst wall as possible, the cyst can be punctured and then rolled up on an endoscopic clamp. Blunt dissection with a pledget can then be used to detach the remaining wall from the pericardium. If dense adhesions are present close to the phrenic nerve it is safer to leave a portion of the cyst wall in place.

Bronchogenic and enterogenous cysts
These are usually located in the visceral mediastinum, and often have thick, vascular adhesions between the cyst wall, and the tracheo-bronchial tree and/or the oesophagus.

Technique
The position of the patient and trocars will depend on the location of the cyst. A 30° optic is preferable as this affords more opportunity to select the easiest direction of dissection at each stage of the procedure. It is sensible to place a bougie in the oesophagus preoperatively as this will help the surgeon to identify and therefore to avoid damaging its wall. As with a pleuropericardial cyst, once the lesion has been emptied, its wall can be rolled up on an Endo-clamp, which will display connective bridges and vessels attached to the mediastinal structures. These can be bluntly dissected and coagulated as appropriate. Removal can be straightforward or, probably depending on previous episodes of inflammation, so difficult as to require sharp dissection in a piecemeal fashion. This is only possible if the cyst is relatively small (<4 cm or so). In this situation it may also be prudent to leave a portion of the wall behind rather than risk damaging a vital structure, eventually coagulating the mucosal layer.[14,15,19,20]

Germ cell tumours

Malignant germ cell tumours are generally treated by neo-adjuvant therapy and open surgical excision. The role of VATS in such cases is therefore mainly diagnostic.

Removal of anterior mediastinal dermoid teratomas using VATS techniques has been reported.[18] The main technical difficulty with this tumour is size which is often too large for a VATS approach.

Diseases of the thymus

Asymptomatic thymic cysts do not usually require to be removed unless imaging techniques are unable to exclude a partially solid and therefore potentially malignant lesion.

Myasthenia without thymoma is currently treated by thymectomy plus radical removal of the fatty tissue of the anterior mediastinum through a median sternotomy[21] or a cervicotomy with sternal split.[22,23] The same kind of operation has been reported recently through a left[5,14,18] or right[24] thoracoscopic approach, and through a cervicotomy plus bilateral thoracoscopic approaches.[25]

A series of 106 consecutive video-assisted thymectomies performed with this technique has been reported: 54 of them thymic hyperplasia, 31 hypertrophy, 17 thymoma and one lymphoma. For non-neoplastic pathology the average operative time was 94 minutes, for Stage 1 thymomas 128 minutes and for invasive thymomas 153 minutes. Conversion into sternotomy was performed three times: one case of thymoma vascular infiltration, one case of cardiomegalia and one of massive pleural adhesions. Average hospital stay was six days. Mortality of this series was zero; the only relevant surgical complication was a phrenic nerve injury in a severely obese patient. This approach allows the radical removal of the fatty tissue from the neck to the diaphragm and of mediastinal pleura from the phrenic nerves to the sternal reflection. The extension and amount of fatty tissue which is capable of resection is exactly the same as in a transsternal maximal thymectomy.[26]

Technique
The patient, ventilated by a double lumen tube, is supine with the back elevated by a support (to increase the intercostal spaces) and arms abducted (Figs. 6.7 and 6.8). Through a five-centimetre cervicotomy the upper thymic lobes are isolated as far as the innominate vein and the pre-tracheal fat is removed. Then, using a hook-shaped lifter inserted behind the manubrium, the sternum is elevated with a 20 kg traction in order to widen the retrosternal space. The left lung is collapsed and three trocars are inserted, two in the inframammary sulcus and one in the second space at the midclavicular line. The mammary vessels and phrenic nerve are identified, and the mediastinal pleura is divided just along the lower path of mammary vessels evidencing the retrosternal lifter, and along the upper path of the phrenic nerve.

Dissection of the thymus starts on the left side from the pericardium and ascending aorta, reaching the innominate trunk. The retrosternal space is totally freed and right mediastinal pleura widely opened. Ports on the right side are symmetrically located and by this approach the mediastinal pleura is incised along the line of the superior vena cava (Fig. 6.15), then the innominate vein is dissected free and the veins of Keines are clipped and cut (Fig. 6.16). Following the phrenic nerves downwards, all the fatty

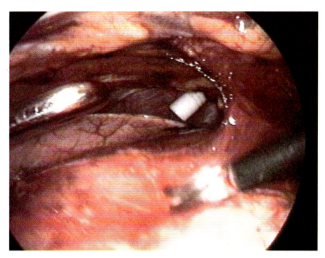

Figure 6.15 *Extended thymectomy: right approach. Both mediastinal pleuras have been resected 'en-bloc' with thymus and fatty tissue. Behind the lifter the left lung can be seen.*

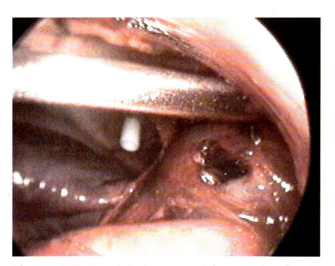

Figure 6.16 *Extended thymectomy: left approach. After the removal of thymus and fatty tissue the contralateral pleural cavity is visible and the innominate trunk is in the foreground.*

tissue which lies on the pericardium as far as the diaphragm is dissected and separately removed through the trocars. Then, pulling the upper thymic lobes which will already have been isolated, the whole gland is removed *en bloc* with the mediastinal pleuras and the remaining fatty tissue. Both pleural cavities are drained.[26]

Thoracoscopic thymectomy for thymoma has been reported[14,27] and heavily criticised.[28,29] It has been observed that this procedure does not allow the surgeon to detect a

limited area of capsular infiltration, and, even dealing with a true stage 1 lesion, a tear in the capsule due to handling could be catastrophic, in view of the well established risk of seeding with these tumours.[29] Furthermore, small stage 1 thymomas can be resected by the only moderately traumatic approach of combined cervicotomy and sternal split.[5] The authors agree with these remarks and their experience is consequently limited to cases with small stage 1 tumours confined within the mediastinal fatty tissue. They started their experience with a monolateral approach, left or right depending on the location of the lesion, performing a radical thymectomy in carefully selected cases. None of their five cases of thymoma had a neoplastic recurrence, but they registered one case of myasthenia onset two years after thymectomy in a patient of this group. He underwent a cervicotomy plus bilateral thoracoscopic mediastinal lipectomy, and a minimal thymic remnant was found at histology. In the light of this experience all the following thymectomies were performed by cervicotomy plus bilateral VATS mainly for myasthenia and in the estimation of the authors this approach represents the highest standard for thoracoscopic thymectomy.

They have found that the combination of right thoracoscopy and mediastinoscopy allows for full access to and surgical control of the thymic space and middle mediastinum. This technique was utilised in cases of suspected relapse of treated lymphoma, and once to remove a mediastinal parathyroid adenoma (Fig. 6.17).

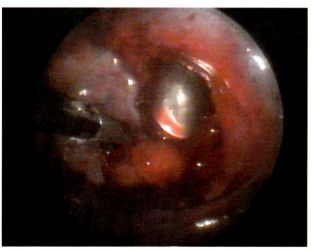

Figure 6.17 *A parathyroid adenoma is being removed through a combined right thoracoscopic and mediastinoscopic approach.*

Lesions of the thoracic outlet

It can be difficult to gain adequate access to the thoracic outlet using open chest surgery unless a highly traumatic extruded lateral thoracotomy or 'T' extruded median sternotomy is used. In the authors' experience, a thoracoscopic approach utilising a 30° optic allows a detailed and precise exploration of this region. Lesions in this area are uncommon but the value of this approach can be judged from the following examples.

- A patient presented with a 4 cm mass at the level of the right thoracic inlet located in the angle between the trachea and oesophagus. The diagnosis could not be made by either needle biopsy or mediastinoscopy but video-assisted biopsy revealed a fibro-microcystic thyroid goitre. Using thoracoscopic techniques it was easy to free the mass up to its upper pole where vessels and a fibrous cord connected it to the right thyroid lobe. The lesion was then removed via cervicotomy together with the right hemithyroid. This is undoubtedly an exceptional application for thoracoscopic surgery and as a note of caution the authors report that in their case, despite careful dissection of the recurrent nerve, a vocal cord palsy occurred. Only two other cases of mediastinal goitre excision using VATS have been reported in the literature but no case details were provided.[30]

- Two patients with an iatrogenic disruption of the trachea arising about 2.5 cm cranial to the thoracic outlet and extending as far as the right main bronchus, were referred to the authors' service and underwent emergency right thoracotomy. The bronchi were intubated selectively from the operative field and the lower thoracic trachea was easily sutured. In order to avoid a cervicotomy the authors completed the upper part of the repair which lay in the extremely narrow space proximal to the first rib (Figs. 6.18–6.19) under video assistance.

In both cases, the postoperative course was uneventful and the functional result excellent. The authors are convinced that video assistance was crucial to managing these cases successfully, and that in favourable cases a short tracheal tear could be repaired solely using video-thoracoscopic techniques.

- Another iatrogenic tracheal lesion was suspected from observation of a minimal air leakage from the cervicotomy during a transhiatal oesophagectomy. By inserting a 30° optic through the cervicotomy a tear of less than 1 mm was brought to light in the distal trachea (Fig. 6.20).

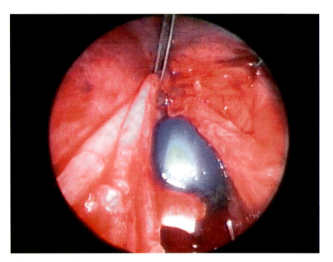

Figure 6.18 *The iatrogenic tracheal tear is shown extending proximally to the thoracic inlet.*

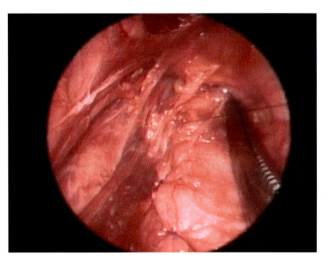

Figure 6.19 *The tear is being repaired by a running suture proximally to the outlet.*

- A 6 cm schwannoma arising from the root of C8 was situated in the left thoracic outlet (Fig. 6.21). After division of the pleura around it and gentle bipolar coagulation of fibrous connections to the first rib, a pedicle of about 2.5 cm in diameter was evident. A suture was then passed through the lesion (Fig. 6.22), grasped with an Endo-clamp and used to provide traction and displacement.

This allowed the authors to look behind the lesion in all directions and therefore to coagulate and dissect the pedicle until the nerve root and vessels were clear enough to be clipped and cut. Haemostasis was completed using bipolar

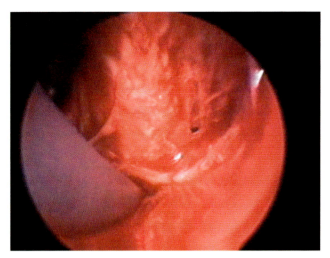

Figure 6.20 *Minimal iatrogenic tracheal tear. A minimal air leakage from the neck after blunt oesophagectomy made the surgeon suspect a tracheal tear, which was confirmed by introducing a 30° optic from the cervicotomy.*

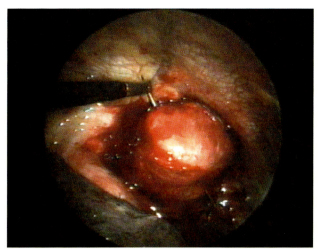

Figure 6.22 *Schwannoma of the left chest wall apex (C8). The lesion is transfixed with a straight needle. The suture will be used for traction and displacement of the mass to dissect its pedicle.*

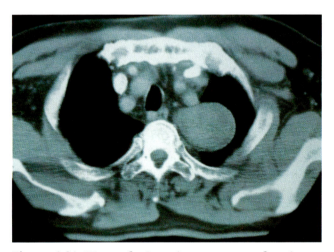

Figure 6.21 *CT scan of a 6 cm schwannoma, rising from the root of C8 and protruding into the left thoracic outlet.*

coagulation, a collagen sponge kept in place with gentle compression with a swab, and fibrin glue.

Neurogenic tumours

Neurogenic tumours can arise anywhere in the chest, but are mainly located along the course of the intercostal nerves, vagi and sympathetic chains. They usually lie in the costo-vertebral sulcus, close to the intervertebral foramina.

Encapsulated neurogenic tumours, especially schwannomas, represent one of the best indications for VATS. Dissection is usually easy and bloodless, as they are not affected by cardiac or pulmonary movement, and generally have a thin pedicle which is easy to dissect. Lesions with a dumbbell shape extension into the vertebral canal, however, require further consideration.

Technique

For lesions of the costo-vertebral sulcus, as for lesions of the spine, oesophagus and thoracic duct, the patient is positioned recumbent at 120° in order to displace the lung anteriorly (Fig. 6.9). The optic is located in the middle axillary line and the operative instruments in the posterior axillary line. A 30° optic will allow the surgeon to look around the pedicle, and to obtain the best possible view of the pedicle structures. Bipolar coagulation is mandatory when working close to the foramina, so as to avoid thermal and electrical injuries to the cord.[5,15] It is helpful to make extensive use of cautery in order to minimise blood oozing, as this can quickly compromise vision in such a restricted field. The pedicle is usually short, and traction is dangerous, so that progress is made in dissecting the pedicle by twisting the mass in either direction in order to gain exposure. If the lesion has a firm capsule, a transfixion suture can be used to grip the mass and can then be passed through the chest wall, thereby sparing a trocar (Fig. 6.22); otherwise one or two endoscopic loops, tied around the base of the lesion, can be used to handle it, while minimizing the risk of rupture. If it is thought that division of the azygos vein would make surgery safer, an Endo-Gia‡ can be used for this but care should be taken not to manipulate the stumps as haemorrhage due to dehiscence of the staple lines has been reported. It is probably safer to staple the vein anteriorly and posteriorly with two Endo-TA‡ instruments and then cut it in the middle. This leaves two long stumps for manipulation and avoids the risk of a tear occurring at the junction with the vena cava.

In case of dumbbell tumours an endoscopic procedure can be performed only if the intervertebral portion does not protrude into the spinal canal. The authors have managed one case using a 5 cm video-assisted thoracotomy in which the tumour was about 5 cm in diameter and the dumbbell approximately 2 cm wide and deep (Fig. 6.23).

In this case, after dissecting all the connections close to the foramen, the authors were able to coagulate around the dumbbell until it was clearly displayed (Fig. 6.24) and then after further gentle dissection popped out revealing the nerve root. On this occasion the view provided by the 30° optic was essential in allowing the pedicle to be clipped and cut without dangerous traction (Fig. 6.25).

Miscellaneous applications

Chylothorax

This condition was discussed in detail in Chapter 5. Surgery to the duct will involve placement of a clip[32] or suture with access being gained via the standard approach for the lower right mediastinum (Figs. 6.5–6.9). Occasionally, if the patient has been given a preoperative fatty meal, the leaking point can be identified by leakage of white chyle but adhesions and pleural thickening commonly obscure the area of leakage. In this situation the pulmonary ligament should be incised so that the duct can be located between the aorta and spine where it is clipped. This dissection has been performed in a case of chylothorax following a traumatic fracture D9–10. As it was impossible to localise the leakage, the thoracic duct and a collateral branch were dissected and clipped (Figs. 6.26–6.27).

‡ United States Surgical Corporation, Norwalk, Conn., USA

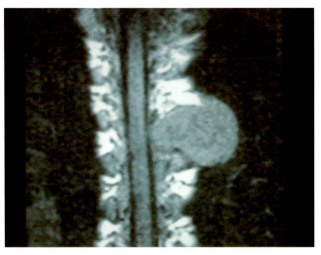

Figure 6.23 *MRI of a 5 cm schwannoma with a 2.5 cm dumbbell intervertebral portion rising from the left T5 root.*

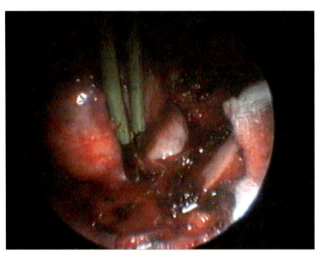

Figure 6.24 *Dumbbell schwannoma of the left paravertebral sulcus (T5). After gentle dissection and bipolar coagulation around the pedicle the dumbbell is peeping out of the foramen.*

Diseases of the spine

Thoracic surgeons may be involved in assisting with the drainage of vertebral abscesses, discectomy and fusion of disc spaces.[33] Thoracoscopic spinal surgery is, however, a highly specialised field and more relevant to neuro- and orthopaedic practice than to cardiothoracic surgery.

Both diagnostic and therapeutic video-assisted procedures for mediastinal non-oesophageal pathology have low complication rates. Sepsis is uncommon as the operative field is not contaminated and most procedures are technically straightforward due to the low vascularity

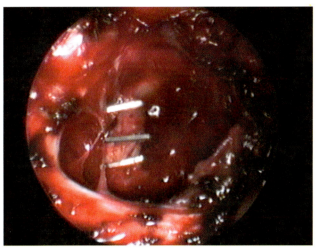

Figure 6.25 *Dumbbell schwannoma of the left paravertebral sulcus (T5). After removal of the lesion the clipped nerve root is evident in the broadened foramen.*

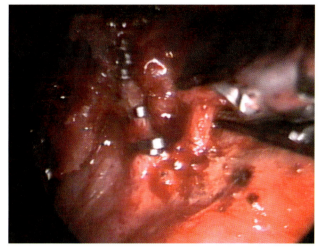

Figure 6.27 *Post-traumatic chylothorax. A collateral lymph vessel has been freed and is being clipped. The leakage will be completely stopped.*

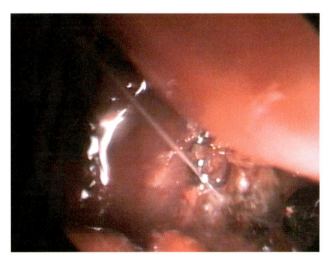

Figure 6.26 *Post-traumatic chylothorax. Through right chest approach the thoracic duct is clipped but a spurt of lymph still occurs.*

of the mediastinal connective tissues combined with the presence of good dissection planes around most benign mediastinal masses. In the authors' view, the use of bipolar cautery is of significant benefit in reducing the risk of inadvertent injury to other structures and in enabling the surgeon to secure a nearly bloodless field thereby optimising the operative view. As with all VATS surgery, should there be any doubts regarding the safety of a mediastinal procedure it is mandatory to convert to an open thoracotomy. If the appropriate indications are followed and correct technique is observed this should rarely be necessary and the patient will have the best possible opportunity to derive the benefits of a minimal access procedure.

References

1 Herman SJ, Holub RV, Weisbrod GL, Chamberlein GW. Anterior mediastinal masses: utility of transthoracic needle biopsy. *Radiology* 1991; **180**: 167–70.

2 Yang PC, Yung CL, Yu CJ *et al.* Ultrasonografically guided biopsy of thoracic tumors. *Cancer* 1992; **69**: 2553–60.

3 Boaron M, Artuso S, Lacava N *et al.* Needle biopsy of anterior mediastinum masses. In: Marx A and Mueller Hermelink HK eds. *Epithelial tumors of the thymus: pathology, biology, treatment.* Plenum Publishing Co. New York, in press, 293–298.

4 Wang KP. Staging of bronchogenic carcinoma by bronchoscopy. *Chest* 1994; **106**: 588–93.

5 Boaron M. Video-assisted thoracic surgery in the diagnosis and treatment of mediastinal lesions. In: Motta G (ed) *Lung cancer: frontiers in science and treatment.* Genoa: Grafica LP 1994: 329–36.

6 Mack MJ, Aronoff RJ, Acuff TE *et al.* Present role of thoracoscopy in the diagnosis and treatment of diseases of the chest. *Ann Thorac Surg* 1992; **54**: 403–9.

7 Landreneau RJ, Hazelrigg SR, Mack MJ *et al.* Thoracoscopic mediastinal lymph node sampling: useful for mediastinal lymph node stations inaccessible by cervical mediastinoscopy. *J Thorac Cardiovasc Surg* 1993; **106**: 554–8.

8 Kleinmann P, Levi JF. Endoscopic procedures in lung and mediastinal surgery. In: Gossot D, Kleinmann P, Levi JF (eds) *Surgical thoracoscopy.* Paris: Springer Verlag 1992: 71–88.

9 Ginsberg RJ. Evaluation of the mediastinum by invasive techniques. *Surg Clin North Am* 1987; **67**: 1025–35.

10 Wihlm JM. La place de la pleuroscopie dans le bilan prè-opératoire du cancer bronchique. *Ann de Chirurgie* 1990; **44**: 139–42.

11 Landreneau RJ, Mack MJ, Hazelrigg SR *et al.* Video-assisted thoracic surgery: a minimally invasive approach to thoracic oncology. *Principle and Practice of Oncology* 1984; **8**: 1–14.

12 Coltharp WH, Arnold JH, Alford WC *et al.* Videothoracoscopy: improved technique and expanded indications. *Ann Thorac Surg* 1992; **53**: 776–9.

13 Hazelrigg SR, Mack MJ, Landreneau RJ. Video-assisted thoracic surgery for mediastinal disease. *Chest Surg Clin North Am* 1993; **3**: 283–97.

14 Acuff TE. Thoracoscopy for mediastinal masses and thymectomy. In: Brown NT (ed) *Atlas of video-assisted thoracic surgery*. Philadelphia: Saunders 1994: 245–9.

15 Gossot D. Abord endoscopique du médiastin. In: *Technique de chirurgie endoscopique du thorax*. Paris: Springer Verlag, 1994: 139–53.

16 Krashna MJ, Mack MJ. Lymph node dissection and staging. In: *Atlas of thoracoscopic surgery*. St Louis: Quality Medical Publishing 1994: 185–94.

17 Casadio C, Giobbe R, Cianci R *et al.* Videothoracoscopy and video-assisted small thoracotomy for the treatment of pulmonary malignancies. *J Cardiovasc Surg* 1994; **35**; 5: 445–8.

18 Roviaro G, Rebuffat C, Varoli F *et al.* Videothoracoscopic excision of mediastinal masses: indications and technique. *Ann Thorac Surg* 1994; **58**: 1679–84.33

19 Lewis RJ, Caccavale RJ, Sisler GE. Imaged thoracoscopic surgery: a new thoracic technique for resection of mediastinal cysts. *Ann Thorac Surg* 1992; **53**: 318–20.

20 Naunheim KS, Andrus CH. Thoracoscopic drainage and resection of giant mediastinal cyst. *Ann Thorac Surg* 1993; **55**: 156–8.

21 Jaretzki A III, Pen AS, Younger DS *et al.* Maximal thymectomy for myasthenia gravis. *J Thorac Cardiovasc Surg* 1988; **95**: 747–57.

22 Levasseur Ph, Le Brigand H. La timectomie par voie cervicale. *Nov Presse Med* 1975; **36**:

23 Paletto A, Maggi G. Thymectomy in the treatment of myasthenia gravis: results in 320 patients. *Int Surg* 1982; **67**: 13–16.

24 Yim AP, Kay RL, Ho JK. Video-assisted thoracoscopic thymectomy for myasthenia gravis. *Chest* 1995; **108**: 1440–43.

25 Novellino L, Longoni M, Spinelli L *et al.* Extended thymectomy, without sternotomy, performed by cervicotomy and thoracoscopic technique in the treatment of myasthenia gravis. *Int Surg* 1994; **79**: 378–81.

26 Novellino L, Longoni M, Spinelli L *et al.* Personal communication: First International Post-Graduate Course of Endocrine Tele-Surgery. February 15th, 1997 Strasbourg, France.

27 Landreneau R, Dowling R, Castillo W, Ferson P. Thoracoscopic resection of an anterior mediastinal tumor. *Ann Thorac Surg* 1992; **54**: 141–4.

28 Pairolero PC. Invited commentary. In: Landreneau R, Dowling R, Castillo W, Ferson P (eds) Thoracoscopic resection of an anterior mediastinal tumor. *Ann Thorac Surg* 1992; **54**: 144.

29 Ginsberg RJ. Thoracoscopy — a cautionary note. Personal communication. *1st Int Symp. Thoracoscopic Surgery*, San Antonio, Te. 1993.

30 Wakabayashi A. Expanded applications of diagnostic and therapeutic thoracoscopy. *J Thorac Cardiovasc Surg* 1991; **102**: 721–3.

31 Peracchia A, Fumagalli U, Rosati R. Thoracoschopishe behandlung von esophagus erkrankungen. *Der Chirurg* 1994; **65**: 671–6.

32 Graham DD, McGahren ED, Tribble CG, Daniel TM, Rodgers BM. Use of video-assisted thoracic surgery in the treatment of chylothorax. *Ann Thorac Surg* 1994; **57**: 1507–12.

33 Mack MJ, Regan JJ, Bobechko WP, Acuff TE. Application of thoracoscopy for diseases of the spine. *Ann Thorac Surg* 1993; **56**: 736–8.

Video-assisted thoracoscopy in the management of spontaneous pneumothorax

7

D.A. Waller and G.N. Morritt

Introduction

Spontaneous pneumothorax occurs in more than seven per 100,000 men and one per 100,000 women per year.[1] Primary spontaneous pneumothorax is caused by rupture of a subpleural bleb in otherwise normal lungs, whereas secondary spontaneous pneumothorax results from underlying lung disease, usually rupture of emphysematous bullae. The aims of treatment are (i) to effect complete re-expansion of the lung by pleural aspiration or intercostal drainage and (ii) to prevent recurrence by causing the visceral pleura to adhere to the chest wall and by controlling the point of air leakage.

Conventional management of pneumothorax has often been restricted to intercostal tube drainage, frequently combined with chemical pleurodesis. This is effective in 60–70% of patients.[2] Surgical intervention is indicated when there is a persisting air leak, the pneumothorax is recurrent or the patient is in a high-risk occupation (e.g. flying or diving).

Conventional surgical treatment has included closure of the parenchymal air leak by suture, staple or ligature together with a procedure to induce pleural symphysis. Parietal pleurectomy has proved superior to pleural abrasion or chemical instillation in preventing recurrence.[3] These procedures are associated with a very low recurrence rate of around 1% when performed via thoracotomy.[4] However, the decision to recommend surgery is often negatively influenced by the postoperative pain and respiratory dysfunction which accompanies thoracotomy. Muscle-sparing incisions have been advocated in an attempt to reduce the trauma of an open surgical approach but still result in impaired respiration[5] and present additional problems with limited surgical exposure.

Thoracoscopic management of pneumothorax

Conventional thoracoscopy has been used for many years to introduce sclerosants into the pleural cavity without subjecting the patient to the trauma of a thoracotomy. The development of endoscopic video imaging equipment and instrumentation has allowed the same range of definitive surgical procedures to be undertaken using minimal access surgical techniques as are available during open thoracotomy. As with open surgery, therefore, video-assisted thoracoscopy is used to identify and seal the air leak and to create pleural adhesions.

Air leak control

The responsible bulla may be ligated with a pretied Roeder knot (Fig. 7.1) using a commercial device[6] (Endoloop†). Alternatively, ablation of blebs has been performed using electrocautery or the carbon dioxide laser.[7] The most widely practised technique, however, is stapled excision bullectomy, usually incorporating wedge excision of the lung apex.

Pleural fusion

Chemical pleurodesis may be performed under video thoracoscopic control and may be advantageous in poor risk

---

†   Ethicon UK Ltd, Edinburgh, Scotland

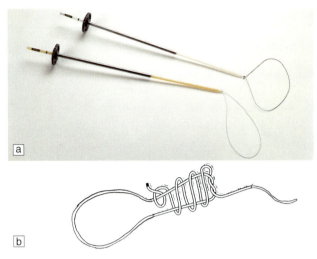

Figure 7.1 *(a) Commercial endoscopic loop applicator utilising a slip knot. (b) Example of hand-tied slip knot (Roeder) which can be created in theatre and pushed into place with a knot pusher.*

patients in whom it can be combined with control of the leaking bulla. The video image can be used to direct sclerosant, particularly kaolin in an even distribution throughout the pleural cavity. Mechanical pleurodesis has been described using several techniques. These include pleural abrasion using a Kittner[#] dissector[8] or a piece of nylon mesh and scarification of the parietal pleura with a Nd:YAG laser.[9] As parietal pleurectomy has the lowest recurrent pneumothorax rate of all the techniques used in open surgery, the authors believe it should be the method of choice for a video-assisted thoracoscopic approach. Methods for stripping the parietal pleura include endosurgical techniques using endoscopic forceps and dissectors,[10] hydrodissection using a Luer-Lock injection needle[11] and pleural elevation with conventional instruments inserted directly under the pleura via a port site. The authors have adopted the latter approach as a simpler and more expeditious method which uses as few specialised instruments and as little operating time as possible.

Operating technique

Anaesthetic technique

Intravenous induction of anaesthesia is preferred as is a double-lumen endobronchial tube and single-lung ventilation.

However, the authors have used endotracheal tubes and high-frequency jet ventilation to one or both lungs if required. Occasionally, in instances of intraoperative desaturation, the operation may be conducted in between periods of bilateral lung ventilation with high concentration oxygen. Perioperative analgesia is greatly improved by the placement of preoperative paravertebral blocks between levels T4 and T8 using 0.25% bupivacaine with adrenaline. Excellent perioperative analgesia has also been obtained by placing extrapleural paravertebral catheters under video control and infusing bupivacaine.[12]

Port placement

With the patient positioned (Fig. 7.2) as for thoracotomy, an initial 2 cm incision is made in the sixth intercostal space just below the tip of the scapula. The pleura is then breached by digital palpation and either a 10.5 mm Thoracoport* or a flexible port (Ethicon Ltd, Edinburgh,

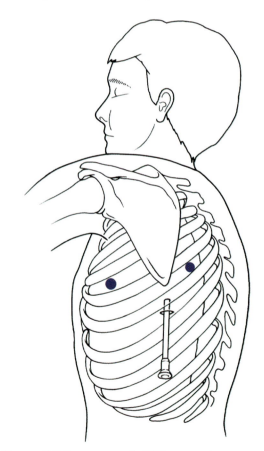

Figure 7.2 *Port positions for VATS pneumothorax surgery.*

O.R. Concepts, Inc. Roanoke, Tex. USA

*   Auto Suture, Ascot, UK

UK) is inserted to allow introduction of the videothoracoscope. The authors have not found it necessary to insufflate carbon dioxide into the thoracic cavity in order to introduce the thoracoscope. Two further incisions are needed to perform an apical bullectomy and parietal pleurectomy. One is placed anterior to latissimus dorsi in the fourth intercostal space and another at the posterior border of this muscle. The authors have modified their original technique to incorporate, as far as is possible, any drain insertion sites. They have also abandoned the use of any ports for the introduction of instruments other than the thoracoscope.

Apical bullectomy

The leaking bleb or bulla (Fig. 7.3) must first be identified. This requires full mobilisation of any pleural adhesions using endoscopic diathermy and shears. Identification of the air leak is facilitated by instillation of saline into the pleural cavity and gentle manual ventilation of both lungs. Once identified, the bleb/bulla is grasped using either an endoscopic grasper or a long Roberts artery forceps.

Bullectomy/blebectomy is performed using an endoscopic linear stapler and cutter (EndoGIA*, Endopath†) (Fig. 7.4) which is inserted alternately via the posterior and anterior incision. Two or three staple lines are often needed to complete the excision.

Pleurectomy

In patients with primary spontaneous pneumothorax where an apical bleb has been identified, an apical parietal pleurectomy is performed. A long Roberts artery forceps (Fig. 7.5) is inserted via the anterior incision into the extrapleural plane under video control. The forceps are advanced towards the apex of the chest, stripping off the parietal pleura with a sweeping motion (Fig. 7.6). Care is taken to keep the pleura intact. This process is then repeated from the posterior incision and may be performed simultaneously by one or two operators. Once the apical pleural sheet has been raised, its edge is grasped by the forceps and the sheet withdrawn from the chest using a twisting motion to wrap the sheet around the forceps whilst applying gentle traction (Fig. 7.7).

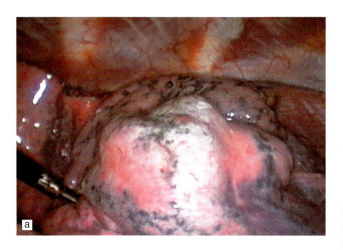

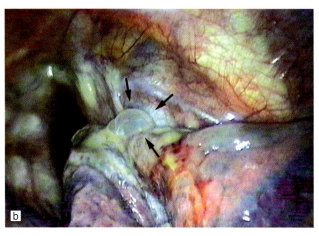

Figure 7.3 *Operative inspection of apex of upper lobe to identify blebs (a) or bullae (b).*

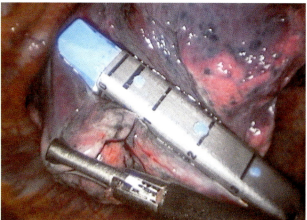

Figure 7.4 *Use of a linear Endo stapler to excise an apex affected by blebs.*

*   Auto Suture, Ascot, UK
†   Ethicon Endo-Surgery

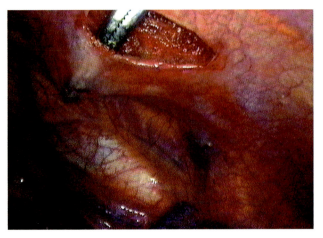

Figure 7.5 *Use of a long Roberts forceps to initiate pleurectomy.*

Abrasion

Abrasion is a reasonable alternative technique for delivering pleural symphysis for patients in whom pleurectomy may be relatively contraindicated, e.g. those with a bleeding disorder. It is particularly relevant when an obvious culprit bulla has been removed. The technique is simple and involves a piece of mesh rolled on a Roberts forceps (Fig. 7.8) which is then used to thoroughly scarify the parietal pleura (Fig. 7.9). Blood in the cavity is suctioned and one apical drain placed under video control. Full reinflation of the lung is achieved under video control and an intercostal multi-holed drain is inserted through the

Figure 7.6 *(a) The curved Roberts forceps are advanced in an extra-pleural plane and used to elevate the parietal pleura. (b) Operative view of pleural elevation.*

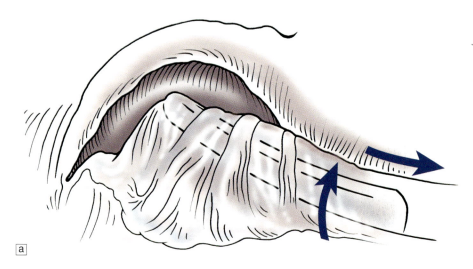

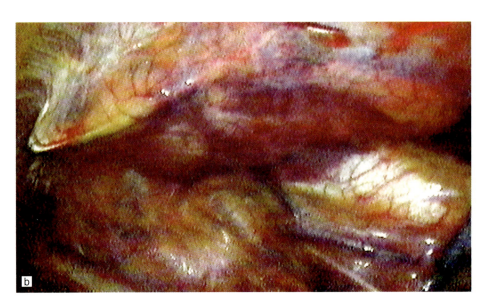

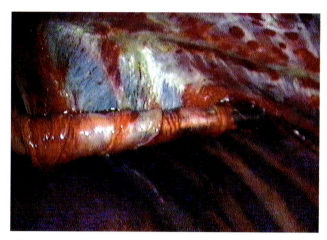

Figure 7.7 *VATS pleurectomy performed by twisting the forceps holding the parietal pleural edge so that the pleura is wound onto the forceps.*

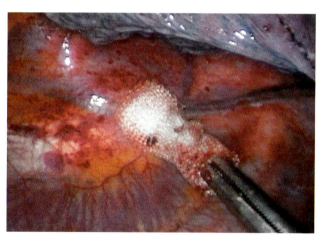

Figure 7.8 *Use of Marlex mesh mounted on Roberts forceps.*

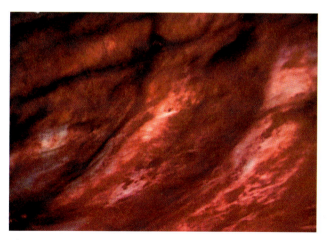

Figure 7.9 *Final appearance after pleural abrasion.*

anterior incision. The other incisions are then closed in layers.

Postoperative care

The drain is placed on suction to 5kPa and a postoperative chest radiograph is obtained at four hours to ensure full re-expansion. The drains are removed when any air leak has ceased and the lung is fully re-expanded. Patients are discharged when apyrexial and pain free on oral analgesics.

Results

Following early reports of the feasibility of treating spontaneous pneumothorax with video-assisted thoracoscopy[6,10,13] the cumulative results of several large series can now be analysed (see Table 7.1).

The authors' initial reported experience with this technique was a series of 18 consecutive patients of which 15 were successfully treated. The median operating time was less than one hour and patients were usually discharged on the fourth postoperative day. The treatment failures were the result of iatrogenic air leak and failure to identify small bullae. Both of these problems could be related to the necessary learning curve for this new technique.[14]

Inderbitzi *et al.* were among the first to report their initial experience with VATS in 79 patients with spontaneous pneumothorax.[15] They used several techniques and found an unacceptably high failure rate of nearly 20% with simple leak ligature using a Roeder knot. Wedge resection and parietal pleurectomy had a 94% success rate and was advocated as the technique of choice. Furthermore, wide excision bullectomy incorporating a generous margin of healthy parenchyma was advised to reduce recurrence. In another large series of 82 consecutive patients Liu *et al.*[16] reported similar problems with slipping of the endoscopic loop ligature and problems of prolonged air leak in patients with diffuse bullous disease. Several series now report excellent long-term follow-up results of VATS for primary spontaneous pneumothorax.[24–30]

Secondary spontaneous pneumothorax

The majority of patients in these initial series have been young and have been treated for primary spontaneous pneumothorax. While the results in this group have been encouraging, doubt still remains about the efficacy of VATS in patients with secondary pneumothorax.[17]

Table 7.1

Results of VATS for pneumothorax

Authors	Patients	PSP: SSP	Lung procedure	Pleural procedure	Mean follow-up (months)	Treatment failure	Mean post-op stay (days)
Andres[24]	54	42:12	–	–	24	4%	5.8
McCarthy[25]	42	–	Staple	Pleurectomy	18	2.5%	5.1
Yim[26]	518	518:0	Staple	Abrasion	20	1.7%	3 (median)
Mouroux[27]	97	75:22	Staple	Abrasion	30	3%	8
Bertrand[28]	163	163:0	Staple	Abrasion	25	4%	6.9
Naunheim[29]	113	83:30	Staple	Abrasion	13	4%	4.3
Waller[30]	150	100:50	Staple	Pleurectomy	32	7%	3 (median)

PSP = Primary spontaneous pneumothorax, SSP = Secondary spontaneous pneumothorax

The authors have attempted to treat patients with secondary pneumothorax using a VATS approach in the belief that these patients stood to benefit most from a minimally invasive technique. In their initial experience[18] they treated 22 patients with pneumothorax secondary to emphysema; 18 were successfully treated. A revisional thoracotomy was required in the remaining four patients due to unstapled air leaks and one of these patients died in respiratory failure. In a comparison with the authors' experience in treating primary spontaneous pneumothorax the operating time was found to be similar and less postoperative analgesia was required but the duration of postoperative air leak (mean 6.3 days) and postoperative stay (9 days) were longer. There were also significantly more treatment failures in the secondary pneumothorax group which were indicative of the diffuse nature of the bullous disease and consequently of the more challenging surgical problem.

Serious anaesthetic problems with high-risk (advanced emphysema) patients undergoing VATS for pneumothorax even in the presence of a contralateral single lung transplant were not observed.[19] In the initial series of 22 patients, inability to tolerate single-lung ventilation, due to desaturation, was noted in five. Intermittent manual ventilation of both lungs or low frequency jet ventilation was necessary to deal with the dilemma of matching the surgical requirements of a partially inflated, quiescent lung and static mediastinum with adequate intraoperative oxygenation.

VATS versus thoracotomy

Although the reported experience of VATS in the treatment of spontaneous pneumothorax has been favourable, the new technique must be compared with the conventional approach via a thoracotomy. There have been several retrospective comparisons of VATS and thoracotomy[20] which have reported a reduction in analgesic requirement and hospital stay in the VATS group. However, their obvious methodological deficiencies make firm conclusions difficult. In an attempt to resolve this problem the authors conducted a prospective comparison of the two methods in both patients with primary and secondary spontaneous pneumothorax.[21]

In the treatment of primary pneumothorax, the use of VATS in comparison to thoracotomy resulted in no increase in operating time, reduced postoperative analgesia and a reduced postoperative stay. Importantly, there was significantly less postoperative respiratory dysfunction following VATS.

In the patients with secondary pneumothorax, operating time was prolonged by the use of VATS and although postoperative analgesic requirement was less, postoperative stay was prolonged. This result relates to the higher number of treatment failures in the VATS group.

Conclusions

Although there are significant apparent advantages when using a VATS approach in the management of spontaneous pneumothorax, further investigation and development is required. As yet, despite present financial restraints, no authors have performed a detailed cost–benefit analysis. Such a study would have to extend beyond the obvious issues of earlier discharge and increased disposables costs to consider additional costs such as timing of return to work, and the costs of late pain and domestic support for the elderly patient in the community.

The elderly emphysematous patient with secondary spontaneous pneumothorax could potentially derive substantial benefit from this form of minimal access surgery. Unfortunately, the diffuse nature of the bullous disease present requires excellent visualisation of the whole lung but this is often difficult to achieve due to the presence of adhesions and conflict with the need to ventilate the lung in order to maintain oxygen saturation. Also, the combination of friable pulmonary parenchyma and multiple staple lines encourages postoperative air leakage. Future developments in this field, therefore, should be orientated towards improving ventilatory techniques so as to maximise the surgical view and to reducing air leakage through staple lines. Technical advances in the use of buttressing materials for endoscopic staplers have been helpful in reducing this problem.

The evidence supporting videothoracoscopic surgery for primary spontaneous pneumothorax is, conversely, more convincing. In this group of patients the goals of future development should lie in improving current technique by further reducing procedure-related pain and in better overall pain control. Fibrin glue[22,23] may represent one method of achieving painless pleurodesis and the use of routine regional anaesthesia with paravertebral catheters placed during the VATS operation may improve postoperative pain. Even on the basis of current experience, it must be appropriate to reassess the indications for surgery in primary spontaneous pneumothorax. In view of the decreased severity of a VATS procedure and the potentially fatal nature of this condition, surgery should now be considered on first presentation rather than after multiple recurrent episodes.

References

1   Melton LJ, Hepper NGC, Offord KP. Incidence of spontaneous pneumothorax in Olmstead County, Minnesota 1950–1974. *Am Rev Respir Dis* 1979; **120**: 1379–82.

2   Elfeldt RJ, Schroeder D, Meinicke O. Spontaneous pneumothorax — considerations on aetiology and therapy. *Chirurg* 1991; **62**: 540–6.

3   Singh SV. The surgical treatment of spontaneous pneumothorax by parietal pleurectomy. *Scand J Thorac Cardiovasc Surg* 1982; **16**: 75–80.

4   Weeden D, Smith GH. Surgical experience in the management of spontaneous pneumothorax 1972–82. *Thorax* 1983; **38**: 737–43.

5   Hazelrigg SR, Landreneau RJ, Boley TM *et al*. The effect of muscle-sparing thoracotomy versus standard posterolateral thoracotomy on pulmonary function, muscle strength and postoperative pain. *J Thorac Cardiovasc Surg* 1991; **101**: 394–401.

6   Nathanson LK, Shimi S, Wood RAB, Cuschieri A. Videothoracoscopic ligation of bulla and pleurectomy for spontaneous pneumothorax. *Ann Thorac Surg* 1991; **52**: 316–19.

7   Wakabayashi A. Thoracoscopic ablation of blebs in the treatment of recurrent or persistent spontaneous pneumothorax. *Ann Thorac Surg* 1989; **48**: 651–53.

8   Melvin WS, Krasna MJ, McLaughlin JS. Thoracoscopic management of spontaneous pneumothorax. *Chest* 1992; **102**: 1875–6.

9   Sharpe DA, Dixon C, Moghissi K. Thoracoscopic use of laser in intractable pneumothorax. *Eur J Cardiothorac Surg* 1994; **8**: 34–6.

10 Inderbitzi RGC, Furrer M, Striffeler H, Althaus U. Thoracoscopic pleurectomy for treatment of complicated spontaneous pneumothorax. *J Thorac Cardiovasc Surg* 1993; **105**: 84–8.

11 Anastasia LF. Method of thoracoscopic pleurectomy. *Ann Thorac Surg* 1994; **57**: 1665–7.

12 Soni AK, Conacher ID, Waller DA, Hilton CJ. Video-assisted thoracoscopic placement of paravertebral catheters: a technique for postoperative analgesia for bilateral thoracoscopic surgery. *Br J Anaesth* 1994; **72**: 462–4.

13 Donnelly RJ, Page RD, Cowen ME. Endoscopy assisted microthoracotomy: initial experience. *Thorax* 1992; **47**: 490–3.

14 Waller DA, Forty J, Yoruk Y, Dark JH, Morritt GN. Videothoracoscopy in the treatment of spontaneous pneumothorax: an initial experience. *Ann R Coll Surg Engl* 1993; **75**: 237–40.

15 Inderbitzi RGC, Leiser A, Furrer M, Althaus U. Three years' experience in video-assisted thoracic surgery for spontaneous pneumothorax. *J Thorac Cardiovasc Surg* 1994; **107**: 1410–15.

16 Liu HP, Lin PJ, Hsieh MJ, Chang JP, Chang CH. Thoracoscopic surgery as a routine procedure for spontaneous pneumothorax. Results from 82 patients. *Chest* 1995; **107**: 559–62.

17 Graham ANJ, McManus KG, McGuigan JA. Videothoracoscopy and spontaneous pneumothorax. *Ann Thorac Surg* 1995; **59**: 266.

18 Waller DA, Forty J, Soni AK, Conacher ID, Morritt GN. Video-thoracoscopic operation for secondary spontaneous pneumothorax. *Ann Thorac Surg* 1994; **57**: 1612–15.

19 Waller DA, Conacher ID, Dark JH. Videothoracoscopic pleurectomy after contralateral single lung transplantation. *Ann Thorac Surg* 1994; **57**: 1021–3.

20 Hazelrigg SR, Landreneau RJ, Mack M *et al*. Thoracoscopic stapled resection for spontaneous pneumothorax. *J Thorac Cardiovasc Surg* 1993; **105**: 389–92.

21 Waller DA, Forty J, Morritt GN. Video-assisted thoracoscopic surgery versus thoracotomy for spontaneous pneumothorax. *Ann Thorac Surg* 1994; **58**: 372–7.

22 Hansen MK, Kruse-Andersen S, Watt-Boolsen S, Andersen K. Spontaneous pneumothorax and fibrin glue sealant during thoracoscopy. *Eur J Cardiothorac Surg* 1989; **3**: 512–14.

23 Hauck H, Bull PG, Pridun N. Complicated pneumothorax: short- and long-term results of endoscopic fibrin pleurodesis. *World J Surg* 1991; **15**: 146–50.

24 Andres B, Lujan J, Robles R *et al*. Treatment of primary and secondary spontaneous pneumothorax using videothoracoscopy. *Surg Lap End* 1998: **8**: 108–112.

25 McCarthy JF, Lannon D, McKenna S, Wood AE. Video-assisted thoracic surgery for spontaneous pneumothorax. *Irish J Med Sci* 1997; **166**: 217–219.

26 Yim AP, Liu HP. Video-assisted thoracoscopic management of primary spontaneous pneumothorax. *Surg Lap End* 1997; **7**: 236–240.

27 Mouroux J, Elkaim D, Padovani B *et al*. Video-assisted thoracoscopic treatment of spontaneous pneumothorax: technique and results of one hundred cases. *J Thorac Cardiovasc Surg* 1996; **112**: 385–391.

28 Bertrand PC, Regnard JF, Spaggiari L *et al*. Immediate and long-term results after surgical treatment of primary spontaneous pneumothorax by VATS. *Ann Thorac Surg* 1996; **61**: 1641–1645.

29 Naunheim KS, Mack MJ, Hazelrigg SR *et al*. Safety and efficacy of video-assisted thoracic surgical techniques for the treatment of spontaneous pneumothorax. *J Thorac Cardiovasc Surg* 1995; **109**: 1198–1203.

30 Waller DA. Video-assisted thoracoscopic surgery for spontaneous pneumothorax — results of a 6 year experience. *Ann R Coll Surg Engl* (in press).

Surgery of bullous-emphysematous lung disease

W.S. Walker

8

Introduction

Bullous-emphysematous lung disease may be regarded as a spectrum of clinical pathology which extends from the single giant bulla at one end to diffuse emphysema at the other (Fig. 8.1). Chronic obstructive lung diseases are common, with US data, for example, indicating that these conditions affect 13.5 million Americans, two million of whom have emphysema, and that they are currently the fourth and also the most rapidly growing cause of morbidity and mortality in the USA.[1,2]

Whereas large bullae have been managed by resection for many years, diffuse emphysema has only recently become amenable to surgical attention with the advent (or reinvention) of lung volume reduction surgery (LVRS). Both types of surgical management can be effectively performed as VATS procedures. The underlying theory, selection criteria and techniques of these two quite different approaches, i.e. bulla excision and lung remodelling, differ appreciably and they will therefore be considered separately.

Diffuse emphysema

Pathological features

Definition

Emphysema may be defined pathologically as enlargement of the air spaces distal to the terminal bronchioles, accompanied by the destruction of the air space (acinar) walls and without obvious fibrosis.[3] Chronic bronchitis is nearly always an associated condition and is a relevant surgical consideration in that these patients produce excessive sputum which is abnormally viscid due to glycoprotein changes and which is usually colonised with *Haemophilus influenzae* and/or *Streptococcus pneumoniae*.

The main pathological structural variants are summarised in Table 8.1. Centrilobular emphysema, which is typically associated with smoking, is the most commonly encountered form of emphysema with only 1% of cases having the panacinar type.[4] These patterns may, however, coexist.

Aetiology

The loss of alveolar elastic fibres in emphysema is well documented.[5] It is hypothesised[6] that the centrilobular pattern of emphysema, which is usually associated with cigarette smoking, results from smoke-induced damage to macrophages lining the terminal bronchioles. These release proteolytic enzymes and chemotactic factors which attract circulating polymorph neutrophils which then release

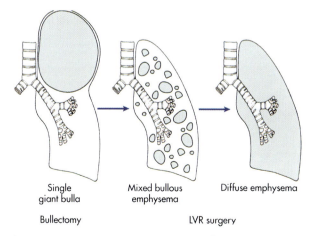

Single giant bulla — Bullectomy

Mixed bullous emphysema

Diffuse emphysema — LVR surgery

Figure 8.1 *Diagrammatic representation of the clinical spectrum of bullous emphysema.*

91

Table 8.1

Emphysema variants

Type	Characteristics
Centrilobular	Acini in the centre of the affected lobule destroyed; the upper lobes are typically more affected; classical smoking-related emphysema
Panacinar	Most of the acini in the lobule are destroyed; distribution favours the lower lobes associated with alpha-1-antiprotease deficiency
Paraseptal	Alveolar disruption distributed in subpleural zone or along fibrous interlobular septa typically in apices; possibly due to congenital abnormal alveoli

elastase. Endogenous proteolytic digestion of lung elastin, collagen and proteoglycans is inhibited by alpha-1-antiprotease which is normally found in serum and airway fluids. Cigarette smoke has powerful oxidant actions, so diminishing locally the effect of this enzyme and leading to maximum damage in the central area of the lobule, i.e. the centrilobular disease pattern common in smokers. Panacinar emphysema is found in patients with alpha-1-antiprotease deficiency which causes the acini to be exposed to the unopposed action of elastase release by circulating polymorphs, thereby accounting for the generalised distribution of disease. Whilst panacinar emphysema appears to be a feature of patients who are homozygous for alpha-1-antiprotease deficiency, heterozygotes are probably at increased risk of smoking-related emphysema.

Pathophysiology

The physiological effects of emphysema may usefully be considered under three headings:

● respiratory work
● haemodynamic effects
● gas exchange.

Respiratory work. Respiratory work is substantially increased in emphysematous patients for whom the oxygen cost of breathing may be several times that of normal controls.[7,8] Various factors contribute to this effect and are summarised below.

Small airway obstruction. The loss of alveolar tissue volume and architecture inherent in emphysema results in diminished elastic recoil and destroys the scaffold-like support to small airways[9] (Fig. 8.2a,b) causing them to become narrowed and tortuous and to collapse prematurely towards the end of expiration. There is, therefore, less force aiding passive expiration and more obstruction to exhalation with consequently increased expiratory work and air trapping which gradually progresses towards hyperinflation.

Stretched respiratory muscles. As the thoracic volume increases, the inspiratory muscles, especially the diaphragm, develop unfavourable length–tension relationships and so become less efficient.[10]

Horizontalised ribs. Chest hyperexpansion causes the ribs to become increasingly horizontal and makes further expansion more difficult.[11]

Positive alveolar pressure at end expiration. Incomplete expiration results in a positive alveolar pressure at end expiration which adds to the respiratory workload.[12]

Reversal of the thoracic recoil effect. Normally, when the forced residual capacity (FRC) is reached, the inward force of the pulmonary elastic recoil is balanced by the outward force of the thoracic cage elastic recoil. In the hyperexpanded emphysematous patient the direction of the thoracic cage elastic recoil is reversed to become an inward-directed force thereby increasing inspiratory work.[11]

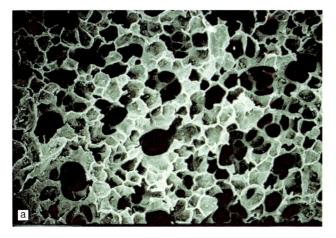

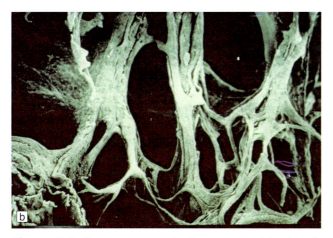

Figure 8.2 *Electron micrographs demonstrating (a) relatively normal alveoli and (b) loss of bronchiolar wall support due to destruction of adjacent alveoli.*

Haemodynamic effects. The haemodynamic consequences of severe emphysema[13,14] contribute to impaired exercise performance. These include:

Restricted diastolic cardiac chamber filling. The mechanical pressure effect of bulky air-trapped lungs causes compression of the cardiac chambers, especially the atria, with consequent impairment of cardiac filling.

Inferior vena cava (IVC) constriction. Flattening of the diaphragm reduces the aperture for the IVC causing partial constriction of the IVC — particularly on exercise.

Pulmonary hypertension. This results from the reduced pulmonary vascular tree. When severe it causes right ventricular failure — the 'blue bloater' syndrome.

Gas exchange. The uneven distribution of emphysematous disease throughout the lung contributes to decreased ventilatory efficiency as measured by carbon monoxide (CO) transfer factor.[15] The more severely emphysematous and bullous areas have a high ventilation/perfusion (V/Q) ratio (i.e. they act as physiological dead space) whereas airway narrowing causes decreased ventilation of better perfused areas. Therefore:

- the patient has to ventilate more than normal to preserve a normal pCO_2 and,
- pO_2 is reduced due to shunt effects.

Lung volume reduction surgery (LVRS)

History of surgical intervention for diffuse emphysema
A variety of diverse surgical approaches have been employed or suggested in the management of emphysema (Table 8.2).[16] Of these, until recently, only pulmonary transplantation has been considered viable. Even this option, however, has been restricted by the shortage of donor organs in comparison to the large number of potential recipients, the inherent difficulties imposed by this demanding form of therapy in an elderly patient group and the uncertain long-term prognosis.

LVRS was originally pioneered by Dr Otto Brantigan and reported initially in 1957[17] with an overall series of 56 patients by 1961.[18] He utilised a multiple wedge resection technique to reduce lung volume in an attempt to improve elastic recoil and diaphragmatic function. This procedure was combined with lung denervation to try to address bronchospasm and hypersecretion. He reported subjective improvement in 75% of patients but did not provide data to support objective improvement and the procedure was associated with a relatively high perioperative mortality of 16%. Given the lack of sophistication in measurement, surgical technology and supportive intensive care at that time, it may well be that his results were far more creditable than was appreciated.

Lung volume reduction (LVR) by laser ablation of emphysematous areas was described in 1991[19] and subsequently[20] with documented modest improvement in the forced expiratory volume in one second (FEV$_1$), forced vital capacity (FVC) and total lung capacity (TLC), but with a perioperative mortality of 21%. The laser reduction technique has been used by others with similar modest improvement in measured indices of respiratory function.[21,22]

93

Table 8.2

Surgical strategies proposed and/or employed in the management of emphysema

Procedure	Rationale
Costochondrectomy Transverse sternotomy }	allow further chest expansion
Thoracoplasty Phrenectomy Pneumoperitoneum Phrenic nerve division }	reduce lung volume
Hilar denervation Procedures }	prevent small airways obstruction
Parietal pleurectomy Kaolin insufflation	promote pulmonary neovascularisation
Lung volume reduction	improve elastic recoil and diaphragmatic function
Lung transplantation	replacement with normal donor lung

Although Brantigan's original work was not pursued for many years, the concept was revisited by Dr Joel Cooper and colleagues who presented their initial experience with 20 patients in 1994.[23] They described bilateral simultaneous LVRS performed through a median sternotomy incision with the parenchymal resection being accomplished using conventional open linear stapling devices. They reported an 82% gain in FEV_1 with a 27% improvement in FVC, 22% fall in TLC and reduction to less than one-third in disability indices. While it is true to say that these results have never been equalled (even by the same surgical team), this experience has formed the basis of and stimulus to all current LVRS, whether through open[24–28] incision or by VATS techniques.[22,27,29–33]

Principles of action of LVR

There remains some debate as to the full mechanisms of action of LVR. The surgical strategy involves excision of the most badly affected areas of emphysematous lung, usually amounting to approximately 25–35% of total lung volume or 50–75 g of tissue per lung. The area removed is predominantly from the upper lobes in patients with centrilobular emphysema but may be from the lower lobes in rare cases of alpha-1-antiprotease deficiency-related panacinar emphysema. The surgical procedure results in an effective reduction in the emphysematous component of the lung and the consequent reversal of many of the adverse features associated with emphysema. Changes identified as being potential beneficial results of LVR surgery are summarised in Table 8.3.

Laboratory data confirm that LVR improves the mechanics of breathing at rest and during exercise with a 49% increase in maximal exercise capacity.[34] LVR improves the ability of the inspiratory muscles to generate force and results in a significant decrease in respiratory drive, decreased mean airway resistance and increased dynamic compliance.[35,36]

Selection criteria

This account presents a synthesis of generally described selection criteria which differ only in minor detail between the various centres describing large series. Indications for and exclusion from surgery are summarised in Tables 8.4 and 8.5 which are derived from the recent American Thoracic Society official statement on LVRS[37] and workshop consensus data reported by Weinmann and Hyatt.[2] The impact of the relative contraindications on clinical outcomes is discussed further in the 'Overall clinical results' section below, where it can be

Result	Functional benefit
Recruitment of previously compressed and underventilated lung	• increased functional lung tissue
Reduced total lung capacity (TLC)	• improved action characteristics of ribs and respiratory muscles • normalised thoracic cage elastic recoil
Reduced physiological dead space	• better ventilation of adjacent lung • improved V/Q matching
Improved pulmonary elastic recoil	• reduced expiratory effort
Removal of narrowed airways	• reduced air trapping • reduced and expiratory airway pressure • reduced respiratory work

Table 8.3

Potential beneficial effects of lung volume reduction surgery (LVRS)

Table 8.4

Indications for surgery

Inclusion criteria

- End stage emphysema refractory to medical management
- Severe dyspnoea
- FEV_1 <35% predicted
- Standard radiological criteria of emphysema:
  - flattened diaphragms
  - hyperexpanded lung fields

Adapted from *Lung Volume Reduction Surgery*. Official statement of the American Thoracic Society.[37]

Table 8.5

Contraindications for surgery

Exclusion criteria

Absolute

Continued smoking
Severe comorbidity
Severe obesity or cachexia

Relative

Age >75 years
Pulmonary hypertension (mean pulmonary arterial pressure >45 mmHg)
Severe hypercapnia ($paCO_2$ ≥50 mmHg)
Diffuse homogenous lung involvement by V/Q or CT scan
End stage disease (FEV_1 <20% predicted; six-minute walk <600 feet)
Inability to undergo pulmonary rehabilitation
Ventilator dependence

Adapted from *Lung Volume Reduction Surgery*. Official statement of the American Thoracic Society[37]; Weinmann and Hyatt 1966.[2]

seen that the adverse impact of these variables is less certain than might be anticipated. These should be viewed, therefore, as strictly relative and interpreted in the context of all available clinical information.

The American Thoracic Society correctly emphasises the need for a multidisciplinary approach to the management of patients undergoing LVR and points to the detailed investigational dataset required to establish suitability for surgery (Table 8.6). The 'typical' patient will have pulmonary investigational data results which are similar to those described by Weinmann and Hyatt (Table 8.7).[2]

Investigational assets will vary between institutions. Basic imaging requires plain chest X-ray (Fig. 8.3), high resolution computed tomography (CT) scan (Fig. 8.4) and

Table 8.6

Basic investigations for screening patients for lung volume reduction surgery (LVRS)

Pulmonary	**Cardiac**
Detailed pulmonary function tests (FEV_1 with reversibilities, FVC, TLC, RV, CO transfer)	ECG
Six-minute walk	LV and RV echocardiography; Doppler estimation of pulmonary arterial pressure
Arterial $pO2$ and $pCO2$	Cardiac catheterisation if ischaemic heart disease suspected
Radiology: – chest films – CT thorax (high resolution / spiral examination)	
V/Q lung scan (presented as separated image sets)	

Adapted from *Lung Volume Reduction Surgery*. Official statement of the American Thoracic Society.[37]

Table 8.7

Typical ranges for baseline pulmonary investigation data in patients selected for LVRS

Test	Result (%) (relative to predicted value)
FEV_1	25–30%
FVC	50–70%
Residual volume	>200%
TLC	130–140%
DLCO	30–40%
Six-minute walk	700–1200 feet

Adapted from Weinmann and Hyatt, 1996.[2]

perfusion/ventilation isotope scanning (Fig. 8.5). Some units will have access to other modalities which may prove to be of value including dynamic magnetic resonance imaging (MRI) and positron emission tomography (PET). Density mask CT imaging, which may be used to show emphysematous areas more clearly (Fig. 8.6), and single photon-emission CT (SPECT) perfusion images[38] can significantly increase the surgeon's understanding of disease distribution. Keenan and colleagues[30] utilised both these techniques. SPECT images can

be presented as three-dimensional reconstructions of lung perfusion allowing the surgeon to determine those areas which may be excised safely without compromising perfused (and therefore functional) lung tissue.

As indicated by the American Thoracic Society, LVRS is not an occasional procedure but rather one which must be undertaken as part of an established programme, with detailed recording of patient data and continuous audit of immediate and late results.

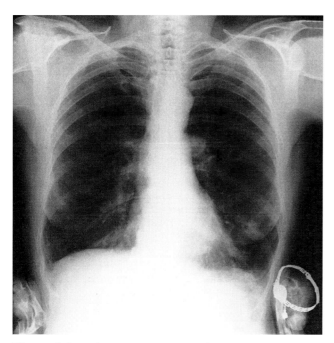

Figure 8.3 *PA chest X-ray in severe emphysema.*

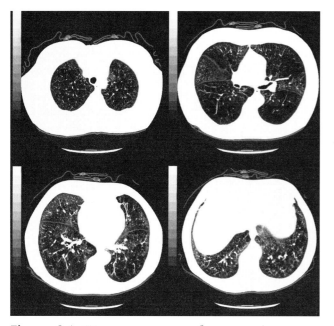

Figure 8.4 *CT scan appearances of severe emphysema at different levels in the chest.*

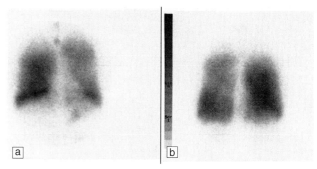

Figure 8.5 *Typical perfusion scan images (a) interior and (b) posterior in emphysema. Note perfusion defect in upper zones.*

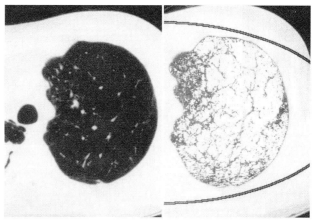

Figure 8.6 *Density mask CT imaging of emphysematous lung (right) compared with conventional CT image (left). (Reproduced from Figure 1, page 311 of Keenan RJ, Landreneau RJ, Sciurba FC et al. Unilateral thoracoscopic surgical approach for diffuse emphysema, J Thorac Cardiovasc Surg 1996; 111: 308–16.)*

Overall clinical results

General data. Several recent series depicting the clinical results obtained with LVRS utilising laser, open stapled and VATS stapled approaches are shown in Table 8.8. These demonstrate modest but significant changes with improvement in FEV_1, decreased TLC and improved dyspnoea status and six-minute walk. The authors usually report a slight reduction in pCO_2 and considerably reduced O_2 and steroid requirement.

Reported complication rates (Table 8.9) are similar across reported data with the headline mortality usually below 6% in most series. There may be a trend for higher reported mortality with open median sternotomy reduction (e.g. Miller and associates 10%[39] and Argenziano and associates 7.1%[40]). There is also, however, evidence that unreported mortality rates may be significantly higher and may approach 50% with bilateral reduction via the median sternotomy route, reflecting the difficulty of achieving good clinical outcomes in poor-risk patients with invasive surgery.[41]

Table 8.8

Results achieved with various types of LVRS

Series	No. in study	Operative technique	Mode	In-patient mortality (%)	FEV₁ (%)	TLC (%)	Six-minute walk (%)	Dyspnoea improvement (various)	In-patient stay (mean days)
Washington University 1996 (Cooper[24])	150	MS Staple	Bilateral	4.0	+51	−14	+16.5*	−1.7 MRCI	13.5
Cleveland Clinic 1997 (Minai[28])	62	MS Staple	Bilateral	4.8	+39	−20.9	+47	−1.0 MRCI	17.9
University of Nevada 1995 (Little[21])	55	VATS YAG Free beam	Unilateral	5.5	+18	–	–	–	–
Multi-institution 1996 (Hazelrigg[29])	141	VATS YAG Contact	Unilateral	5.7	+13.7	−6.5	+29.2	'Minor'	12 (median)
University of Pittsburgh 1996 (Keenan[30])	57	VATS Staple YAG Free beam	Unilateral	3.4	+27	−6.8%	+14	+0.3 Total Disability Index	17
Lung Center Orange, California 1996 (McKenna[22])	33	VATS YAG Contact vs	Unilateral	0	+13.4	–	–	1+ in 8/33 MOS − 36	11
	39	VATS Staple	Unilateral	2.5	+33	–	–	1+ in 26/39 MOS − 36	13
Saint Louis University USA 1996 (Naunheim[32])	50	VATS Staple	Unilateral	4	+33.8	–	+19.7	0.68−>1.1 Mahler	13.1
University Hosp. Zurich 1997 (Stammberger[33]) ++	42	VATS Staple	Bilateral	0	+43	−8.2%	+27.4	−1.9 MRC	13

*patients had undergone extensive preoperative pulmonary rehabilitation; ++ six-month data

MS = Median sternotomy; VATS = Video-assisted thoracic surgery; YAG = neodymium: yttrium-aluminium-garnet, MRCI = Medical Research Council Index.

Table 8.9

Typical complication rates for LVRS

Complication	Rate (%)
Reventilation	6
Bleeding	6
Pneumonia	14
Air leak >7 days	30–50
Mortality	≤6

The most significant complication is undoubtedly postoperative air leakage. This prolongs chest intubation, hospital stay and the risk of inanition-associated secondary morbidity including hypostatic pneumonia and venous thrombosis. Air leak arises from two sources: torn pulmonary parenchyma and leakage at the resection staple line or laser ablation/shrinkage zone. Parenchymal lacerations can be avoided by careful handling of the lung but it has proved more difficult to prevent staple line leakage which occurs around the staples due to the poor sealing qualities of emphysematous lung tissue. Alternative strategies include: buttressing the staple line with bovine pericardium[42] or polytetrafluoroethylene[43] and the application of tissue glue to the resection line. Comparison between several large series (Table 8.10) does not suggest a marked improvement with the use of buttress material which does, however, add significantly to operative costs.

Comparative surgical studies

Laser versus stapled resection. The large multi-institutional series reported by Hazelrigg and colleagues[29] demonstrated that the results of laser therapy were less rewarding than those generally reported with stapled resection (Table 8.8). Keenan and colleagues[30] abandoned laser-only treatment early in their experience citing a high incidence of cardiopulmonary complications and prolonged hospital stay. McKenna[22] in a prospective randomized study comparing VATS stapled resection with contact Nd:YAG (neodymium:yttrium-aluminium-garnet) laser found a greater incidence of late postoperative pneumothorax following laser treatment (6/33 vs 0/39, p = 0.005), better elimination of oxygen dependence with staples (87.5% vs 52%, p = 0.02) and better FEV_1 improvement with staples (32.9% vs 13.4%, p = 0.01).

VATS versus open approach. This issue was addressed by Kotloff and colleagues[27] who compared the results obtained with stapled bilateral LVR in 80 patients operated via a median sternotomy approach with those in 40 patients undergoing bilateral VATS procedures. The mortality was lower in the VATS group (total in patient mortality: median sternotomy 13.8%, VATS 2.5%, p = 0.05). There was no difference in air leakage, in patient stay and either mean postoperative FEV_1, FVC, residual volume (RV) and six-minute walking test or the change in these data in comparison with the preoperative values. They concluded that a VATS approach was associated with a significantly lower incidence of respiratory failure and a trend towards decreased mortality, which may make VATS the preferred technique particularly for high risk patients.

These findings were confirmed by Wisser and colleagues[44] who compared stapled reduction in 15

Series	Use of pericardial strips	Incidence (%)
Cooper[24]	Yes	46
McKenna[22]	Yes	48
Naunheim[32]	No	30
Stammberger[33]	No	50

Table 8.10

Effect of pericardial strip use on incidence of prolonged air leak (>7 days)

sternotomy cases with 15 bilateral VATS cases. They found no significant differences in perioperative outcomes or functional result at three months. They did, however, observe that whereas the VATS groups had a substantially increased FEV_1 at one month, the maximal improvement in FEV_1 in the open group took three months to develop. They attributed this to less discomfort in the VATS group and, given equal results with the less invasive approach, have now adopted the VATS approach as their procedure of choice.

Unilateral versus bilateral reduction. McKenna[31] analysed 166 consecutive patients undergoing VATS stapled LVR, of which 87 were unilateral and 79 bilateral. There was no significant difference in operative mortality (3.5% unilateral vs 2.5% bilateral), LOS (11.4 +/− 1 unilateral vs 10.9 +/− 1 bilateral) or morbidity. Elimination of O_2 dependence (36% unilateral vs 68% bilateral, p < 0.01) and steroid dependence (54% unilateral vs 85% bilateral, p = 0.02), and FEV_1 increase (57% bilateral vs 31% unilateral, p < 0.01) were significantly better with bilateral procedures. He also reported that poor-risk patients had the same perioperative mortality in either group but an increased one-year mortality with unilateral reduction due to a greater incidence of death from respiratory failure in that group. He concluded that bilateral VATS reduction was superior to unilateral reduction, had the same operative risk and gave equivalent results to open reduction via a median sternotomy.

Kotloff[45] also compared unilateral (26 patients) with bilateral (86 patients) VATS reduction and confirmed better results with the bilateral approach. FEV_1 tested at three to six months (25% improvement bilateral vs 16% unilateral, p < 0.001), six-minute walk and reduction in RV were all superior in the bilateral group.

No useful data are available comparing open unilateral reduction with bilateral open reduction.

LVR versus lung transplantation. Gaissert and colleagues[46] compared patients undergoing open median sternotomy stapled LVR against single lung transplant and double lung transplant procedures. They found much better improvement in lung function with transplant but a higher one year mortality with transplant (LVR 1/33; SLT 4/39; BLT 4/25). Exercise tolerance was improved by 28% in LVR cases as compared to 47% and 79%, respectively, for single and double lung transplant cases. They concluded that LVR could be a valid alternative to transplantation in selected patients and had the potential advantage of allowing access to therapy faster than transplant, possibly as an intervening step.

Guided versus standardized resection. In theory, the V/Q scan and CT images enable the surgeon to identify the most severely damaged and most poorly perfused areas of lung which may then be resected. In practice, the necessary resection is often a 'U' shaped resection of either upper or lower lobar tissue in centrilobular or panacinar emphysema, respectively.

Travaline and colleagues from Temple University School of Medicine, Philadelphia[47] compared bilateral apical (guided) and targeted non-apical (unguided) resection and found no statistical difference between either method in morbidity, six-minute walking distance, FEV_1 increase, change in RV/TLC ratio, and fall in pCO_2.

In summary, the available comparative data suggests that for LVR:

- stapled resection is superior to laser shrinkage
- bilateral reduction is superior to a unilateral approach
- VATS reduction is at least as effective as open reduction and operative mortality is probably less
- reduction is less effective than transplant but is associated with a lower late mortality and could be used as a temporising measure
- apical resection is as effective as multiple 'targeted' resections.

Absolute value of LVRS. *Comparison with rehabilitation*: The most obvious therapeutic question is the comparison between LVRS and rehabilitation. Cooper, for example[24] achieved a 29.6% increase in six-minute walk with intensive preoperative pulmonary rehabilitation alone — a finding which has been confirmed in randomised prospective studies.[48] Others have cogently argued that the scientific evidence supporting LVRS is currently lacking.[49]

Preliminary data is available from one prospective randomised comparison of 105 patients receiving either LVRS or rehabilitation.[50,51] This study showed that in contrast to rehabilitation, LVRS resulted in a significant improvement across all quality-of-life and sickness-impact profile categories, with improved lung function, gas exchange and exercise ability at three months in the LVRS group. At present a multi-institution study comparing LVRS with rehabilitation is planned in the USA but such a trial may be difficult to establish, and may report outmoded data by the time it comes to fruition given the current rate of development in surgical practice.[52]

Cost effectiveness. Little data is available regarding cost effectiveness, but Bailey and colleagues from the University of Michigan[53] compared healthcare costs between 15 operated emphysema patients (one year pre- and one year post-surgery) with the care costs for 30 unoperated patients (one year pre- and one year post-rehabilitation). They found that the costs of surgery would be recovered after three years of non-surgical treatment. This study is flawed, however, as the rehabilitation group were surgery rejects and therefore potentially worse patients than the surgical group. In addition, the study was not randomised.

Duration of surgical benefit. The extent to which the benefits of LVRS will be maintained is unknown. Cooper's group[24] reported that improvement was sustained at up to two years (e.g. FEV_1: preoperative value 0.83, one year value 1.33, at two years value 1.25 — i.e. still up by 25% over preoperative value). LVR, however, may simply have a 'reset' effect after which gradual decline continues (Fig. 8.7), as others[54] have noted a gradual drift in benefit by two years with the FEV_1 slipping from +30% at six months to +13.8% at two years. Interestingly, Brenner and colleagues[70] recently reported a study reviewing the rate of FEV_1 change following LVRS in which they compared the outcomes after stapled and laser resection. This confirmed the superior initial result with a stapled approach and also showed that the long-term rate of decline was greatest for the stapled group. The longevity of surgical benefit will only

be resolved after the passage of several more years when a large amount of cohort follow-up data should have become available.

Risk analysis. *Predictors of poor outcome.* Hypercapnia and particularly poor preoperative pulmonary gas transfer or performance status are generally accepted as indicators of raised operative risk. Keenan[30] found preoperative hypercapnia ($pCO_2 = 50$ mmHg) and DLCO (25%) were significant risk factors for adverse outcome with unilateral VATS LVRS. Szekely[54] in a study of 47 Massachusetts General Hospital patients undergoing LVRS found that in-patient death was strongly associated with preoperative $pCO_2 = 45$ mmHg (p = 0.012) and the inability to walk at least 200 m in six minutes before or after preoperative pulmonary rehabilitation (p = 0.004). Raised preoperative pCO_2 was also associated in this study with a prolonged in patient stay >21 days (p = 0.0002).

These findings have been challenged by Argenziano,[40] who compared high and low risk groups within a series of 85 patients undergoing LVRS at Columbia University Medical School. A variety of highly invasive techniques have been used by this group including sternotomy, unilateral and bilateral thoracotomy and even clamshell incisions. Despite this, severe hypercapnia did not preclude successful LVRS and the 'high risk' patients (hypercapnia, steroid dependence, profound pulmonary dysfunction and inability to complete rehabilitation) had the same operative mortality (7%) and equal functional benefit to low risk patients.

Coincident disease. Given the linkage between smoking and emphysema it is perhaps surprising that reported cardiorespiratory comorbidity is remarkably modest in most series of LVRS cases. Concurrent non-small cell bronchogenic carcinoma was found by McKenna[55] in 11 of 325 LVRS cases (3.4%), all of whom underwent successful combined lobectomy. McKenna observed that LVRS candidates should be carefully evaluated for concurrent masses (16% overall incidence in this series) but commented also that the ability to perform LVRS may now allow previously inoperable bronchogenic carcinoma cases to undergo resection.

Concurrent significant coronary artery disease, defined as angiographic evidence of coronary stenosis >50%, has been identified in 22% of patients eligible for LVRS.[33]

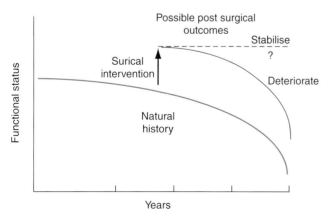

Figure 8.7 *Diagrammatic representation of the possible impact of LVRS on long-term lung function.*

VATS stapled LVR

Range of procedures. VATS stapled LVR procedures have been described using various operative strategies:

- unilateral
- staged sequential
- bilateral simultaneous (lateral approach)
- bilateral simultaneous (anterior approach).

In a sense the ability to perform unilateral *or* bilateral LVR is a specific advantage of VATS resection. Some surgeons[30,32] have taken the view that it is safer to operate on one side and then wait to see how the patient progresses. The second side may be reduced as an interval procedure some months later if the patient wishes to proceed to further surgery and it is clinically indicated. This approach limits the dangers of persistent air leakage to one side and may also have economic advantages with regard to surgical staple costs. In my experience, less than one third of patients express the desire to proceed to further surgery having gained a significant and adequate improvement with surgery to the worse side. Others have demonstrated that a bilateral approach is feasible[27,31,33,44,56] and clearly the total benefit is increased. It is probable that access to the posterior aspects of the lung[31] — and particularly the lower lobe — is better with a lateral approach,[33] but apical resection is certainly possible from an anterior submammary approach,[33,56] and presents a similar aspect to that obtained at median sternotomy.

Pulmonary lobectomy has occasionally been undertaken during VATS LVRS for concurrent carcinoma.[55] This would be an option also for a totally destroyed lobe but there is some dispute as to whether lobectomy should ever be performed simply for presumed lobar replacement by emphysema as it is believed that there is always functioning lung at the hilum.[57]

Preoperative preparation. The value of an extended pulmonary rehabilitation programme is not generally accepted but there is no doubt that it is essential to optimise the patient's pulmonary status prior to surgery. After preliminary tests (Tables 8.4, 8.5, 8.6 and 8.7) have indicated that a patient is a suitable candidate for surgery, the author's team has found that an initial assessment admission to the surgical unit is very helpful. The patient can be seen for physiotherapy assessment, instructed in breathing exercises and led through a programme of general exercises designed to improve overall fitness. Emphysema patients are almost always deconditioned. They can improve their performance and fitness levels and consequently their self-confidence significantly with help, advice and encouragement. During this admission the patient is instructed regarding the nature (and difficulties) of the postoperative period and the need for co-operation with postoperative physiotherapy and mobilisation is emphasised. The rapport established during this admission with the physiotherapy and nursing teams contributes greatly to this process.

After discharge, in the interval before surgery, the patient's progress is monitored by telephone and by outpatient visits as required. This supportive process helps to maintain the patient's morale and enthusiasm.

The preoperative assessment admission also provides a useful opportunity to assess general medical issues, notably ischaemic heart disease, and to optimise management. Oral steroid therapy worsens wound healing and the author's unit therefore commences a weaning programme aimed at either tailing it off completely or reducing it to a modest level (<10 mg prednisolone/day) for at least two weeks prior to surgery.

Procedure

Anaesthesia

Anaesthesia for bullous-emphysematous lung disease can be a challenging and occasionally alarming experience for the anaesthetist who has the difficult task of balancing the ventilatory requirements of a patient with very poorly functioning air-trapped lungs against the surgeon's desire for single lung ventilation and modest mediastinal movement.

Double lumen selective tracheobronchial intubation is required as single-lung ventilation is necessary during large portions of the procedure. The capnograph usually shows a square wave trace due to slow washout of CO_2 instead of the normal saw-tooth wave and, as one-lung ventilation begins, it is almost always necessary to accept some degree of permissive hypercapnia. Air-trapping may make it difficult to adequately ventilate the patient using a mechanical ventilator and gentle hand ventilation can then be the best method for portions of the procedure. If the patient becomes excessively hypoxic, oxygenation can be improved by insufflating the collapsed lung with a gentle continuous oxygen stream. This tends to be less disruptive than intermittent ventilation, which may ruin the surgical view by causing the lung to re-expand.

VATS LVRS spares the patient the pain of a major thoracic incision but adequate analgesia is vital in order to promote postoperative cough function. Epidural analgesia with bupivacaine is frequently employed to good effect, particularly when bilateral reduction is performed, but it does carry associated problems with reports of gastrointestinal stasis, urinary retention and hypotension. The author has found patient-controlled analgesia supplemented with intercostal nerve blocks to be a simple and effective approach. Non-steroidal analgesics can have a valuable morphine-sparing effect but they should be used cautiously in elderly patients and are precluded by impaired renal function.

Positioning and ports. *Lateral approach.* The patient is positioned in a classical lateral decubitus thoracotomy position. Port site positions vary somewhat but in general a three-port approach is usually employed providing the classical triangular arrangement. Variations include the addition of a small (5.5 mm) port, which Stammenberger[33] found helpful; and Naunheim[32] described occasionally extending a port incision sufficient to allow the simultaneous passage of two instruments.

The author has found it helpful to make the first port incision in the submammary area in approximately the 5th interspace in the nipple line. If this port is made as a slit of about 3 cm, the chest can be entered under direct vision, thereby ensuring meticulous haemostasis and avoiding pulmonary injury. The lung can be seen to fall away and this is then confirmed by inserting the videothoracoscope in order to ensure that the other intended port sites are free of adhesions. This slit provides a convenient mini 'utility' incision through which large (60 mm) endostaplers or ring forceps can be introduced and as a route for removing the excised lung tissue. A posterior port is generally placed approximately 2 cm below and posterior to the tip of the scapula, where it provides good access to the posterior aspects of the lung. If the resection is only to be from the lower lobe, this port can be moved two interspaces lower. A third port is located in the 7th interspace in the mid lateral line (Fig. 8.8). This lower port is used alternately with the posterior port for insertion of the videothoracoscope during the procedure and for insertion of 36 FG drain at the end. Port tubes are used for the lower and posterior port sites, both to allow the videothoracoscope to be inserted and to facilitate passage of smaller staplers (30/35 mm), as the interspaces are relatively narrow at these sites.

Anterior approach. The patient is positioned supine with both arms extended over the head (Fig. 8.9) or abducted. Surgical access is improved by placing inflatable bags under each scapula so that the operated side can be elevated and by rotating the operating table away from the surgeon. Vigneswaran[56] describes the use of a three-port technique. Ports are fashioned anteriorly and posteriorly in the submammary line. A third port is placed anteriorly at the

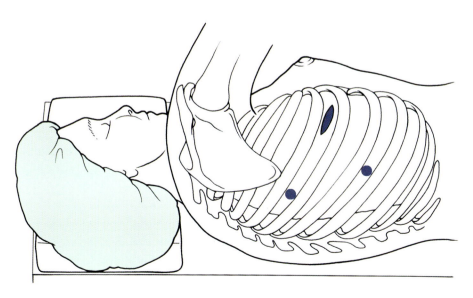

Figure 8.8 *Suggested port arrangement and patient positioning for VATS LVRS via a lateral approach.*

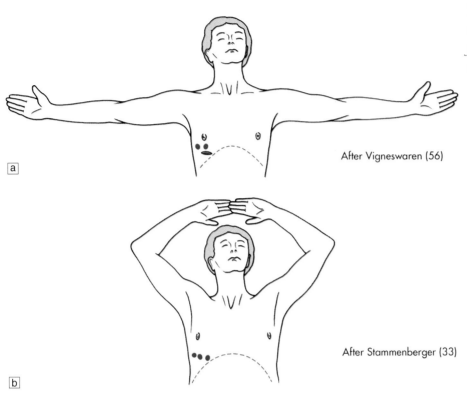

Figure 8.9 *Suggested port arrangement and patient positioning for VATS LVRS via an anterior approach.*

After Vigneswaren (56)

a

After Stammenberger (33)

b

level of the diaphragm and provides access for large staplers through the rather wider anterior intercostal gap at this level. Stammenberger[33] utilises the same port sites whether operating from a lateral or a supine position with three 11.5 mm trocars placed in the 7th or 8th intercostal space and a 5 mm trocar in the 4th.

Although an anterior approach can be used for upper and middle lobar resections, access to the posterior and/or lower zones is probably superior via a lateral approach.[33]

Operative technique. The great majority of patients undergoing LVRS will have predominant centrilobular emphysema and will require upper zone volume reduction. In practical terms this involves a hockey stick or inverted 'J'-'U'-shaped resection commencing with the middle lobe or lingula and passing around the apex and down the posterior aspect of the upper lobe. Resection of 25–35% of lung volume or, typically, approximately 50–75 g weight per lung is generally described, although this is essentially a guide to the total amount to remove rather than a means of planning the actual staple line. As discussed previously, there is little evidence to suggest that an entirely 'targeted' resection

comprised of multiple wedges of supposedly worse tissue offers any functional advantage over a more stylised 'J' excision; but it is obviously important to scrutinise the CT and perfusion images in case there are any other areas outwith the proposed resection which should be reduced. Similarly, at the time of surgery the lung should be inspected for particularly diseased areas.

With bilateral resection it is prudent to operate on the less affected side first so that it is not necessary to utilise the worse lung for single lung ventilation after it has been reduced. Adhesions are frequently present, particularly at the apex and often to the mediastinum. They should be carefully divided using cautery, taking care to avoid injury to the brachial plexus or phrenic nerve. Division of adhesions has several advantages. It helps the lung to expand properly at the end of the procedure, makes it possible to inspect the whole lung for disease distribution and for concurrent pathology such as nodules, and makes it much easier for the surgeon to manipulate the lung. Endoscopic staplers, particularly 45 mm and 60 mm size, are difficult to manoeuvre within the chest and it is often helpful to adjust the shape of the staple line by orientating the lung within the jaws of the stapler. Handling of pulmonary tissue should be restricted to those portions which will ultimately be removed. There is usually marked air-trapping and both vision and handling are facilitated by deliberately perforating the lung in a portion intended for removal as this allows the lung to deflate.

If pericardial (Fig. 8.10) or PTFE strips are used to buttress the staple line, a 4.8 mm (green) cartridge should be used whereas a 3.5 mm (blue) cartridge is sufficient if the staples are used without buttressing. Manoeuvrability issues often determine that a combination of 60 and 30/45 mm staplers is best. Cooper[24] has moved from multiple wedge excisions towards an attempt to create one staple line on the basis that this approach reduced the tension on staple lines. In the author's experience, a 'Y'-shaped staple line often results in less tension than a linear one when a large apical area is being excised (Fig. 8.11). Where possible, crossed staple lines should be avoided as the lung tends to leak more at the crossover site. If desired, tissue glue can be applied along the staple lines at the end of the procedure (Fig. 8.12). An effective flexible applicator can be made by cutting a double lumen central venous pressure catheter prior to the proximal orifice. This provides two channels through which the glue components can be injected and allows them to mix at the cut end as the glue flows onto the staple line.

When the reduction has been completed, some authors test the staple lines by forcibly inflating the lung under water[32] and then restaple, glue or suture any leaking points. The author's team has been concerned that this manoeuvre may create leaks at the staple line and has realised a reduced

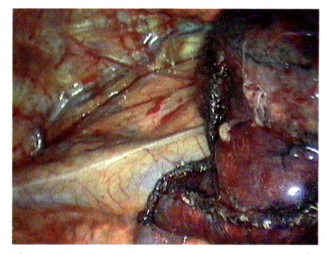

Figure 8.11 *'Y'-shaped staple lines created with excision of a broad apical area.*

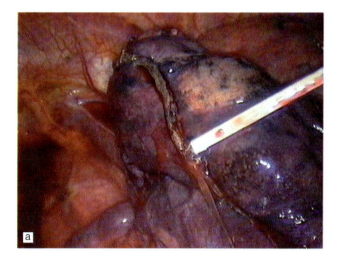

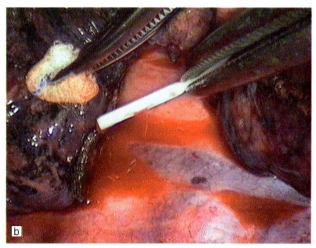

Figure 8.12 *Use of tissue glue delivered through a double lumen CVP catheter to seal different portions of lung volume staple lines.*

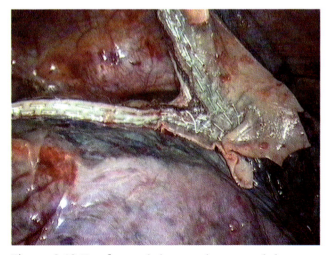

Figure 8.10 *Use of pericardial strips to buttress staple line.*

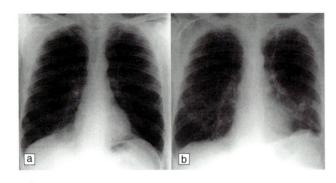

Parameter	(a) Preoperative	(b) Postoperative
FEV$_1$*	0.5	1.0
FVC*	2.95	3.75
Ratio*	16.9%	26.7%
RV	6.02	4.76
TLC	9.4	8.31

(*Measured after inhaled bronchodilator)

Figure 8.13 *(a) Pre- and (b) postoperative chest X-rays and pulmonary function data in a bilateral VATS LVRS patient.*

leakage rate by simply reconnecting the lung to the ventilator after suctioning the bronchus clear of secretions. The lung re-expands very effectively and gently within several minutes due to air-trapping. The author's team routinely divides the pulmonary ligament at the end of the procedure in order to promote re-expansion of the lower lobe. An apical pleural tent has been recommended[24] when there appears to be a particularly large apical space. Subcutaneous emphysema is more common with a VATS approach and may be reduced by careful suturing of the port sites.[44] One or two large calibre (36 FG) drains are inserted through port sites at the end of the procedure.

Postoperative management. As previously noted, adequate analgesia and intense physiotherapy are the essentials of postoperative management. Routine antibiotic and thromboembolism prophylaxis should be given and

standard postoperative monitoring should include O$_2$ saturation, regular arterial blood gas estimations (for the first few hours) and continuous ECG. In some patients sputum retention will occur due to the combination of pain, debilitation and bronchitic hypersecretion in which case a minitracheostomy is a valuable procedure.

Air leakage is often brisk in the immediate postoperative period. Practice varies regarding the use of drain suction. Recommendations include using this routinely, when the postoperative film shows a pneumothorax >30%, or not at all. There is some evidence that suction may prolong late air leakage. Occasionally, a disasterous or very persistent air leak will require re-exploration — typically in about 6% of cases. Late persisting air leak i.e. >7 days will occur in approximately half the patients; in this situation it may be appropriate to consider converting the patient to a Heimlich valve drain system as this will allow more rapid mobilisation.

Long-term follow-up (Fig. 8.13) is an essential component of any LVRS programme in order to allow audit and consequent modification in technique and/or selection based on clinical outcomes and complications.

Giant bullae

Large bullae or discrete bullous complexes, as distinct from multiple small bullae integrated with generalised emphysematous lung disease, are relatively rare. Wakabayashi,[58] for example, reported that giant bullae constituted less than 3.5% of his bullous-emphysematous case volume, and it is likely that the total surgical experience in this area is now considerably less than that gained with lung reduction surgery over the last four years.

Pathological considerations

All three types of emphysema may be associated with pulmonary bullae which are defined structurally as emphysematous spaces greater than 1 cm in diameter in the inflated lung and usually outlined by curved hairline shadows.[59] A more functional classification[60] with clinical relevance divides bullae into three groups (Table 8.11). Group I patients and some of those in Group II may be appropriate candidates for surgery. Bullae in Group III cases may, however, serve to prevent hyperexpansion of adjacent destroyed lung and removal of these is unlikely to yield good clinical results. Subpleural apical microbullae or blebs which

Table 8.11

Clinical classification of bullae

Group	Characteristics
I Bullae associated with well-preserved underlying lung parenchyma	• broad base, often single e.g. 'giant' bulla • compression of adjacent lung
II Bullae associated with diffuse emphysema	• multiple • variable size
III Air space created by loss of parenchyma	• often segmental or lobar • air space replaces lung • no compression

After Witz and Roeslin 1980.[60]

are typically associated with primary spontaneous pneumothorax (see Chapter 7) are associated with paraseptal emphysema.[61] Wakabayashi identifies two structural types of giant bullae — those with smooth walls and those with trabecular elements.[58]

Large bullae are not perfused and are rarely ventilated (<10%). They do not, therefore, generally produce ventilation/perfusion mismatch problems unless there is compression of adjacent lung tissue. The clinical condition of the patient is determined by the general effects of underlying emphysema and pulmonary hyperexpansion and by those directly related to the bulla itself (Table 8.12). The benefit associated with bulla resection derives mostly from the improved function associated with recruitment of previously compressed adjacent lung. There will also, however, be gains in pulmonary function derived from the reduction in overall lung volume and the consequent reversal of the deleterious effects of hyperexpansion (Table 8.3).

Indications for surgery

In contrast to the surgery of diffuse bullous-emphysematous lung disease, the indications for surgical intervention in patients with a giant bulla or large bullous complex — although relative — are established. These have been well detailed in excellent reviews by Deslauriers.[16,62] Current possible indications are summarized in Table 8.13. If surgery is to be undertaken with a view to improving or maintaining pulmonary function, i.e. for

Table 8.12

Clinical effects of an isolated large bullous complex

A. Space-occupying lesion effects

Compression of adjacent lung:
  loss of respiratory exchange volume
  shunt (V/Q mismatch) in compressed lung

Haemodynamic effects:
  effects of pulmonary hyperexpansion

B. Impaired elastic recoil

Bulla has no elastic recoil and so worsens expiratory function

C. Secondary pathology

Pneumothorax
Mistaken intubation
Infection
Haemoptysis (rare)

dyspnoea or in a relatively asymptomatic patient with giant bulla, it is essential to demonstrate evidence of marked

107

Table 8.13

Indications for surgery in giant bullous disease

Intervention status	Indication
Prophylactic	Single large bulla: • >50% of hemithorax • compression of adjacent lung • increasing size
Elective therapeutic	Dyspnoea, chest pain (rare): • large bulla with evidence of pulmonary compression • decreasing FEV$_1$ on serial review Recurrent pneumothorax Concurrent indication: • adjacent nodule
Urgent therapeutic	Pneumothorax: • large persisting air leak Infection: • failure to resolve with conservative therapy

compression of adjacent lung tissue. Without this feature there is much less reason to be confident that surgery will result in a useful benefit to the patient (Table 8.14 and Fig. 8.14).[63]

In rare instances, further second-line tests may be helpful. Right heart catheterisation and pulmonary angiography are indicated if there is evidence of significantly elevated pulmonary artery pressure and surgery is still contemplated. Pruning of the distal arterial tree would effectively preclude operative intervention, but elevated pressure associated with distortion or compression would not. Coronary angiography should be performed when significant ischaemic heart disease is suspected.

Compression of adjacent lung is suggested on plain chest X-ray and CT scan by increased vascular markings indicating crowding and by relatively increased tissue density. Angiography is the most accurate determinant of vascular compression but it is not generally necessary to

undertake this simply to establish that compression is present.

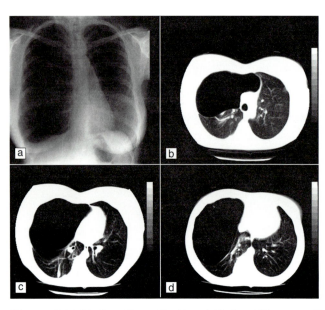

Figure 8.14 *(a) Chest X-ray; (b), (c) and (d) show CT images, all of a giant right bulla, with significant compression of the remaining lung.*

Table 8.14 *First line assessment investigations for giant bulla*

Test	Purpose
PA and lateral chest X-rays (Fig. 8.14a) CT of thorax (Fig. 8.14b, c and d) V/Q scan	Establish anatomical situation
Blood gases Detailed spirometry CO transfer Walking test	Define baseline pulmonary function status
ECG Echocardiography Exercise ECG	Screen for pulmonary hypertension and coronary artery disease

Surgical management

Open resection was originally accomplished using a mass ligature technique. In many centres this became superceded by the use of surgical staplers which had the specific advantage of allowing resection where there was not a pedunculated base to the bulla.

The principles of open stapled resection[62] are essentially those employed during a VATS procedure and are worth repeating here as a guide to the intended procedure. Pedicled bullae can be stapled or ligated. A large broad-based bulla is opened, redundant wall excised and the wall edges are then grasped with tissue forceps so as to include normal tissue at the base of the bulla. A linear stapler is then applied below the tissue forceps. This seals the base of the bulla together with a strip of normal parenchyma while the free walls serve to buttress the staple line.

VATS approaches

The first thoracoscopic approach to bullae utilised lasers to shrink large bullae.[19,20] This could then be supplemented by stapler excision of remaining bullous tissue if necessary. Shrinkage has also been achieved with the argon beam coagulator[64] but this is probably less effective and appears to be associated with more tissue disruption than the Nd:YAG laser.[65] Early studies[20] confirmed that, as previously described with open resection, optimal results were associated with radiological crowding of adjacent structures, suggesting local compression of adjacent lung. Stapled resection[66,67] is probably the commonest approach whether in isolation or in combination with laser therapy; it is reported to be associated with satisfactory results. As might be expected in patients with advanced emphysema, in-patient stay can be prolonged. Ishida and colleagues[67], for example, contrasted the 4.7 day median in-patient stay in 44 patients undergoing VATS bleb resection with the 11.3 day median stay in six patients undergoing VATS resection of giant bullae. Liu and colleagues[68] have recently described a large series of VATS bullectomies for bullous-emphysematous lung disease utilising endoscopic Roeder knot loops. They treated 79 patients with a mean age of 64 years. The mean in-patient stay of 9.5 days with no mortality and 82% of the patient had improved dyspnoea status postoperatively. Whilst many of these patients may have been in the category of LVR rather than true large

bullae, these authors' experience suggest that endoloops may provide a much cheaper alternative to endoscopic staplers.

As a matter of historical interest, one of the earliest techniques for dealing with giant bullae described nearly 50 years ago by Head and Avery remains a useful minimal access approach for patients unlikely to be able to sustain a major thoracic procedure. This utilises a modified version of the Monaldi procedure which originally comprised suction tube drainage of an intrapulmonary tuberculous abscess. When applied to a giant bulla,[69] a rib resection is created over the bulla (under local anaesthesia if necessary) and a purse-string suture is used to suture the parietal pleura to the bulla wall in order to prevent pneumothorax. A drain catheter is then inserted into the bulla and attached to an underwater seal which is placed on suction for one or two weeks. During this time the bulla involutes around the drain. The suction is removed and, if the bulla remains collapsed, the drain is withdrawn.

Technique of VATS management of giant bulla

Anaesthesia. Most of the remarks made concerning the anaesthetic management of LVR are equally pertinent to the surgery of large bullae. Double lumen intubation is essential and if this cannot be achieved it is best to convert to an open procedure.

There are, however, differences. Chiefly, the bulla is said to pose a risk of pneumothorax at the time of induction of anaesthesia, thereby restricting use of nitrous oxide and positive pressure ventilation. As noted previously, however, less than 10% of bullae are directly ventilated and this concern may, therefore, be more theoretical than real. Also, in Type I bullae where the remaining lung function is virtually normal there should be little problem with single lung ventilation, in contrast to the problems encountered in LVR cases.

Positioning and port sites. The patient is positioned in the lateral decubitus position. As with LVR, a triangular port arrangement is appropriate, with the posterior and inferior port sites being placed higher or lower on the chest wall depending upon the location of the bulla(e). The author would recommend strongly that the third port is a 3 cm mini-utility incision in the submammary area. Apart from the advantages this port offers in terms of inserting large staplers and conventional instruments, it also facilitates ligation of bullae using a slip knot introduced through the port and tightened using a knot pusher. The lower central port serves as the drain site following surgery.

Procedure. Adhesions must be divided, after which the pleural cavity and lung should be inspected to confirm the preoperative findings. Vision is often completely obscured by a tense giant bulla (Fig. 8.15); in which case this should be punctured (Fig. 8.16) so that a good view can be obtained. A decision should then be taken regarding the best management strategy for the bulla(e).

Pedicled bullae may be stapled or ligated according to preference. Although some descriptions suggest that it is acceptable to leave the ligated bulla *in situ*, the author's team is concerned that that may predispose to infection, and it will certainly obscure the operative field to some extent.

Large broad-based bullae may be contracted by beam or, preferably, contact laser therapy. Wakayabashi[58] then describes laser excision of the bulla walls using a laser scalpel and emphasises the need for haemostasis of vessels running in the bulla wall. His technique utilises endoscopic suturing to place multiple sutures in the base of the bulla which seal any bronchial communications. These are more frequent in patients with trabeculated bullae. Whilst this technique has been shown to work effectively, the mean operating room time of 3.6–4.7 hours may be considered excessive by many.

Stapled closure offers a more expeditious method of dealing with bullae, and a technique which is entirely analogous to established practice in open surgery. The bulla will normally have already been punctured and should be opened longitudinally. The edges are partially trimmed but left

sufficiently long to allow their use as traction handles. An endoscopic grasper is used to elevate the edges towards one end and an endostapler is then placed at the base of the bulla where it joins normal lung tissue. This manoeuvre is really only feasible in a well deflated lung which will allow the stapler to be partially slipped down onto more normal underlying lung at the junctional zone (Fig. 8.17). As previously noted, the choice of staple leg length will depend on whether or not buttress strips of pericardium are used and on the quality of the remaining lung. If strips are used and/or if the remaining lung is of good quality a 4.8 mm (green*) cartridge should be used. Otherwise a 3.5 mm (blue*) cartridge is sufficient.

Closure. The pulmonary ligament should be divided to mobilise the lower lobe. It is reasonable to immerse the lung

* Colour-size coding correct at time of going to press.

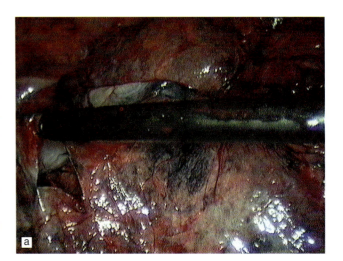

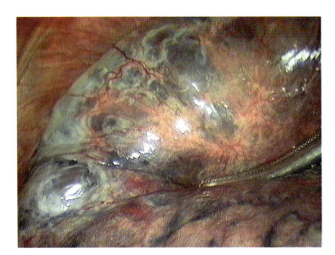

Figure 8.15 *Operative appearance of giant bulla completely obscuring view.*

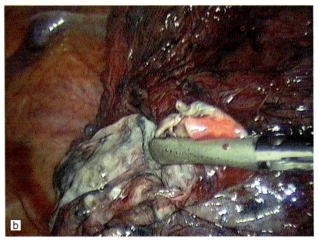

Figure 8.16 *Operative view in same patient as Figure 8.15, (a) during and (b) after bulla has been punctured.*

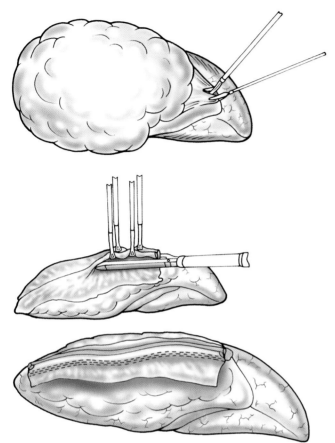

Figure 8.17 *Diagrammatic representation of the method of using an endostapler to seal a large bulla at the base.*

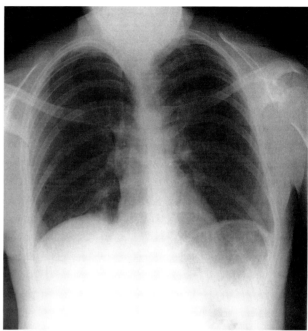

Figure 8.18 *Some patient as in Fig. 8.14: early postoperative appearance following VATS bullectomy. Right lung has re-expanded.*

under saline and inflate the lung to 20 or 30 cm water pressure in order to test for leaks because the quality of the pulmonary tissue is generally better than with LVR cases and the risk of a secondary tear is consequently reduced. Either external suture, glue or further staples may be used to control unexpected air leaks. If a large residual air space exists after resection of the bulla, consideration can be given to elevating the apical pleura so as to create a pleural tent. This adjunctive procedure does not reduce excessive air space but does allow the visceral and parietal pleurae to come into apposition, thereby promoting adhesion and sealing of raw surfaces, which may speed re-expansion. In the author's experience a single large 36 FG drain is usually sufficient.

Postoperative management. As with LVR cases, the role of suction is controversial. The author believes that it should be used if the immediate postoperative film shows that the lung is not well inflated (i.e. more than a 25% peripheral pneumothorax is present). If suction is applied, a further chest film should be reviewed about four hours post surgery and if there is minimal air leakage and the lung is well inflated, it may then be discontinued. Suction is usually uncomfortable or frankly painful, so that morphine consumption is reduced and cough function is improved if it is not used. Pain control is an important component in securing good compliance with physiotherapy and should be efficiently managed. Drain removal is usually possible within a few days of surgery as the quality of the underlying lung parenchyma is generally good (Figure 8.18) and parenchymal air leakage often seals relatively promptly.

Long-term results. Whereas the long-term results of LVR remain to be established there is good data on the outcome of bullectomy. This has been summarised by Deslauriers[16] who notes that bullectomy for Type I bullae has an excellent long-term outlook, with well sustained gains following resection. The results with Type II are less good, with postoperative gains being sustained for five years or so. Type III cases exhibit a steady and marked decline in pulmonary function with no preservation of gain at two years and marked continuation of loss of pulmonary function. These data demonstrate that it is the nature of the remaining lung tissue which determines the long-term result, however good the surgical excision of the bulla(e).

Conclusions

LVRS has refocused clinical attention on a group of patients previously regarded with little interest and offered no hope. The long-term outcome of this procedure is uncertain and many issues remain to be resolved including optimum selection, cost–benefit arguments and the most effective methods of producing an airtight suture line. Nonetheless, the results can be highly gratifying for both patient and surgeon. VATS management of giant bullous lung disease represents the videothoracoscopic application of established open surgical techniques, stapling, ligation and laser shrinkage.

The use of a minimal access approach in either context allows the surgeon to offer the same procedure as would have been performed at open surgery. Given the debilitated nature of patients undergoing either form of surgery, it is difficult to see on what basis open resection can reasonably be advocated when the available evidence would suggest that a VATS approach offers equal functional results with reduced chest wall trauma and pain.

References

1   Lung Disease Data 1995. New York, NY: American Lung Association, 1996. Epidemiology and Statistical Units.

2   Weinmann GC, Hyatt R. Evaluation and research in lung volume reduction surgery. *Am J Resp Crit Care Med* 1996; **154**: 1913–18.

3   American Thoracic Society. Chronic bronchitis asthma and pulmonary emphysema: a statement by the Committee on Diagnostic Standards for Nontuberculosis Respiratory Diseases. *Am Rev Respir Dis* 1962; **85**: 762–8.

4   Snider GL. Emphysema: The first two centuries and beyond. An historical overview with suggestions for future research: Part 2. *Am Rev Respir Dis* 1992; **146**: 1615–22.

5   Snider GL. Emphysema: The first two centuries and beyond. An historical overview with suggestions for future research: Part 1. *Am Rev Respir Dis* 1992; **146**: 1334–44.

6   Flenley DC. *Respiratory Medicine;* Ballière Tindall, London, 1981. Chapter 9: Chronic Bronchitis and Emphysema.

7   Otis OB. The work of breathing. *Physiol Rev* 1954; **34**: 449–58.

8   Fleury B, Murciano D, Telamo C et al. Work of breathing in patients with chronic obstructive pulmonary disease in acute respiratory failure. *Am Rev Respir Dis* 1985; **131**: 822–7.

9   Lamb D, McLean A, Gillooly M et al. Relationship between distal airspace size, bronchiolar attachments and lung function. *Thorax* 1993; **48**: 1012–17.

10   Sharpe JT. The respiratory muscles in chronic obstructive pulmonary disease. *Am Rev Respir Dis* 1986; **134**: 1089–91.

11   Tobin MJ. Respiratory muscles in disease. *Clin Chest Med* 1988; **9**: 263–86.

12   Sciurba FC, Rogers RM, Keenan RJ et al. Improvements in pulmonary function and elastic recoil after lung volume reduction surgery for diffuse emphysema. *N Engl J Med* 1996; **334**: 1095–9.

13   Nakhjavan FK, Palmer WH, McGregor M. Influence of respiration on venous return in pulmonary emphysema. *Circulation* 1966; **33**: 8–16.

14   Butler J, Schrijen F, Henriquez A, Polu JM, Albert RK. Cause of the raised wedge pressure on exercise in chronic obstructive pulmonary disease. *Am Rev Respir Dis* 1988; **138**: 350–4.

15   Riley RL, Cournand A. Analysis of factors affecting partial pressures of oxygen and carbon dioxide in gas and blood of lungs: theory. *J Appl Phys* 1959; **4**: 77–101.

16   Deslauriers J. History of surgery for emphysema. *Sem Thorac Cardiovasc Surg* 1996; **8**: 43–51.

17   Brantigan OC, Mueller E. Surgical treatment of pulmonary emphysema. *Am Surg* 1957; **23**: 789–804.

18   Brantigan OC, Kress MB, Mueller EA. The surgical approach to pulmonary emphysema. *Dis Chest* 1961; **39**: 485–501.

19   Wakayabashi A, Brenner M, Kayaleh RA et al. Thoracoscopic carbon dioxide laser treatment of bullous emphysema. *Lancet* 1991; **337**: 881–3.

20   Brenner M, Kayaleh RA, Milne EN et al. Thoracoscopic ablation of pulmonary bullae; radiographic selection and treatment response. *J Thorac Cardiovasc Surg* 1994; **107**: 883–90.

21   Little AG, Swain JA, Nino JJ et al. Reduction pneumoplasty for emphysema: early results. *Ann Surg* 1995; **222**: 365–74.

22   McKenna RJ, Brenner M, Gelb AF et al. A randomized prospective trial of stapled lung reduction versus laser bullectomy for diffuse emphysema. *J Thorac Cardiovasc Surg* 1996; **111**: 317–22.

23   Cooper JD, Trulock EP, Triantafillou AN et al. Bilateral pneumectomy (volume reduction) for chronic obstructive pulmonary disease. *J Thorac Cardiovasc Surg* 1995; **109**: 106–19.

24   Cooper JD, Patterson GA, Sundaresan RS et al. Results of 150 consecutive bilateral lung volume reduction procedures in patients with severe emphysema. *J Thorac Cardiovasc Surg* 1996; **112**: 1319–30.

25   Miller JL, Lee RB, Mansour KA. Lung volume reduction surgery: lessons learned. *Ann Thorac Surg* 1996; **61**: 1464–9.

26   Szekaly LA, Oelberg DA, Wright C et al. Preoperative predictors of operative morbidity and mortality in COPD patients undergoing bilateral lung volume reduction surgery. *Chest* 1997: 111: 550–8.

27   Kotloff RM, Tino G, Bavaria JE et al. Bilateral lung volume reduction surgery for advanced emphysema. A comparison of median sternotomy and thoracoscopic approaches. *Chest* 1996; **110**: 1399–406.

28   Minai O, Mehta A, Arroliga A et al. Lung volume reduction surgery for end-stage emphysema (Abstract). *Am J Resp Crit Care Med* 1997; **155**: Part 2 Supplement; A608.

29   Hazelrigg S, Boley T, Henkle J et al. Thoracoscopic laser bullectomy: a prospective study with three-month results. *J Thorac Cardiovasc Surg* 1996; **112**: 319–27.

30   Keenan RJ, Landreneau RJ, Sciurba FC et al. Unilateral thoracoscopic surgical approach for diffuse emphysema. *J Thorac Cardiovasc Surg* 1996; **111**: 308–16.

31   McKenna RJ, Brenner M, Fischel RJ, Gelb AF. Should lung volume reduction for emphysema be unilateral or bilateral? *J Thorac Cardiovasc Surg* 996; **112**: 1331–8.

32   Naunheim KS, Keller CA, Krucylak PE et al. Unilateral video-assisted thoracic surgical lung reduction. *Ann Thorac Surg* 1996; **61**: 1092–8.

33   Stammberger Uz, Thurnheer R, Bloch KE et al. Thoracoscopic bilateral lung volume reduction for diffuse pulmonary emphysema. *Eur J Cardiothorac Surg* 1997; **11**: 1005–10.

34   Benditt JO, Wood DE, McCool FD, Lewis S, Albert RK. Changes in breathing and ventilatory muscle recruitment patterns induced by lung volume reduction surgery. *Am J Resp Crit Care Med* 1997; **155**: 279–84.

35   Teschler H, Stamatis G, el-Raouf Farhat AA et al. Effect of surgical lung volume reduction on respiratory muscle function in pulmonary

emphysema. *Eur Resp J* 1996; **9**: 1779–84.

36 Tschernko EM, Wisser W, Hofer S *et al*. The influence of lung volume reduction surgery on ventilatory mechanics in patients suffering from severe chronic obstructive pulmonary disease. *Anesth Analg* 1996; **83**: 996–1001.

37 American Thoracic Society. Official Statement on Lung Volume Reduction Surgery. *Am J Resp Crit Care Med* 1996; **154**: 1151–2.

38 Wallis JW, Miller TR. Volume rendering in three-dimensional display of SPECT images. *J Nucl Med* 1990; **31**: 1421–30.

39 Miller DL, Dowling RD, McConnell JW, Skolnick JL. Effects of Lung volume reduction surgery on lung and chest wall mechanics. *Ann Thorac Surg* (in press).

40 Argenziano M, Moazami N, Thomashow B *et al*. Extended indications for lung volume reduction surgery in advanced emphysema. *Ann Thorac Surg* 1996; **62**: 1588 97.

41 Naunheim KS, Ferguson MK. The current status of lung volume reduction operations for emphysema. *Ann Thorac Surg* 1996; **62**: 601–12.

42 Cooper JD. Technique to reduce air leaks after resection of emphysematous lung. *Ann Thorac Surg* 1994; **57**: 1038–9.

43 Vaughn CC, Wolner E, Dahan M *et al*. Prevention of air leaks after pulmonary wedge resection. *Ann Thorac Surg* 1997; **63**: 864–6.

44 Wisser W, Tschernko E, Senbaklavaci Ö *et al*. Functional improvement after volume reduction: sternotomy versus videoendoscopic approach. *Ann Thorac Surg* 1997; **63**: 822–8.

45 Kotloff R, Tino G, Hansen-Flaschen J *et al*. Short-term functional outcomes following unilateral vs bilateral lung volume reduction surgery (LVRS). *Am J Resp Crit Care Med* 1997; **155**: Part 2 Supplement; A602.

46 Gaissert HA, Truloch EP, Cooper JD *et al*. Comparison of early functional results after lung volume reduction or lung transplantation for chronic obstructive pulmonary disease. *J Thorac Cardiovasc Surg* 1996; **111**: 296–307.

47 Travaline M, Furakawa S, Kuzma AM *et al*. Comparison between bilateral apical vs targeted nonapical resection during lung volume reduction surgery(LVRS)[Abstract]. *Am J Resp Crit Care Med* 1997; **155**: Part 2 Supplement; A603.

48 Ries AL, Kaplan RM, Limberg TM, Prewitt LM. Effects of pulmonary rehabilitation on physiologic and psychosocial outcomes in patients with chronic obstructive pulmonary disease. *Ann Intern Med* 1995; **122**: 823–32.

49 Make BJ, Fein AM. Is volume reduction surgery appropriate in the treatment of emphysema ? [Editorial]. *Am J Resp Crit Care Med* 1996; **153**: 1205–7.

50 Kuzma AM, Reese L, O'Brien G, Furukawa S, Criner GJ. Prospective randomized trial of intensive rehabilitation (R) vs lung volume reduction surgery (LVRS) in severe COPD. *Am J Resp Crit Care Med* 1997; **155**: Part 2 Supplement; A603.

51 Criner GJ, Cordova FC, Furukawa S *et al*. A prospective randomized trial comparing bilateral lung volume reduction surgery (LVRS) to pulmonary rehabilitation in severe COPD. *Am J Resp Crit Care Med* 1997; **155**: Part 2 Supplement; A606.

52 Snider G. Health-care technology assessment of surgical procedures. The case of reduction pneumoplasty for emphysema. *Am J Resp Crit Care Med* 1996; **153**: 1208–13.

53 Bailey TM, Martinez FJ, Lowenbergh N *et al*. Lung volume reduction surgery (LVRS) short- and long-term cost effectiveness of patients with chronic airflow obstruction (CAO) [Abstract]. *Am J Resp Crit Care Med* 1997; **155**: Part 2 Supplement; A604.

54 Szekely L, Oelberg D, Wright C *et al*. Long-term follow-up of pulmonary function following bilateral lung volume reduction surgery. *Am J Resp Crit Care Med* 1997; **155**: Part 2 Supplement; A608.

55 McKenna RJ, Fischel RJ, Brenner M, Gelb AF. Combined operations for lung volume reduction surgery and lung cancer. *Chest* 1996; **110**: 885–8.

56 Vigneswaran WT, Podbielski FJ. Single-stage bilateral, video-assisted thoracoscopic lung volume reduction operation. *Ann Thorac Surg* 1997; **63**: 1807–9.

57 Gaensler EA *et al*. Surgical management of emphysema. *Clinics in Chest Medicine* 1983; **4**: 443.

58 Wakabayashi A. Thoracoscopic technique for management of giant bullous lung disease. *Ann Thorac Surg* 1993; **56**: 708 12.

59 CIBA Guest Symposium Report: Terminology, definitions and classification of chronic pulmonary emphysema and related conditions. *Thorax* 1959; 14: 286.

60 Witz JP, Roeslin N. La chirurgie de l'emphysème bulleux chez l'adulte: ses résultats éloignés. *Rev Fr Mal Respir* 1980; **8**: 121.

61 Cosio MC, Majo J. Overview of the pathology of emphysema in humans. *Chest Surg Clin N Am* 1995; **5**: 603–21.

62 Deslauriers J, Leblanc P, McClish A. *General Thoracic Surgery*, 3rd Ed, Lea & Febiger, Philadelphia, London, 1989. Ed Shields TW, Chapter 65, Bullous and bleb diseases of the lung: 727–49.

63 Gunstensen J, McCormack RJM. The surgical management of bullous emphysema. *J Thorac Cardiovasc Surg* 1973; **65**: 920.

64 Lewis RJ, Caccavale RJ, Sisler GE. VATS-Argon beam coagulator treatment of diffuse end-stage bilateral bullous disease of the lung. *Ann Thorac Surg* 1993; **55**: 1394–9.

65 Sawabata N, Nezu K, Tojo T, Kitamura S. In vitro comparison between argon beam coagulator and Nd:YAG laser in lung contraction therapy. *Ann of Thorac Surg* 1996; **62**: 1485–8.

66 Yim AP, Ho JK. Video assisted thoracoscopic staple resection of a giant bulla. *Aus & New Zealand J Surg* 1996; **66**: 495–7.

67 Ishida T, Kohdono S, Fukuyama Y *et al*. Video-assisted thoracoscopic surgery of bullous and bleb disorders of the lung using endoscopic stapling device. *Surg Laparosc Endosc* 1995; **5**: 349–53.

68 Liu HP, Chang CH, Lin PJ, Chu JJ, Hsieh MJ. An alternative technique in the management of bullous emphysema. Thoracoscopic endoloop ligation of bullae. *Chest* 1997; **111**: 489–93.

69 MacArthur AM, Fountain SW. Intracavity suction and drainage in the treatment of emphysematous bullae. *Thorax* 1977; **32**: 668.

70 Brenner M, McKenna RJ, Gelb AF, Fischel RJ, Wilson AF. Rate of FEV_1 change following lung volume reduction surgery. *Chest* 1998; **113**: 652–9.

Pulmonary wedge biopsy: technique and application to interstitial lung disease

9

S. W. Fountain

Introduction

Lung resection using thoracoscopic techniques became possible with the development of the linear endoscopic staple gun. Although the use of conventional staplers inserted through small incisions under video imaging had previously been described by Lewis *et al.*[1] this technique was only an intermediate step between conventional open lung biopsy and the truly minimally invasive video endoscopic procedures commonly used today.

Whether a small wedge of lung is being excised for diagnostic purposes, or a discrete lesion is being resected therapeutically, the fundamental technique is the same. The procedure is essentially simple and technically straightforward, provided appropriate selection criteria are observed and the surgery is undertaken in a controlled situation by a surgical team with the skill and experience to handle problems, and which is familiar with standard open thoracic surgical techniques.

Preoperative selection

The indications for diagnostic lung biopsy in patients with an apparently solitary nodule are dealt with in detail elsewhere (Chapter 10). The need for a CT scan to localise a discrete lesion is obvious, but identifying the lesion may still be difficult if it cannot be visualised on the surface of the lung. Various methods to aid identification have been described[2] and are discussed in Chapter 10, including needle localisation and ultrasound, but inserting a finger through a port site or passing an instrument over the lung to detect changes in tissue density are probably the most useful. CT is also invaluable for selecting sites for diagnostic biopsy. Careful scrutiny of the CT in such cases bearing in mind the constraints of the technique is essential in planning. As with open diagnostic biopsy, the most diseased area may not be the best to biopsy as pathological examination of the tissue obtained may show only terminal fibrotic changes. At the other extreme, ostensibly normal areas should be avoided. It is desirable to take more than one biopsy if the appearances are particularly heterogeneous. The crucial difference in site selection between open and VATS biopsy is that, in the latter, the lung cannot easily be palpated for subtle abnormalities such as 'grittiness' and thus the site or sites must be selected preoperatively on the basis of CT appearances. Fissures can usually be seen on the 'soft' CT cuts and this too gives a guide to the most suitable areas (Fig. 9.1). Staple guns are difficult to apply to the convex surfaces of the lungs, particularly if they are stiff and non-compliant. As the staple leg length is fixed, attempts to biopsy deep into the lung, where the tissue becomes progressively thicker along the length of the cut, will lead to unsatisfactory staple closure, with fired but loose staples at the periphery and unclosed or cut-through staples more centrally. This creates a ragged section line and large areas of damaged pulmonary parenchyma which bleed and leak air. It is therefore advisable to excise only superficial discrete lesions and always to take diagnostic biopsies along fissures if possible,

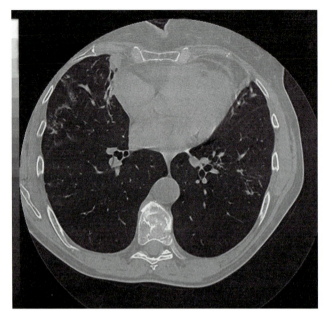

Figure 9.1 *CT scan showing interstitial disease most marked along superior surface of middle lobe.*

preferably from superior surfaces as the histopathogists may have difficulty in making a diagnosis from biopsies taken from dependent parts of the lung (e.g. the inferior surface of the lingula or middle lobe).

Video endoscopic pulmonary wedge resection

Anaesthesia, positioning, port placement

The operative requirements for VATS lung biopsy are listed in Table 9.1. General anaesthesia utilising a double lumen endotracheal tube is required. The patient should be placed in the appropriate lateral position and the anaesthetist asked to clamp off the upper lung and open the appropriate limb of the endotracheal tube to air. (It is often said that this should take place at the outset, partly to assess the patient's tolerance of single lung ventilation and partly to allow absorptive atelectasis to take place. While the former point is valid, the latter is not. Collapse will not occur until the intrapleural vacuum has been broken, whether the lung is being ventilated or not. This may be achieved by inducing a pneumothorax with a needle and syringe, but only if there are no adhesions, an impossible assessment to make pre-operatively. A better plan is to induce the pneumothorax with the first incision or port site in the manner described below.)

Table 9.1

Requirements for VATS lung biopsy

	Requirements
Preoperative	• Chest radiograph • Computed tomography scan (CT) • Respiratory function tests • Consent by patient to proceed to open biopsy if necessary
Intra-operative	• An anaesthetist experienced in managing patients with poor lung function undergoing pulmonary surgery • Single lung ventilation • Ability to monitor oxygen saturation continuously and arterial blood gases at frequent intervals • A video camera and videothoracoscope which can be completely sterilised • A varied supply of linear endoscopic stapling guns • Thoracoscopic atraumatic lung-grasping forceps and scissors with diathermy • A powerful suction device
Postoperative	• Nursing staff experienced in the management of patients with intercostal tube drains

The operator generally stands behind the patient with the assistant in front and the monitor located above the patient's head. For lesions or areas at the base of the lower lobes, it may be more satisfactory for the operator to stand in front of the patient, with the video monitor behind the patient's feet. For some areas of the left lung, it may be easier for a right-handed operator to stand in front of the patient. The closest approximation to perfection is obtained for a right-handed operator when trying to resect a wedge or biopsy from the apex of the lower right lobe (Fig. 9.2).

Port positions need to be chosen carefully to enable the lung resection to be as easy as possible, whether for a discrete lesion or a diagnostic biopsy. Port incisions are made approximately in the posterior, mid and anterior axillary lines, although the increasing depth of the interspaces anteriorly makes it easier to site the anterior port in the most convenient position. A physical port is used for the thoracoscope but the other two port sites are often best left as simple incisions. In obese patients, however, a port will allow easier passage of the endostapler. (The actual interspace or interspaces chosen will depend on the site of the area to be resected but it should be remembered that, if it is necessary to convert a VATS procedure to a thoracotomy, incisions in the same interspace will be easy to join up.) Operating instruments are introduced through the anterior and posterior ports and the assistant holds the video thoracoscopy in the mid axillary port.

Technique

Even with two open ports and a good single lung ventilation, the lung will take several minutes to collapse. During this time the appearance of the lung should be studied and a general inspection of the pleural cavity carried out. When collapse has occurred, running an instrument over the surface of the lung will give the best approximation to palpation available. Hard masses can usually be identified if they are fairly superficial and even a degree of 'grittiness' may be appreciated. The surgeon should grasp the portion of the lung to be excised with a ring forceps or grasper (Fig. 9.3) passed through either the posterior or anterior port. Both the operator and the assistant should work in the same direction and look at the monitor placed directly above the operative field.

The staple gun is then introduced through the opposite port and fired to create the first portion of the wedge (Fig. 9.4). The positions of the graspers and the stapling instrument are then reversed so that the second firing is towards the first (Fig. 9.5). The exact number of firings will depend on the area of the lung to be resected. Staple lines can be crossed, as the design of the instruments allows this, but no gap must be left between them. Making sequential firings in the same direction ('orange peeling') is sometimes unavoidable, particularly in small patients, but it will yield much less useful lung for diagnostic biopsy purposes and cannot be used for resecting a discrete lesion as an inadequate depth of parenchyma is obtained.

Having excised the specimen of lung tissue, this should be extracted through the anterior port as the interspace is widest. A solitary lesion should be placed into a polythene bag prior to extraction in order to prevent possible implantation of malignant cells. Such a lesion may also require division away from the operating table so that specimens may be sent separately to histopathology and

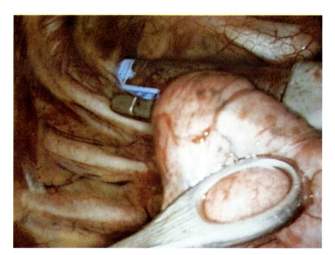

Figure 9.2 *A wedge resection of the apex of the right lower lobe being performed. In this instance the grasping instrument has been inserted through the posterior and the staple gun through the anterior port.*

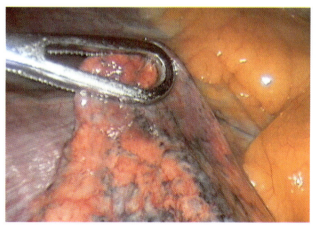

Figure 9.3 *Use of ring forceps to elevate a portion of lung (in this case the anterior basal segment of the left lower lobe) to be biopsied.*

bacteriology. Specimens of lung taken for presumed interstitial lung disease should be inflated with formalin in saline solution so as to preserve parenchymal architecture and aid diagnosis.

The staple lines (Fig. 9.6) and port sites should be checked for haemostasis and a single intercostal drain is then inserted through the anterior port. This can be guided under video imaged control into the optimum position. The lung is then reinflated and the port sites closed.

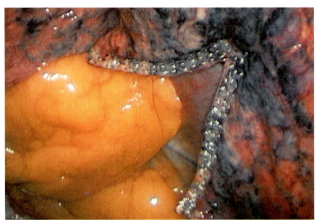

Figure 9.6 *Completed staple lines after endoscopic lung biopsy.*

Post-operative management

Although this kind of procedure is much less traumatic than its open equivalent, postoperative pain can be expected for the first 48 hours. The insertion of large instruments through small interspaces is traumatic to skin, muscle and intercostal nerves. Local anaesthetic agents may be injected directly into port sites or into the appropriate space posteriorly. Alternatively, local anaesthetic can be infused subpleurally into the paravertebral gutter.[3] These methods, combined with the use of non-steroidal analgesics should reduce or obviate the need for opioids in the immediate postoperative period. The need for an intercostal drain in straightforward cases is debatable, but if there is no air leak, and a chest radiograph taken in the recovery area shows full expansion of the lung, the drain can certainly be removed at that stage.

VATS wedge biopsy of lung can be a simple procedure, and fit patients need be in hospital for no more than about 24 hours following surgery. Without due care in performing the technique, however, the development of complications can quickly erode and nullify the advantages of the minimally invasive procedure.

Special cases and complications

Patients with poor lung function

In the early days of thoracoscopic lung biopsy, it was a widely held belief amongst chest physicians that, because the technique was minimally invasive, it could be applied to patients who were not fit for an open lung biopsy. In fact, the elements of the procedure which make it hazardous to the sick patient are not altered by performing it

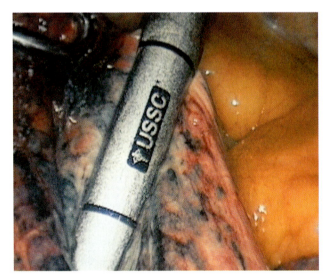

Figure 9.4 *Use of endoscopic staple gun to create first section line for endoscopic lung biopsy.*

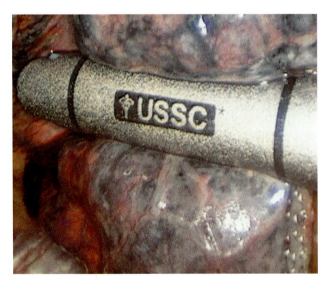

Figure 9.5 *The creation of a second section line for endoscopic lung biopsy. The staple gun has been introduced through the opposite port and is here applied at 90° to the base of the first staple line.*

thoracoscopically, apart from the reduced need for postoperative opioids. The patient must still be fit for single lung anaesthesia and so an individual in respiratory failure on a ventilator will not be suitable. Similarly, an oxygen-dependent but self-ventilating patient is unlikely to tolerate this kind of anaesthetic. Two alternatives may however make the procedure possible in such cases:

1. High-frequency ventilation

With this mode of ventilation, when a pneumothorax is induced, the lung adopts a roughly 50% inflated position while maintaining adequate oxygenation. The action of the high-frequency jet causes it to 'shiver' but this does not inhibit the use of the standard operative technique described above.

2. Carbon dioxide insufflation

Thoracoscopic surgeons discovered at an early stage that the use of a sealed port system with carbon dioxide insufflation, as used for laparoscopic surgery, was unnecessary if single lung ventilation was available. For complex video-assisted thoracic procedures, the use of utility incisions, and the capacity to employ conventional instruments is essential, but a wedge biopsy can be carried out using a sealed port system. Laparoscopic ports are used and CO_2 is insufflated to a pressure of 8 mmHg. This creates sufficient lung compression for the procedure to be performed, but it is crucial not to injure the lung or absorption of the CO_2 may ensue.

The importance of meticulous technique in patients with poor lung function cannot be over-emphasised. The vast majority of patients referred for diagnostic lung biopsy will have undiagnosed interstitial disease and will show the features of a restrictive ventilatory abnormality with a diffusion defect: they will have small, stiff lungs. Such lungs will be difficult to reinflate after being collapsed and high airway pressures may be required. A pneumothorax will be poorly tolerated and may tip the patient into respiratory failure. It is therefore vital to pay attention to detail in positioning staples to ensure that there is no air leak.

Adhesions

Adhesions do not preclude thoracoscopic biopsy in all cases, but they do make it more difficult. So long as they are not present at the first port site and are not too extensive, they should not present an insuperable problem. If they are encountered at the first port site and cannot be separated by gentle digital dissection, an alternative port of entry should be sought. Any lung injury should be closed by stapling the damaged area. Adhesions visualised through the videothoracoscope should be divided by sharp dissection using diathermy scissors. Gentle traction on the lung to identify the tissue plane and tear avascular adhesions may be helpful but bleeding points need to be identified and coagulated quickly (see below). In most circumstances, when carrying out a diagnostic or wedge excision biopsy, division of adhesions can be kept to a minimum. Because of the necessity to use sharp dissection and diathermy, division of adhesions to the mediastinum should be avoided if possible.

Staple failure

Although instrument failure is well reported, most cases where staples fail to be applied correctly will be due to operator error. Mention has already been made of the difficulties which can be encountered when trying to take deep biopsies. All staple guns are designed to be applied along tissue of uniform thickness. It may, be necessary therefore, to pre-crush the edge of the area to be resected in order to create tissue of uniform thickness. A vascular clamp without much curve, such as an aortic cross clamp, is a suitable instrument for such a manoeuvre. It may also be used to calibrate the thickness of the tissue edge — a useful procedure when a biopsy of fibrotic lung is being undertaken. Staples are usually available with three different leg lengths: 3.0 mm, 3.5 mm and 4.8 mm, and staple size calibrators are available. These instruments have parallel jaws, however, and are not of much use for lung work, but a feel for the thickness of a tissue edge using a vascular clamp can soon be gained with experience and the appropriate staple size selected. For most biopsies the correct size will be 3.5 mm.

If comprehensive staple failure does occur, it may be possible to reapply another row deep to the first but, as the cause of failure is likely to be excessive tissue thickness, this is unlikely to work and conversion to an open technique is indicated.

Bleeding

A collection of blood within the pleural space will absorb light and make any VATS procedure more difficult. It is rarely possible to apply pressure to a bleeding area as it is in open surgery and, because of the narrow angle of view of videothoracoscopes, it is easy not to notice bleeding a short distance away from the operative field. So it is vital to ensure all bleeding is stopped instantly by active measures even if the loss appears minimal.

If major bleeding occurs, the procedure should be 'converted' immediately. For most diagnostic and wedge biopsy procedures, it is probably not necessary to have a thoracotomy set of instruments open, but they must be readily available in the operating theatre, and all staff present need to be prepared and sufficiently experienced to undertake a thoracotomy.

Indications for diagnostic lung biopsy

Diagnostic lung biopsy is usually undertaken for interstitial lung disease or suspected disseminated malignancy.

Patients with interstitial lung disease usually present with shortness of breath on exertion, a dry cough, or both. A plain chest radiograph may be normal or show fine reticular shadowing. Occasionally, multiple small, ill-defined abnormalities not quite amounting to discrete lesions may be seen. CT scanning shows the nature and the distribution of the abnormalities much more clearly and, using the latest techniques in scanning, many radiologists now confidently diagnose interstitial disease on scanning alone. Tests of respiratory function commonly show a restrictive defect with a reduction in diffusion. A number of different diseases can give rise to this pattern and, despite advances in CT technology, most physicians prefer a histological diagnosis on which to base therapy.

Patients with suspected malignancy may or may not be short of breath and may have no abnormality of lung function. X-rays and CT scans tend to show a more nodular pattern, i.e. diffuse disease and nodules which are widespread and superficial.

Percutaneous lung biopsy using a fine-needle aspiration technique for cytological examination, or a cutting needle for core biopsy histology, has been shown to give good diagnostic yield for discrete lesions[4,5] but is not of much value for interstitial disease. Transbronchial biopsy is moderately successful in diagnosing interstitial lung disease, particularly sarcoidosis[6], but its success rate of 40–60% does not match the over 90% diagnostic accuracy

Table 9.2

Contraindications to VATS lung biopsy

- Patient unfit for general anaesthetic
- Adhesions precluding development of a plane between pleural surfaces
- Inability to pass double lumen endotracheal tube (relative)
- Inability to tolerate single lung ventilation (relative)

of open lung biopsy.[7] The diagnostic yield of a VATS biopsy equates with that of the open procedure and thus the indications for both open and VATS biopsy are essentially the same.[8,9]

The contraindications have been indicated above and are summarised in Table 9.2.

Results

Standard open lung biopsy procedure constitutes major surgery. It leaves a scar, causes pain, temporarily exacerbates the breathing difficulties of individuals with severe symptoms and usually requires a prolonged in-hospital stay. These problems are not completely obviated by using a minimally invasive technique, but for most patients the procedure trauma and postoperative pain and disability, and length of hospital stay, are reduced.

Several substantial series of VATS lung biopsies have now been published and a summary of the results is presented in Table 9.3.[8–13] It is for the most part a safe, simple procedure. The risks are essentially the same as for open biopsy and are related to the patient's state of health rather than to the procedure, as can be seen from scrutiny of the above series, most of which compared open to VATS biopsies in similar patient groups. The results show a high diagnostic yield indicating that the lack of 'feel' for the lung enjoyed at open biopsy does not impair diagnostic accuracy. A typical range of histological results is shown in Table 9.4.

Attempts have also been made to compare the costs.[14] Most methods of estimating the cost of an in-patient stay are probably inaccurate but procedure costs are easier to quantify and the price of disposable instruments is exact. It has been the experience of most groups that in-patient stay following a VATS lung biopsy

Table 9.3

Summary of results of VATS lung biopsy

Source	Number	Mean age	M:F	Yield (%)	Mortality (%)	Morbidity (%)	Post-op stay (days)
Trivedi[8]	67	56.1	1.1:1	97	0	3	2.0
Carnochan[9]	25	57.5	14:11	96	0	0	1.4
Ferson[10]	47	51.9	24:23	100	6.3	–	4.9
Kadokura[11]	71	56.9	37:34	100	8	15	–
Mouroux[12]	41	55.2	23:18	97	4	5	5.5
Ravini[13]	65	39.0	33:32	98	0	5	4.7

Table 9.4

Histological diagnosis in 65 cases of VATS lung biopsy (Trivedi et al.)

Histology	% of cases
Cryptogenic fibrosing alveolitis	42
Extrinsic allergic alveolitis	12
Sarcoidosis	8
Bronchiolitis obliterans organising pneumonia	8
Metastatic carcinoma	12
Non-Hodgkin's lymphoma	3
Other	12
Non-diagnostic/normal	3

is reduced by one-third when compared to open biopsy. It should be possible to use conventional or purpose-built reusable instruments for virtually every step in a VATS lung biopsy apart from the stapling, and to use two or three firings of one staple gun. At this level, the procedure is cost effective.

References

1   Lewis RJ, Caccavale RJ, Sisler GE, Mackenzie JW. Video-assisted thoracic surgical resection of malignant lung tumours. *J Thorac Cardiovasc Surg* 1992; **104**: 1679–87.

2   Mack MJ, Murray JG, Ostma TW *et al*. Percutaneous localisation of pulmonary nodules for thoracoscopic lung resection. *Ann Thorac Surg* 1992; **53**: 1123–24.

3   Soni AK, Conacher ID, Waller DA, Hilton CJ. Video-assisted thoracoscopic placement of paravertebral catheters: a technique for postoperative analgesia for bilateral thoracoscopic surgery. *Br J Anaesth* 1994; **72**: 462–4.

4   Todd TRJ, Weisbrod G, Tao LC *et al*. Aspiration needle biopsy of thoracic lesions. *Ann Thorac Surg* 1981; **32**: 154–61.

5   Burt ME, Flye MW, Webber BL, Path FF, Wesley RA. Prospective evaluation of aspiration needle, cutting needle, transbronchial and open lung biopsy in patients with pulmonary infiltrates. *Ann Thorac Surg* 1981; **32**: 148–53.

6   Wall CP, Gaensler EA, Carrington CB, Hayes JA. Comparison of transbronchial and open biopsies in chronic infiltrative lung diseases. *Am Rev Respir Dis* 1981; **123**: 280–5.

7   Gaensler EA, Carrington CB. Open biopsy for chronic diffuse infiltrative lung disease: clinical, roentgenographic and physiological correlations in 502 patients. *Ann Thorac Surg* 1980; **30**: 411–26.

8   Trivedi UH, Millner RWJ, Griffiths EM, Townsend ER, Fountain SW. Three year review of video-assisted thoracoscopic lung biopsy. *Thorax* 1994; **49**: 1060P.

9   Carnochan FM, Walker WS, Cameron EWJ. Efficacy of video-assisted thoracoscopic lung biopsy: an historical comparison with open lung biopsy. *Thorax* 1994; **49**: 361–3.

10 Ferson PF, Landreneau RJ, Dowling RD *et al*. Comparison of open versus thoracoscopic lung biopsy for diffuse infiltrative pulmonary disease. *J Thorac Cardiovasc Surg* 1993; **106**: 194–9.

11 Kadokura M, Colby TV, Myers JL *et al*. Pathologic comparison of video-assisted thoracic surgical lung biopsy with traditional open lung biopsy. *J Thorac Cardiovasc Surg* 1995; **109**: 494–8.

12 Mouroux J, Clay-Meinesz C, Padovani B *et al*. Efficacy and safety of video thoracoscopic lung biopsy in the diagnosis of interstitial lung disease. *Eur J Cardiothorac Surg* 1997; **11**: 22–6.

13 Ravini M, Ferraro G, Barbieri B *et al*. Changing strategies of lung biopsies in diffuse lung diseases: the impact of video-assisted thoracoscopy. *Eur Resp J* 1998; **11**: 99–103.

14 Hazelrigg SR, Nunchuk SK, Landreneau RJ *et al*. Cost analysis for thoracoscopy: thoracoscopic wedge resection. *Ann Thorac Surg* 1993; **56**: 633–5.

Thoracoscopic management of the solitary pulmonary nodule

10

M. J. Mack

Introduction

There are many diagnostic modalities for the definitive diagnosis of the indeterminate solitary pulmonary nodule. While there are multiple non-invasive or minimally invasive diagnostic tests, the definitive diagnosis, or the assurance that malignancy does not exist, often remains elusive. Although the surgical removal of lung nodules is highly accurate in determining a definitive diagnosis, the morbidity of a thoracotomy is significant, especially in the context of benign disease.[1] Thoracoscopy has recently been introduced as a diagnostic and occasionally therapeutic modality in the management of indeterminate lung nodules,[2] but sufficient experience has now been gained to define appropriate case selection and the proper application of this procedure.[3] This chapter will identify the role of thoracoscopy or video-assisted thoracic surgery (VATS) in the diagnostic algorithm for the management of a solitary pulmonary nodule.

Diagnostic management

By definition, a solitary pulmonary nodule is a single, intrapulmonary, spherical lesion that is well circumscribed. The incidence is approximately 150,000 newly-detected nodules annually in the USA[4] and, depending upon the population surveyed, approximately 40–50% of the solitary nodules will prove malignant. There are multiple risk factors that enhance the probability that a nodule is malignant, including:

- increasing age of the patient
- diameter of the nodule
- amount of cigarette-smoking
- the nature of the edge of the lesion on X-ray, and
- the absence of calcification.[5,6]

Optimal management dictates that unless the nodule can be demonstrated to have a high probability of being benign, surgical removal is mandatory.

There are numerous diagnostic tools for obtaining the definitive diagnosis of the indeterminate nodule (Table 10.1).

The management algorithm for a solitary nodule discovered on a chest X-ray is as follows:

A careful examination of the chest X-ray should determine whether or not calcification is present. If the calcification is diffuse, central, popcorn, or laminar in configuration it can confidently be assumed that the nodule is benign.[5] If calcification is not apparent on the chest X-ray, it can occasionally be detected by fluoroscopy or computerized tomography (CT). A nodule density of at least 200 Hounsfield units on the CT scan is indicative of the presence of calcium and therefore of a benign lesion.[7] If calcification is not present, then a detailed search for the existence of previous X-rays is indicated. If the nodule can be demonstrated to have been present for a minimum two-year period, with no evidence of growth, it can be considered benign.[6]

Clinical evaluation of the patient is also important. In those less than 35 years old, with no previous history of

Table 10.1

Diagnostic tools for the indeterminate solitary lung nodule, ranked by degree of invasiveness

- Examination of X-ray characteristics for signs of benignancy
- Clinical history
- Review of previous chest X-rays
- Computerised tomography
- Observation with serial chest X-rays or CT scans
- Positron emission tomography (FDG-PET scan)
- Sputum cytology
- Bronchoscopy
- Fine-needle aspiration biopsy
- Thoracoscopy
- Thoracotomy

malignancy and a non-smoking history, the risk of malignancy is less than 1%.[5] Since the risk of the nodule being malignant is so low, an observation-only approach is appropriate in this setting. On the other hand, the index of suspicion and risk of malignancy must be substantially greater in a 65-year-old cigarette smoker.

The next consideration is the size of the nodule. If the nodule is 3 cm or more in diameter, the likelihood of malignancy is 93–99%[8]; further nonsurgical diagnostic evaluation only serves to delay definitive surgical treatment. Likewise, determination of the characteristic (the appearance) of the edge of the nodule where it interfaces with the surrounding lung parenchyma is important. An irregular-shaped nodule with a spiculated or fuzzy margin (Fig. 10.1) should also be managed directly by surgery without delay for further diagnostic testing.

When considering further diagnostic testing, the following question should first be asked: What result will allow the patient to avoid a surgical intervention? The only acceptable answer to that question is: a specific benign diagnosis. A diagnosis of malignancy, 'no malignancy seen', or 'non-specific benign diagnosis' all require surgical intervention. Therefore, unless there is a significant chance of obtaining a *specific benign diagnosis* by day test, the test should not be performed.

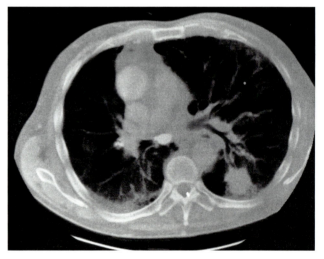

Figure 10.1 *CT scan demonstrating a 3 cm irregular nodule in the superior segment of the left lower lobe in a 65-year-old smoker.*

For example, the diagnostic yield of sputum cytology is very low and ranges from 15–19% in peripheral nodules.[5] Sputum cytology and cultures seldom demonstrate benign disease. The diagnostic yield of bronchoscopy ranges from 20–80%, depending upon the location and size of the nodule in the lung[4], but only 10% of surgically demonstrated benign nodules are able to be diagnosed by bronchoscopy.[9] The probability of obtaining a specific benign diagnosis is, therefore, very low with either of these tests and a diagnosis of malignancy makes surgical intervention mandatory anyway, so why perform the tests?

The same logic holds true for transthoracic needle aspiration biopsy. The sensitivity for malignancy from needle aspiration biopsy ranges from 64–97%, with a false positive rate of 1–3%, and a false negative rate, in the presence of malignancy, of 3–11%.[10,11] With smaller nodules the yield is lower. In multiple series in the literature, including those by Khouri and Calhoun, the incidence of obtaining a specific benign diagnosis ranges between 4–14% of all patients biopsied.[12,13] Although the test is simple to perform, has a low complication rate, and has a significant diagnostic yield in malignancy, the chance of obtaining a specific benign diagnosis is distressingly low. At the present time, the authors believe that the role for transthoracic needle aspiration biopsy is to demonstrate malignancy in a patient who is *not* a candidate for surgical resection or to diagnose malignancy when metastatic disease is suspected.

Standard surgical procedure for diagnosing an indeterminate nodule is a limited thoracotomy. Although the diagnostic yield is virtually 100%, there is the well-known morbidity of a rib-spreading thoracotomy incision.[1] Thoracoscopy has been demonstrated as effective in diagnosing the indeterminate nodule. In the authors' series of 242 patients, the nodule was able to be located in all but two patients who required conversion to an open thoracotomy to locate and resect the nodule.[3] A definitive diagnosis was obtained in all patients, with minimal morbidity. As well as being diagnostic, the procedure is often therapeutic, and in 10% of the patients in this series the thoracoscopic resection was also the definitive surgical procedure because of the inability of the patient to tolerate a lobectomy due to poor pulmonary function. Another 12% underwent conversion to an open procedure for a more extensive resection. To sum up, thoracoscopy has the following advantages:

● it is minimally invasive
● it has a high diagnostic yield, and
● it can be therapeutic.

For these reasons thoracoscopy has assumed a more prominent role in the diagnosis of the indeterminate solitary pulmonary nodule in the author's practice. The other diagnostic procedures have assumed a less important role, unless metastatic disease is suspected and the patient is unable to tolerate a surgical procedure. However, further studies with positron emission tomography (PET) scanning may eventually change the role of thoracoscopy. Early results with F-18 fluorodeoxyglucose tracer (FDG-PET) scanning for the diagnosis of the indeterminate nodule are quite encouraging.[14,15] A sensitivity of 95–100%, with a specificity of 86–90%, indicate an enhanced role for PET scanning in the management of the indeterminate nodule. However, this would require confirmation in other studies and the availability of the scanner.

Patient selection

Indeterminate nodules which are suitable for thoracoscopic resection are less than 3 cm in diameter and located in the outer third of the lung parenchyma. Lesions larger than 3 cm are virtually always malignant and there can be difficulty extracting nodules of this size through the chest wall. Therefore, one should proceed directly to formal lung resection (Fig. 10.1). Roviaro has shown that there is a significant role for thoracoscopy in the staging of lung cancer prior to resection.[16] He has been able to reduce the negative thoracotomy rate in his institution from 19% to 6% by using this technique to demonstrate previously unsuspected pleural metastases prior to thoracotomy.

Nodules located in the more central portions of the lung are difficult to find and to resect by thoracoscopic techniques, and in this situation an alternative approach, e.g. needle aspiration biopsy or thoracotomy, should be considered (Fig. 10.2). However, careful examination of the CT scan may demonstrate that a nodule, which on initial cursory examination was felt to be deep within the lung, is in fact adjacent to an interlobar fissure and therefore able to be located at the time of thoracoscopy (Fig. 10.3).

Nodules less than 1 cm and not immediately adjacent to the surface of the lung, may also prove difficult to detect. If a nodule is more than 2 cm from the closest lung surface and/or less than 1 cm in diameter, a preoperative needle localization technique may be able to detect the nodule at the time of thoracoscopy.[17] Some nodules, although small, are very close to the surface of the lung and through a properly placed trocar site, a digit can be introduced and the

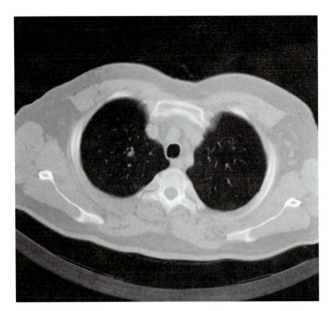

Figure 10.2 *CT scan showing a 1cm nodule approximately 2 cm from the nearest pleural surface. Preoperative needle localisation is indicated. Thoracotomy is probably the best approach for location and resection.*

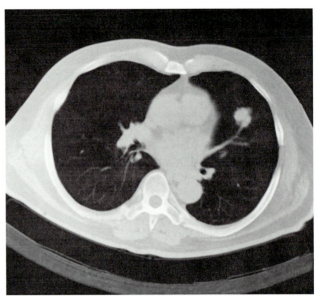

Figure 10.4 *This nodule can be detected by digital palpation through a trocar site.*

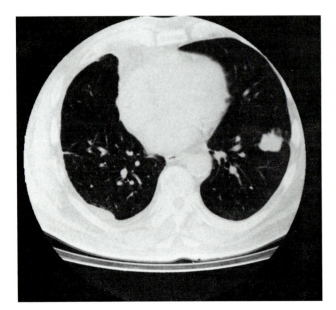

Figure 10.3 *This nodule is abutting the visceral pleura in the fissure and can be detected in the fissure at time of thoracoscopy.*

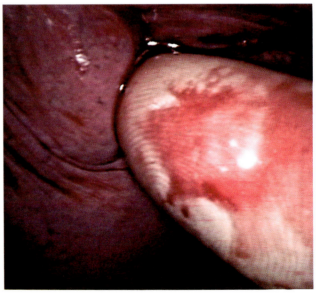

Figure 10.5 *Digital palpation of the lung to detect the lung nodule in Fig. 10.4.*

lung palpated to locate the target lesion (Figs. 10.4, 10.5). The accompanying illustrations (Figs. 10.6–10.8) demonstrate a number of nodules which lend themselves easily to thoracoscopic location and resection, as well as some which should undergo needle localisation.

Localisation techniques

Careful preoperative assessment of the CT scan will determine those nodules which are easy to locate and resect by thoracoscopic techniques and those that would be more

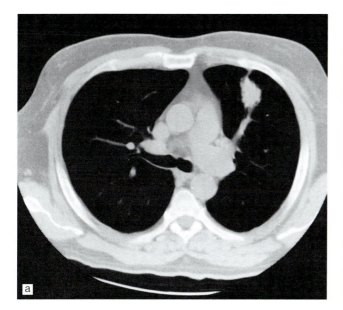

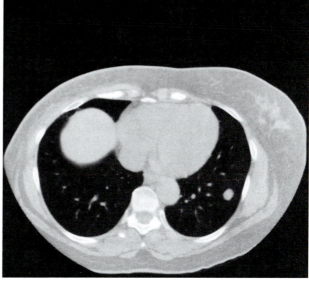

Figure 10.7 *This nodule is large enough and sufficiently close to the pleura to detect at thoracoscopy.*

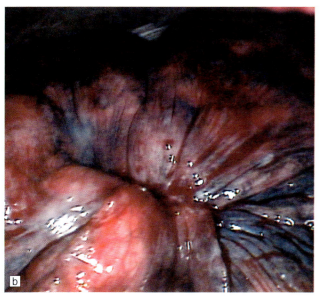

Figure 10.6 *(a) Visceral pleural involvement from this nodule will render it easy to detect visually at thoracoscopy. (b) Thoracoscopic appearance of this nodule.*

Figure 10.8 *This nodule is too small and deep to be reliably detected and should undergo preoperative needle localisation.*

difficult. Nodules anticipated to be difficult should undergo preoperative needle localisation. In the authors' current experience, this constitutes less than 5% of all patients undergoing diagnostic resection of a lung nodule. Preoperative needle localisation is best accomplished under CT guidance in the X-ray department immediately before operating. A hook wire similar to that used for localising occult breast lesions can be accurately placed within 1 cm of the target nodule (Fig. 10.9). The wire is then taped in place and the patient transported to the operating room. Inadvertent dislodgement of the hook wire from the lung occasionally occurs, and a small amount (0.01 cc) of methylene blue should therefore be injected through the needle prior to placement of the hook wire (Fig. 10.10). If

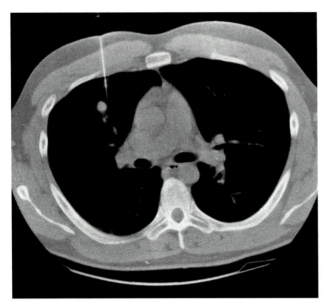

Figure 10.9 *Preoperative needle localisation of a deep lung nodule.*

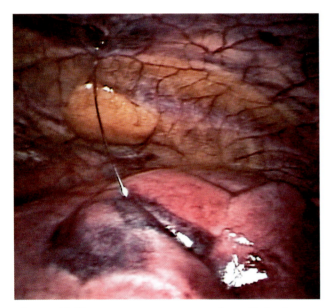

Figure 10.10 *Intraoperative appearance of a needle localisation. Note the methylene blue staining at the base of the wire.*

the hook wire dislodges from the lung when the lung is collapsed upon entry to the chest the methylene blue staining of the surface will still indicate the area of the lung to be resected. It should again be emphasised that by a variety of manoeuvres discussed under 'operative technique', the overwhelming majority of lung nodules can

be located and resected without preoperative localisation. If the nodule cannot be located by any of the methods described, an open procedure is required. Under no circumstances should a patient who is brought to the operating room for the diagnosis of an indeterminate nodule leave the operating room without that nodule being located and diagnosed.

Operative technique

As is standard with all thoracoscopic procedures, resection of the indeterminate nodule is performed under general endotracheal anaesthesia with the ipselateral lung collapsed. Patients are positioned in a lateral position (Fig. 10.11) and fully 'prepped'. A computerised tomogram showing the location of the target nodule must be present in the operating room and trocar placement is planned on the basis of these films. This is the first step in a carefully-planned approach to the detection of lung nodules thoracoscopically (Table 10.2). Careful examination of the preoperative CT scan aids the identification of proper landmarks within the chest cavity and on the chest wall, such that the general area of lung containing the nodule can be localised to within a few square centimetres. In most circumstances, the initial trocar is placed in the sixth or seventh intercostal space in the mid-axillary line. Two more trocars are placed in the fifth or sixth intercostal space in the anterior and posterior axillary lines in the traditional inverted triangle configuration (Fig. 10.12). One of these trocar sites should be shifted so that it overlies the part of the lung anticipated to contain the nodule. This, of course, presents difficulty when the nodule is beneath the scapula or is on the medial aspect of the upper lobes; then, a trocar site should be placed as near as possible to the target nodule.

Once the first trocar has been placed, visual inspection of the thoracic cavity should be performed. Nodules that involve the visceral pleura are easily identified on the initial exploratory thoracostomy. Visual inspection can still be helpful for nodules that do not involve the visceral pleura. As resorptive atelectasis occurs, effacement of the lung around a subpleural nodule takes place. It is often possible to identify visually a subpleural nodule as this effacement occurs (Fig. 10.13).

If the nodule is not found during the visual inspection, instrument palpation is the next technique. By running an

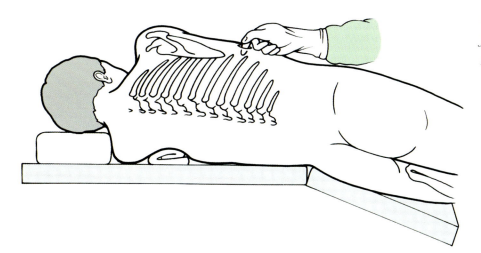

Figure 10.11 *Patient positioning for thoracoscopic resection of pulmonary nodule.*

- Preoperative and intraoperative examination of the CT scan

- Visual inspection of the lung surface

- Instrument palpation

- Digital palpation

- Preoperative needle localisation

- Carefully planned 'blind' resection

- Conversion to open procedure

- Intraoperative ultrasound

Table 10.2

Localisation techniques for lung nodules

instrument across the surface of the lung under which the target lesion is anticipated to be located, the surgeon can detect a subtle change in tissue texture. With experience, this technique of instrument palpation can be surprisingly sensitive. If these methods do not work an index finger can be placed through the closest trocar site. Most areas of the lung can be palpated by a properly placed trocar site adjacent to the suspect area of lung. Digital palpation will reveal the location of most nodules which cannot be detected by the methods described earlier. If the surgeon's finger is not long enough to palpate the collapsed lung, a lung-grasping instrument placed

through another trocar site can often be used to bring the lung into range.

By the use of these techniques, over 95% of properly selected nodules (i.e. nodules ≥1 cm diameter located subpleurally or adjacent to a fissure) can be located for thoracoscopic resection. In the few instances in which the nodule is too small or soft to be located, a blind resection of lung may be necessary. It should be emphasised that by careful examination of the preoperative CT scan and the identification of proper landmarks within the chest cavity and on the chest wall, the general area of lung containing the nodule can be localised to within a few square centimetres.

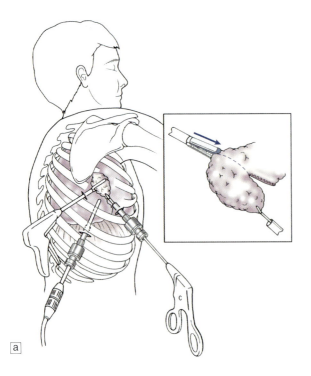

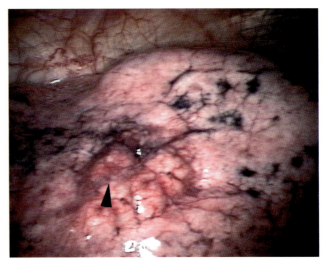

Figure 10.13 *Effacement of the atelectatic lung around the lung nodule (arrow) seen on the CT scan in Fig. 10.7.*

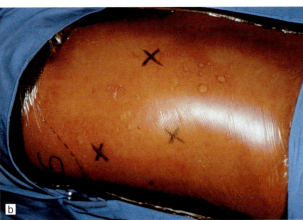

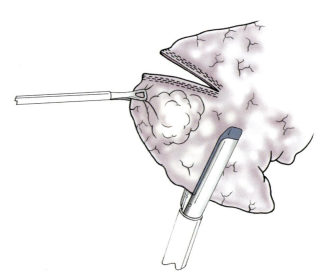

Figure 10.12 *(a) Schematic representation of trocar placement in an inverted triangle for thoracoscopic lung resection. (b) Patient is properly positioned with anticipated trocar sites marked for thoracoscopic pulmonary nodule resection.*

Figure 10.14 *Endoscopic stapler resection of a lung nodule. Stapler and grasping instrument are alternated between opposite trocar sites to complete resection.*

Also, if a nodule cannot be located or a firm identification made, conversion by a limited thoracotomy should occur so that a potentially malignant lesion is not missed.

Once the target nodule has been identified, the resection procedure can begin. Most nodules are amenable to excision with a stapler. Using an endoscopic stapling device placed through one of the portals, a wedge resection is undertaken which should include a margin of at least 1 cm around the

nodule. By alternating placement of the stapler through separate trocar sites as illustrated in Figure 10.14, the appropriate angles for stapler placement can be found to resect most nodules.

Numerous options for endoscopic staplers now exist. The initial stapler available was the EndoGIA* which

---

* Auto Suture, US Surgical, Norwalk, CT

staples and resects a portion of lung 30 mm in length. Two staple sizes are available including 2.5 and 3.5 mm length of staple legs for resection of thin and thicker segments of lung tissue, respectively. A 60 mm gas-powered version of the EndoGIA is also available; however, the length and size are such that manoeuvrability in the chest is difficult and there is very little role for this length stapler in thoracoscopic lung resection.

More recently, the Endocutter[†] endoscopic stapler has become available. The advantage of this stapler is that it is available in 35 and 45 mm lengths allowing resection of larger portions of lung tissue with less staple firings required. The 45 mm length is an optimal one for use in the chest cavity. It is available in 3.5 and 4.8 mm stapler lengths. An additional advantage is that the jaws of the stapler open wider than earlier versions allowing easier application, especially on bulky portions of lung tissue. This stapler has become our standard stapler for endoscopic pulmonary resection.

Another, flexible version of the stapler has also become available. This device, the Endoflex[†], allows the stapler jaws to articulate within the chest cavity. This minimises the limitation placed on stapler application by the rigidity of the chest wall. To date this is available in only 30 mm lengths and the jaws do not open nearly as widely on the 45 mm application. It has become our standard stapler for managing the pulmonary vessels and bronchus for VATS lobectomy, but has limited usage at present for lung resection.

There have been recent reports concerning tumour seeding in the chest wall following extraction of unprotected specimens.[18,19] Once the wedge of lung tissue that includes the nodule has been resected, it should therefore be placed in an endoscopic specimen bag (Fig. 10.15) in order to minimise the risk of seeding tumour along the trocar site.

The specimen should be sent for frozen section examination and if the nodule is demonstrated to be a primary lung malignancy, and the patient has sufficient pulmonary function to tolerate a formal lung resection, a lobectomy is undertaken. The author currently prefers to perform this lobectomy by VATS technique. However, if the surgeon is more comfortable with an open technique, conversion to a muscle-sparing thoracotomy is possible. If

†   Ethicon Endosurgery, Cincinnati, OH

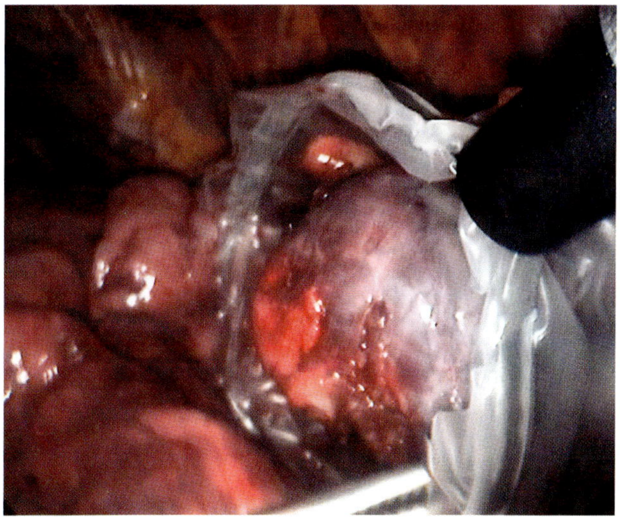

Figure 10.15 *Specimen suspected of containing malignancy is placed in a protective pouch for extraction through the chest wall.*

the nodule is a primary lung cancer and the patient has poor pulmonary function which precludes a more extensive lung resection or if the lesion is a metastasis, the procedure is terminated at this point. Similarly, if the nodule is benign, the procedure is also terminated. Air leaks are found by immersing the staple line in fluid instilled into the chest cavity and inflating the lung under direct vision. A small chest tube (20 or 24 Fr) is then placed through one of the anterior trocar sites and the lung is re-expanded. The remaining trocar sites are closed with subcuticular sutures. The chest tube which has been placed to a water seal bottle is checked under positive pressure for an air leak. If no air leak exists and a chest X-ray showing full expansion of the lung is obtained in the recovery room, the chest tube can be removed immediately. If any air leak persists, the chest tube is continued until that air leak ceases, which is usually within 24 hours. As soon as the chest tube can be removed, the patient may be discharged from hospital.

Results

In the series of 242 consecutive patients with indeterminate lung nodules who underwent thoracoscopic excisional biopsy as the primary method of diagnosis[3], thoracoscopic wedge resections of the nodules were performed using the endoscopic stapler alone in 72%; in the remaining patients, Nd:YAG laser or both stapler and laser were used. In this reported series, a definitive diagnosis was obtained in all patients, although two patients required conversion to open thoracotomy because of inability to locate the nodule, which was malignant in both cases. A benign diagnosis was obtained in 52% of patients and a malignant diagnosis in 48%. All those with primary lung cancer having adequate pulmonary reserve (29 patients) underwent a formal open lung resection during the same procedure. There was no mortality and significant morbidity was limited to atelectasis in three patients (1.2%), pneumonia in two patients (0.8%) and a prolonged air leak more than seven days in four patients (1.6%). The average hospital stay for patients having thoracoscopy only was 2.4 days.

Since this series, the author's experience has continued with virtually the same results, although the author now uses only an endoscopic stapler to perform the wedge resection. By proper case selection it has been possible to locate the target nodule in all patients. At the present time, preoperative needle localisation techniques are used in less than 5% of patients. Of course, the author uses clinical judgement when selecting candidates for thoracoscopy. For example, if a patient is a heavy cigarette smoker and has a new nodule on a chest X-ray with a ragged edge, this will in all likelihood represent a carcinoma. In this situation, if the patient is able to tolerate a formal lobectomy, this would not be preceded by a thoracoscopic wedge resection. The author also proceeds immediately to lobectomy (either by open or VATS technique) without preceding thoracoscopic excisional biopsy if the hilum is free of tumour.

Discussion and future direction

The success of thoracoscopy in diagnosing indeterminate solitary pulmonary nodules has made this the author's primary diagnostic modality for such lesions. Transthoracic needle aspiration biopsy is reserved only for those patients who are felt not to be candidates for operative resection or those with a strong likelihood of having metastatic disease or primary small cell carcinoma of the lung. In the author's opinion, although the yield of transthoracic needle aspiration biopsy is high in malignancy, the yield of a specific benign diagnosis that would avoid an eventual operation is so low as to not justify routine use of transthoracic needle aspiration biopsy.

The author is gaining experience using FDG-PET imaging accurately to differentiate malignant from benign solitary pulmonary nodules. The tracer F-18 fluorodeoxyglucose (FDG) with positron emission tomography has proved quite accurate in detecting malignancy in solitary pulmonary nodules. A series recently reported shows a sensitivity of 95–100% and specificity ranging from 86–90% with FDG-PET scanning.[14,15] If subsequent studies support the initial promising early results, there may be an increased role for PET scanning as against thoracoscopy.

Another development that offers some promise is interventional magnetic resonance imaging (MRI). In this technique an operative MRI scanner is used to present a real-time image of a lung nodule. Although this technology is in the very early stages, it offers the promise of being able to use the magnetic resonance image rather than the traditional visual image to view the surgical field. If this technology can be perfected, the surgeon will truly develop 'X-ray vision' and the occult lung nodule will no longer be occult.

At the present time, thoracoscopy has significantly enhanced the diagnosis and management of the indeterminate pulmonary nodule, and the author continues to be encouraged by experience and results.

References

1 Ginsberg RJ, Hill LD, Eagan RT et al. Modern thirty-day operative mortality for surgical resections in lung cancer. *J Thorac Cardiovasc Surg* 1983; **86**: 654–8.

2 Mack MJ, Aronoff RJ, Acuff TE et al. The present role of thoracoscopy in the diagnosis and treatment of diseases in the chest. *Ann Thorac Surg* 1992; **54**: 403–9.

3 Mack MJ, Hazelrigg SR, Landreneau RJ, Acuff TE. Thoracoscopy for the diagnosis of the indeterminate solitary pulmonary nodule. *Ann Thorac Surg* 1993; **56**: 825–32.

4 Lillington GA. Management of solitary pulmonary nodules. *Dis No* 1991; **37**: 271–318.

5 Midthun DE, Swensen SJ, Jett JR. Clinical strategies for solitary nodules. *Ann Rev Med* 1992; **43**: 195–208.

6 Steele JD, Buell P. Asymptomatic solitary pulmonary nodules. Host survival, tumor size and growth rates. *J Thorac Cardiovasc Surg* 1973; **65**: 140–51.

7 Zerhouni EA, Stitik FP, Siegelman SS et al. CT of the pulmonary nodule: a cooperative study. *Radiology* 1986; **160**: 319–27.

8 Swenson SJ, Jett JR, Payne WS, Viggiano RW, Paiolero PC, Trastek VF. An integrated approach to evaluation of the solitary pulmonary nodule. *Mayo Clin Proc* 1990; **65**: 173–86.

9 Fletcher EC, Levin DC. Flexible fiberoptic bronchoscopy and brush biopsy in the diagnosis of suspected pulmonary malignancy. *West J of Med* 1982; **136**: 477–83.

10 Levine MS, Weis JM, Harrell JH, Cameron TJ, Moser KM. Transthoracic needle aspiration biopsy following negative fiberoptic bronchoscopy in solitary pulmonary nodules. *Chest* 1988; **93**: 1152–5.

11 Westcott JL. Direct percutaneous needle aspiration of localized pulmonary lesions: results in 422 patients. *Radiology* 1980; **137**: 31–5.

12 Khouri NF, Stitik FP, Erozan YS *et al*. Transthoracic needle aspiration of benign and malignant lung lesions. *Am Roentgenology* 1985; **144**: 281–8.

13 Calhoun P, Feldman PS, Armstrong P *et al*. The clinical outcome of needle aspirations of the lung when cancer is not diagnosed. *Ann Thorac Surg* 1986; **41**: 592–6.

14 Gupta NC, Frank, AR, Dewan NA *et al*. Solitary pulmonary nodules: detection of malignancy with PET with 2-[F-18]-fluoro-2-deoxy-D-glucose. *Radiology* 1992; **184**: 441–4.

15 Gupta NC, Dewan NA, Frank A. Diagnostic evaluation of suspected solitary nodules (SPN) using PET FDG imaging. *Chest* 1993; **104**: 119S.

16 Roviaro GC, Varoli F, Rebuffat C *et al*. Videothoracoscopic staging and treatment of lung cancer. *Ann Thorac Surg* 1995; **59**: 971–4.

17 Mack MJ, Gordan MJ, Postma TW *et al*. Percutaneous localization of pulmonary nodules for thoracoscopic lung resection. *Ann Thorac Surg* 1992; **53**: 1123–4.

18 Walsh GL, Nesbitt JC. Tumor implants after thoracoscopic resection of a metastatic sarcoma. *Ann Thorac Surg* 1995; **59**: 215–6.

19 Fry WA, Siddiqui A, Pensier JM, Mostafavi H. Thoracoscopic implantation of cancer with a fatal outcome. *Ann Thorac Surg* 1995; **59**: 42–5.

Major pulmonary resection

W.S. Walker

11

Introduction

In conventional thoracic surgical practice, access for major pulmonary resection is gained through a formal thoracotomy incision held open by a mechanical rib retractor. The most common approach, a standard posterolateral thoracotomy, provides excellent exposure — but at the cost of a highly destructive incision which causes major soft tissue damage and ligamentous disruption, and often results in neuropraxic injury to the intercostal nerves. Postoperative pain is intense. Apart from causing distress, this restricts chest wall movement, resulting in impaired pulmonary expansion.[1] Muscle-sparing thoracotomy causes less muscle trauma and is associated with reduced immediate pain, but has not been shown to produce any significant improvement in postoperative pulmonary function.[2] Furthermore, as rib separation is not different from a standard thoracotomy, ligamentous and neuropraxic pain are not improved. Conversely, the surgeon's vision is somewhat restricted by the necessarily reduced exposure and there is a 4–23% incidence of wound seroma formation.[2] Either form of thoracotomy is highly traumatic and can be associated with significant depression of aspects of cell-mediated immunity[3] probably related to cytokine activation.

It is common for post-thoracotomy patients to complain of wound discomfort for some weeks after surgery. In many cases, pain will fade away over 2–3 months but in others this does not occur. These individuals suffer from chronic post-thoracotomy pain syndrome, an affliction which may last for many years and which can significantly degrade quality of life. Estimates of the incidence of post-thoracotomy pain syndrome vary in the literature, reflecting the degree to which data is actively sought; chronic pain sufficient to interfere significantly with quality of life probably occurs in 25–40% of patients, while pain of crippling intensity occurs in at least 5%.[4]

Most patients undergoing major pulmonary resection do so in the context of malignant pulmonary disease. Unfortunately, many ultimately will not be cured of their condition. It is tragic that open thoracotomy will subject these patients to a very painful operative procedure and a high risk of subsequent severe chronic wound pain which may well marr the limited time remaining to them.

Against this background, a video-assisted thoracic surgery (VATS) approach to major pulmonary resection offers potentially outstanding patient benefits.

This chapter provides an overview of the VATS techniques currently used to perform pulmonary lobectomy, bilobectomy and pneumonectomy. The operative technique for the commonest approach — total endoscopic hilar dissection — is described here in detail, together with outcome data based on experience reported in the literature and results derived from the author's first 130 major VATS pulmonary resections using this technique.

Development of video-assisted major pulmonary resection

Video-assisted dissectional pulmonary lobectomy was first performed in 1991 and initially described by Roviaro and colleagues.[5] Several further accounts were soon published describing small series of patients undergoing lobectomy, some with quite different operative techniques,[6–11] and pneumonectomy was reported shortly afterwards.[7,8,12] Since these initial descriptions, a variety of papers have confirmed that VATS lobectomy is feasible and safe,[13] but the published data regarding VATS pneumonectomy is modest,[21–24] suggesting limited overall experience.[7,8,12,17,22] This may reflect the fact that pneumonectomy is often dictated by hilar involvement which itself militates against a thoracoscopic approach, but it probably also reveals the need for further instrument development to cope with safety and technical aspects of this procedure.

Philosophical approach

Basic principles

Major pulmonary resection is most likely to be undertaken for malignant disease. Evaluation of patients for surgery and the discipline of pre- and intraoperative staging applies equally to a VATS procedure as to open surgery. It is also essential that any operation carried out thoracoscopically does not differ in completeness from an open procedure. The choice of procedure selected should not be influenced and the adequacy of resection should not be jeopardised by a predilection for a VATS approach.

VATS surgery involves dissection of major vessels and presents a definite risk of intra-operative haemorrhage from inadvertent vascular damage. The surgeon, therefore, must always consider the safety margin available not only at the outset of surgery but continuously during the procedure.

Conversion to thoracotomy

It follows from the preceding considerations that circumstances may dictate conversion to open thoracotomy. Review of current published series suggests a rate for conversion to open thoracotomy of 10–30% for major VATS pulmonary resection. Whilst this rate will clearly vary with experience, it is also influenced by the nature of the cases attempted so that direct comparison between centres is difficult. The fact remains, however, that even in 'expert' hands an appreciable conversion rate exists. This event, therefore, should not attract criticism directed at either the VATS approach or at the surgeon. It is important to appreciate that when conversion is deemed necessary, it does not represent failure but rather an

intelligent selection of the optimum approach for the patient.

Furthermore, appropriate placement of the thoracoscopic incisions will ensure that conversion simply results in much the same wound as would otherwise have been made prior to the advent of thoracoscopic techniques. The patient still gains from the opportunity afforded the surgeon to inspect the pleural cavity before electing to create an open thoracotomy. If conversion has occurred after a portion of the procedure has been completed thoracoscopically, the author has found that it is often possible to complete the surgery through a more limited open thoracotomy than would normally have been used. This is obviously beneficial to the patient and results from the fact that much of the mobilisation and dissection of structures will have been accomplished already.

Adopting a general policy of pre-resectional videothoracoscopic evaluation at the time of any proposed major pulmonary resection has considerable merit even when a thoracoscopic resection is not contemplated. The surgical team gains experience in thoracoscopic assessment and evaluation, and the patient benefits as the videothoracoscopy may demonstrate a contraindication to resection such as pleural seedlings or direct tumour spread (Fig. 11.1). Adopting this policy as routine has been shown virtually to abolish the irresectability rate in patients scheduled for major pulmonary resection.[17]

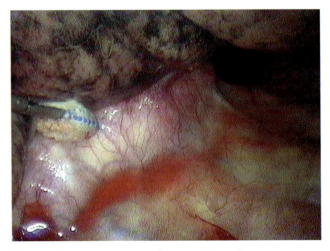

Figure 11.1 *Operative view of inoperable bronchogenic carcinoma detected at preliminary videothoracoscopy — direct spread of tumour onto the lateral aortic wall.*

Selection of patients for VATS major pulmonary resection

General considerations

Suitability for pulmonary resection

A VATS approach involves less operative trauma and offers an easier postoperative course to patients undergoing major pulmonary resection so that some discretion can be exercised when selecting patients. Marginal patients, therefore, can be offered surgery. In general, however, the conventional criteria for pulmonary resection must still be considered when selecting patients for videothoracoscopic lobectomy or pneumonectomy. The loss of functioning lung tissue is no different to an open procedure so that quality of life will still depend on adequate residual lung function. Similarly, if conversion is necessary, the patient must have sufficient cardiovascular reserve to sustain an open resection. It is important, therefore, for all patients to ascertain whether:

- pulmonary reserve is adequate, and
- cardiac status is acceptable

according to standard unit selection protocols for the intended extent of major pulmonary resection. Similarly, in cases of malignant disease, the standard oncological criteria for resection apply. The surgeon should ensure that:

- local resectability is confirmed, and
- distant spread is excluded.

The primary lesion

The requirement to deliver a lobe or lung containing a mass through a small intercostal incision with either no or very limited rib retraction imposes an upper size limit of about 6 cm diameter for a pulmonary lesion. Tumours which involve the chest wall are not suitable for VATS techniques as chest wall resection may be required. A large central mass is not suitable for VATS resection as it may impede access to the major vessels and therefore pose a significant operative risk.

Mediastinal lymph nodes

The management of the mediastinal nodes at the time of major pulmonary resection remains controversial. The choice lies between mediastinal node sampling or clearance.

It is beyond the scope of this chapter to debate the relative merits of these options but a VATS approach can be entirely compatible with either philosophy.

The author's mediastinal assessment protocol for all potential VATS major resection cases with malignant disease specifies both CT scan of thorax and mediastinoscopy. This policy utilises the CT scan to ensure that the pulmonary lesion is solitary and as a guide to specific areas of interest for the subsequent mediastinoscopy. Lymph node size may not be an accurate predictor of potential involvement by metastatic disease[23] and the author's team therefore undertakes mediastinoscopy without regard to a specific node diameter. This form of detailed assessment is intended to ensure that N2 and N3 cases are excluded and further detailed mediastinal lymph node sampling is undertaken at the time of resection to finalise the mediastinal staging.

Some surgeons proceed direct to thoracotomy with block dissection of the lymph nodes for patients with mediastinal lymph nodes below 1–1.5 cm in diameter on CT scan. This form of management is perfectly compatible with a VATS approach, as a thoracoscopic mediastinal block dissection can certainly be combined with either VATS lobectomy or pneumonectomy. Resection of large or matted mediastinal nodes is, however, likely to be difficult, hazardous and inappropriate for thoracoscopic techniques. Consequently, a VATS approach is not suitable for patients with known or suspected N2 disease. Although it is possible, the author would not recommend thoracoscopic mediastinal block dissection if a detailed preoperative mediastinoscopy has been performed, as the mediastinoscopy leads to considerable mediastinal fibrosis, matted nodes and increased vascularity of the mediastinal tissues.

Adhesions

Intrapleural adhesions increase the difficulties of surgery, by limiting working space and vision and by tethering the lobe(s), thereby impeding mobility. The degree of interlobar fusion is important also as thoracoscopic lobar resection is easier when the fissures are well developed. An incomplete fissure will require a more complex and time-consuming procedure as the surgeon may need to adopt different operative strategies depending upon the precise anatomical situation. Both intrapleural and interlobar adhesions, therefore, present relative contraindications to VATS

137

resection. They may be divided thoracoscopically but this requires appropriate experience and adequate available operating time.

Selection criteria for VATS lobectomy

The indications and contraindications for VATS lobectomy are summarised in Tables 11.1 and 11.2. In broad terms, the aim is to select either benign disease, Stage I (T1 or 2, N0) or early Stage II (T1 or 2, intrapulmonary N1) cases. This criteria may require intraoperative frozen section analysis of

nodes present at the lobar bronchus section line and elsewhere in the pulmonary hilum and mediastinum.

Selection criteria for VATS pneumonectomy

The criteria given for VATS lobectomy are generally relevant for patients undergoing VATS pneumonectomy, but in some instances pneumonectomy may be indicated by intra-operative findings at the time of anticipated lobectomy. Additional indications and contraindications are listed in Table 11.3.

Table 11.1

VATS lobectomy: indications

Known benign disease

Bronchiectasis
Lobar destruction (pneumonia, infarction)
True benign neoplasm <6 cm too centrally placed to allow safe wedge resection

Presumed or confirmed primary malignant disease

Peripheral lesion (clinical T1 or T2 status) which is solitary on pulmonary CT scan
Localised intrabronchial lesion
Negative mediastinoscopy and mediastinal CT scan (clinical N0 or N1 status)

Solitary metastatic malignant disease

Definite single lesion after period of review and fine cut CT scan
Primary tumour type compatible with solitary metastasis (renal, colon)

Table 11.2

VATS lobectomy: contraindications

Relative

Patients with radiographic evidence of intrapleural adhesions
Those on significant antiplatelet medication (may cause oozing)
Gross obesity (chest wall thickness may exceed port length)

Absolute

Large masses (>6 cm)
Central hilar lesions
Lesions which are adherent to the chest wall
Air trapping (if excessive this precludes adequate space in which to operate)

Indications

- Proximal, small, largely intrabronchial growth not suitable for sleeve resection
- Involvement of several lobes across fissure(s) by a malignant lesion
- Attachment of tumour to the main pulmonary artery within the hilum

Contraindications

- Inadequate length of main PA available to allow safe thoracoscopic placement of a proximal vascular clamp (as with hilar fixity, this is likely to occur with a centrally-placed hilar lesion)

Table 11.3

VATS pneumonectomy: selection criteria additional to those applicable to lobectomy

Technique of VATS major pulmonary resection

At present, at least three different techniques have been developed to perform video-assisted major pulmonary resection. These may be classified as:

- Video-imaged total endoscopic resection with individual dissection of hilar structures
- Video-imaged endoscopic mass section of hilar structures
- Mini-thoracotomy with video assistance.

Video-imaged total endoscopic resection with individual dissection of hilar structures

This approach involves detailed dissection and control of each hilar structure in turn in a manner which is entirely analogous to a standard open lobectomy or pneumonectomy. The procedure is visualized entirely by video screen and a rib retractor is not employed. Several authors[5,7,9–12,14,17–22] have described variations of this thoracoscopic technique, which may be viewed as the application of minimal access surgery to classical thoracic hilar and mediastinal dissection. In addition to performing an anatomical hilar dissection, it is possible to clear or sample ipselateral mediastinal nodes and subcarinal nodes (Fig. 11.2).

Video-imaged endoscopic mass section of hilar structures

In this technique the procedure is imaged by video screen. However, the hilar structures are not taken individually but rather en masse using stapling devices. Lewis[6,15,16,24] has so far been the only author to advocate this technique, known as simultaneously stapled (SIS) resection or, more recently, as VATS non-rib–spread simultaneously stapled VATS–SS resection. It has been criticised because the proven techniques for safe hilar dissection and nodal clearance have been ignored. Lewis, however, describes excellent results and now has probably the largest single experience of VATS lobectomy. He argues that for appropriate cases his approach confers the advantages of minimal access surgery and that simultaneous stapling of the hilar structures is safer than individual dissection. Mediastinal node dissection may be performed following the lobectomy but detailed sampling is usually undertaken.

Mini-thoracotomy with video assistance

Whereas the preceding techniques employ video imaging and avoid the use of a rib spreader, an alternate strategy has been described by Giudicelli and colleagues[8,13] and latterly by

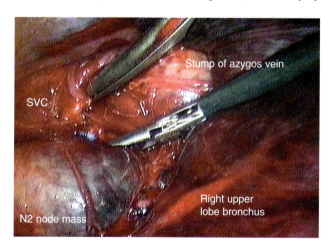

Figure 11.2 *Mediastinal nodes being sampled/cleared at endoscopic hilar dissection.*

Naruke.[25] This technique utilises a mini-thoracotomy held open by a retractor as the main route for vision and surgery, the latter being performed with conventional and specially modified instruments. The videothoracoscope is used to provide supplementary vision and illumination. These authors have demonstrated that it is possible to perform a thorough hilar and mediastinal dissection directly through the mini-thoracotomy. This technique, however, may perhaps be described as an extreme variation of a muscle-sparing thoracotomy rather than true endoscopic surgery. The methods of thoracic access are reduced as opposed to minimal, and the need for rib separation by a retractor for the duration of the procedure may obviate some of the potential benefits to be gained. Also, this approach fails to use the opportunity provided by videothoracoscopic technology for detailed visualisation of the hilar structures with the added benefits of magnification and excellent visualisation of the apical and basal regions.

Incisions

All current techniques for VATS pulmonary resection employ two or three ports and a short 5–8 cm intercostal 'access' or 'utility' incision which is used for the insertion of large instruments and for removal of the specimen. The placement of the access thoracotomy varies (Fig. 11.3). Kirkby and associates[9,14] locate this somewhat posteriorly below the tip of the scapula. Giudicelli and colleagues[8,13] advocate an incision in the 5th interspace posterior to the midaxillary line and Lewis,[6,15,16,24] McKenna[11] and Roviaro and colleagues[5,7,17] an incision in the 4th intercostal space in the anterior axillary line. The author[10,18–21] favours an inframammary incision on the basis that the intercostal space is widest at this point and because this incision can be rapidly linked to the thoracoscope port site if a formal thoracotomy is required, thereby creating a standard lateral thoracotomy (Fig. 11.4).

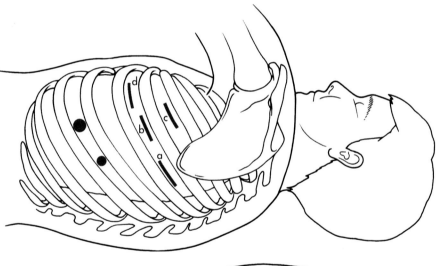

Figure 11.3 *Location of utility or access incisions as described by various groups.*

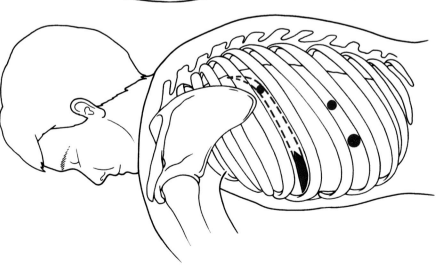

Figure 11.4 *Conversion to open thoracotomy by linkage of a submammary access incision with the posterior videothoracoscope port.*

Operative technique for video-assisted total endoscopic major pulmonary resection

This account is based on the author's experience of over 130 major pulmonary resections at the time of writing. It incorporates improvements and some variation from the original description.[10] Whilst there are differences in detail from the technical descriptions published by others with experience of the endoscopic hilar dissection technique, the general outlines are largely equivalent. The basic guiding principles, of safety and analogous practice to open thoracic surgery with detailed exposure of hilar structures and effective nodal clearance, remain consistent.

Anaesthesia and preparation

The patient is positioned, anaesthetised and draped as for a standard posterolateral thoracotomy (Fig. 11.5). It is helpful to elevate the bridge on the table to open the interspaces in the operative field. A double lumen endotracheal tube is used and invasive radial arterial pressure, cutaneous O_2 saturation, end tidal CO_2 and ECG are monitored continuously. A large intravenous cannula is placed to provide vascular access for rapid transfusion in case of intraoperative haemorrhage and a full thoracotomy tray with a selection of vascular clamps is open and available by the operating table.

Incisions

Access is gained for lobectomy using three 1–2 cm stab incisions and one 4–5 cm submammary anterior intercostal incision (Fig. 11.6). If pneumonectomy is to be performed, one inferior stab incision is omitted.

The thoracoscope is inserted through the upper posterior stab incision, which is placed approximately 1 cm below and posterior to the lower pole of the scapula. This site provides an excellent general view of the chest with several specific advantages. The view obtained is broadly similar to that presented to the surgeon at a standard posterolateral thoracotomy, thereby preserving the anatomical relationships assimilated from open procedures. It also aligns with the oblique fissure to give a good view for fissural dissection. It is not usually necessary to move the thoracoscope from this port as, with appropriate manipulation of the thoracoscope and lung, the relevant structures can all be brought into good view.

The inferior ports provide intra-operative access for dissection instruments and endostaplers, and are used at the end of the procedure for apical and basal intercostal drain placement. If a pneumonectomy is to be performed, one inferior port is created through which a single drain is inserted at the end of the procedure. The inferior port(s) are generally placed about two interspaces below the level of the submammary incision, but the exact position(s) can be best assessed intra-operatively in relation to the shape of each

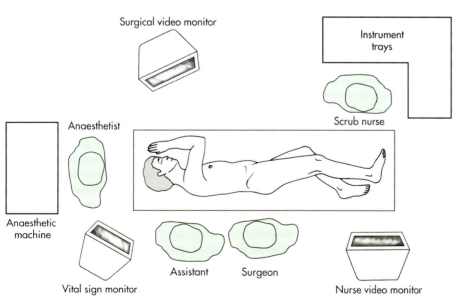

Figure 11.5 *Patient positioning and monitor arrangement for endoscopic hilar dissection lobectomy.*

Surgical video monitor

Instrument trays

Anaesthetist

Scrub nurse

Anaesthetic machine

Vital sign monitor

Assistant

Surgeon

Nurse video monitor

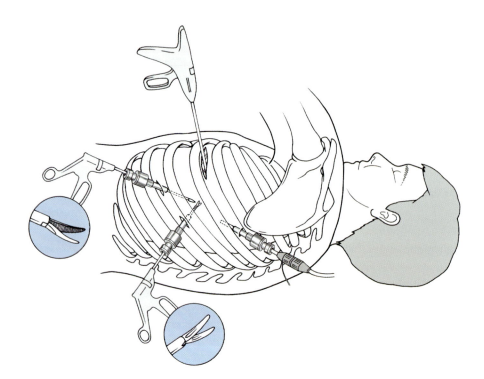

Figure 11.6 *Arrangement of port sites for endoscopic hilar dissection lobectomy.*

patient's chest cavity and the intended procedure can be determined.

The anterior submammary incision functions as a further port for instrument insertion during the operation and for specimen removal at the end. This enlarged port provides sufficient room to insert large instruments such as the Endo-GIA 60 endostapler, conventional staplers normally used in open surgery and conventional long vascular clamps.

Imaging

The operative field for major pulmonary resection is relatively large, and therefore frequent reorientation of the thoracoscope is required to provide adequate coverage. It is also necessary to move the thoracoscope closer or further from the operative field depending on the nature of the dissection being undertaken at any given time. The author has found that it is easiest for the individual holding the thoracoscope to cope with these requirements when using a 0° instrument. Others[11] have found a 30° thoracoscope helpful when visualising anterior vessels.

A high specification camera system is required to provide the detailed visualisation of the hilar structures necessary in performing thoracoscopic dissection. Similarly, a high resolution video monitor using RGB or component signal input is indicated for optimal detail. The monitor is positioned towards the head of the table, opposite the surgeon and assistant/camera person and angled towards them so that they can view the image comfortably. A similar slave monitor is positioned on the surgeon's side of the table at the level of the patient's hips for the scrub nurse, second assistant if one is present and the anaesthetist (Fig. 11.5).

General aspects of operative technique in video-assisted major pulmonary resection

Ensuring good vision

Safe and effective surgery requires the best possible visualisation of the operative field. The general operative principles which support that aim are:

- maintaining collapse of the lung
- minimising ooze, and
- intelligent manipulation of the hilar structures.

It is not necessary to use elevated intrapleural pressures by insufflation of CO_2 as the non-ventilated lung will collapse satisfactorily on exposure to the atmosphere provided there is no intrabronchial obstruction. It does, however, take a few minutes to collapse and it is helpful to ask the anaesthetist to stop ventilating the operative lung when commencing draping. If the anterior access incision is created first this allows the pleura to be entered under direct vision with minimal risk of parenchymal damage. The surgeon can then determine whether the lung has fallen away from the chest wall and, if adhesions are present, divide these sufficiently to allow the posterior thoracoscope port to be created safely. When the thoracoscope has been inserted, all the intrapleural adhesions should be divided as it is important to have a fully mobile lung before starting hilar dissection. Suction should be performed below the surface of any fluid collection, and it can be helpful to clamp the endobronchial lumen leading to the operated lung so that the reduction in intrathoracic pressure does not cause the lung to reinflate.

Intrapleural adhesions and the pulmonary ligament are divided using a cautery to minimise bleeding. Venous congestion is a nuisance during dissection as it promotes oozing from raw parenchymal edges; it is therefore convenient to divide the lobar vein(s) last. If minor bleeding does occur, pressure can be applied using a swab mounted in a sponge-holding forceps which is introduced through the access incision. Spilt blood and ooze overlying a dissection area can be cleaned away in a similar manner.

It is necessary to manipulate the lung in order to provide the best view of a structure or the ideal angulation for section. This can be achieved initially by grasping the lung with sponge-holding or ring forceps and folding it in the appropriate direction. Once the bronchus has been cleared of surrounding tissue a sling can then be passed around it and used to provide an alternate method of reorientating the lobe or lung.

Dealing with cancer

For those patients with known or possible malignancy, management must not be compromised by a minimal access approach. There are, however, specific advantages to a VATS resection. The surgeon can discover unforeseen causes of inoperability such as pleural seedlings or extensive local tumour spread, thereby avoiding a pointless thoracotomy. There is also the opportunity to confirm operability in marginal cases who might tolerate lobectomy but not pneumonectomy.

Detailed assessment must be performed to define the correct operative procedure and one must be ready to accept the need to proceed to an open resection, where appearances indicate that a complex surgical procedure is likely to be required, rather than try to make the procedure fit the surgical approach. With endoscopy, the opportunity exists to take frozen section samples from a pulmonary mass or abnormal hilar tissue. It can be difficult to identify small intraparenchymal lesions thoracoscopically. Accurate preoperative localisation by CT, needle localisation, dye injection or even ultrasound have all been found helpful[27–30] but, unless the lesion is quite obviously in a particular lobe, e.g. in the very apex of an upper lobe, it is essential that the surgeon can confidently identify it. Digital palpation through the access incision is useful in assessing lesions and guiding biopsy (Fig. 11.7). If necessary, the lobe can be pushed forwards with an instrument to reach the palpating finger. Another useful technique is to roll across the lobe with a peanut pledget on a Roberts forceps (Fig. 11.8). If the lesion cannot be clearly identified, this is an absolute indication to convert to an open thoracotomy.

Assessment of possible hilar fixity is important in deciding whether to proceed to an open operation. The mediastinum can be inspected and the pleura incised to allow further pre-resectional sampling of nodes if desired.

The physical constraints of VATS procedures reduce handling of a tumour but at delivery the author believes that it is essential to place the specimen in a polythene bag prior to pulling it out of the access incision in order to avoid the risk of tumour implantation.[31] As a further precaution the pleural cavity and ports should be thoroughly lavaged with sterile water at the end of the procedure.

Technique

Dissection of structures is performed using a combination of sharp dissection with endoscopic scissors and blunt dissection with a pledget mounted on a Roberts forceps, which is also a source of tactile feedback when assessing lesions. Blunt dissection is particularly useful when dissecting around the pulmonary vessels, and for sweeping tissue along the lobar bronchus peripheral to the line of intended bronchial division so that all the bronchial nodes can be included in the operative specimen — much as one would do in an open procedure. It is often convenient to pass large conventional instruments through the access incision when trying to encircle a large structure. Long, gently- or acutely-curved vascular clamps can be particularly helpful

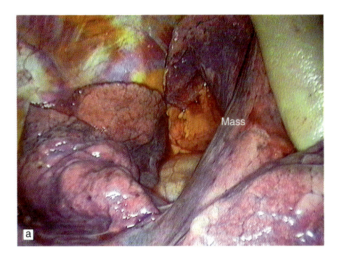

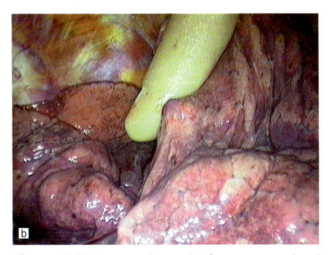

Figure 11.7 *Operative photograph of peri-operative digital palpation of an intraparenchymal pulmonary nodule. The palpating finger is swept over the mass from one side (a) to the other (b) of the nodule.*

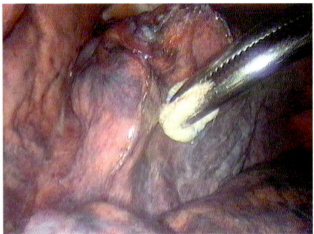

Figure 11.8 *Operative photograph of use of peanut pledgets mounted on Roberts forceps to 'finger' a pulmonary lesion.*

lubricating jelly to which surplus fired staples adhere, thereby reducing the number of free staples lying in the operative field.

Bronchial arteries should be clipped rather than cauterised prior to division in order to avoid damage to the bronchus. Mediastinal node dissection is facilitated on the right by division of the azygos vein and it is easier to clear subcarinal nodes if a traction sling has been passed around the main bronchus so that it can be elevated. At pneumonectomy, therefore, the bronchus should not be divided until the subcarinal nodes have been cleared or sampled as preferred. In keeping with standard open surgery, the middle and lower lobes can be tied together after right upper lobectomy through the access thoracotomy, and the pulmonary ligament may be incised after resection of either upper lobe to encourage expansion of the residual lung.

Vessels

Placement of a vascular clamp across a major vessel, either a lobar vein or main stem pulmonary artery, prior to division (Fig. 11.9) is an essential feature of safe practice in thoracoscopic surgery.[32] This protects the patient against the possibility of massive intra-operative blood loss in the event of malfunction of a stapling device or laceration of the vessel at the time of ligature or stapling. In general, endostaples are the safest method of control for most vessels. Ligature is appropriate for very small vessels and clips may be applied to small systemic and pulmonary artery branches but, in the author's experience, these may either cut through the pulmonary artery branch or be pulled off by swabs. Dissection

for this purpose. In general, a silastic sling should be passed around a structure prior to attempting division, as this enables the structure to be manoeuvred and facilitates further clearing of tissue. Meticulous haemostasis is essential to avoid oozing, and small bleeders can be controlled by diathermy or pressure.

Endoscopic stapler cartridges should be chosen with the correct staple leg length for the tissue which is to be divided, and care must be taken to ensure that cartridges are correctly loaded. It is particularly important to ensure that any free staples are not allowed to come between the jaws when they are closed as this will cause the instrument to misfire. A useful technique is to coat the instrument with a water-soluble

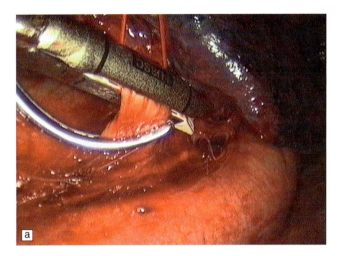

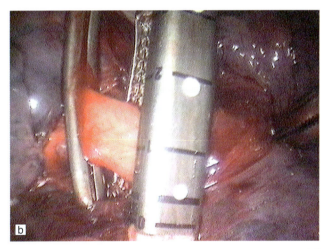

Figure 11.9 *Vascular clamp placed across (a) upper left pulmonary vein and (b) right pulmonary artery at level of lower lobe, prior to firing vascular stapler.*

of the lobar pulmonary artery branches has to be based on a comprehensive understanding of the anatomy of the branches of the pulmonary artery and the possible variations[30], notably the right upper lobe posterior segmental artery and the lingular artery, both of which may arise lower than expected from the main trunk or from lower lobar branches.

One particular hazard in patients with inflammatory disease (either primary or associated with a malignancy) is the presence of lymph nodes along the pulmonary sheath which have become adherent to the underlying artery. If nodes do not sweep away when the sheath has been opened, it is prudent to proceed to an open thoracotomy so that the opportunity for optimal vascular control is present if the vessel should rupture.

Fissures

In the author's early experience, sharp dissection of a fused pulmonary fissure resulted in marked postoperative air leakage. This is unfortunate as leakage prolongs the period during which intercostal drainage is necessary and so prevents earlier discharge. The author, therefore, has abandoned sharp dissection of fissures in VATS cases in favour of using endostaplers to divide areas of fissural fusion. Air leakage may be further reduced by buttressing the staples with pericardial strips.[31]

Bronchi

Bronchial division and control is also best achieved in VATS cases by the use of endostaplers. Segmental bronchi can be secured with a blue cartridge (3.5 mm) and lobar or main bronchi with a green (4.8 mm) cartridge. Ideally, the stapler should cross the bronchus at a right angle and, as the endostaplers do not currently roticulate, this may require manipulation of the bronchus to achieve this relative orientation (Fig. 11.10). Occasionally, reinforcing sutures may be placed if testing underwater demonstrates a leak through the suture line, but this is rare. It has been suggested that segmental branches should be divided rather than lobar branches[9] but in most instances direct section of the lobar bronchi is easily achieved. In the case of a right lower lobectomy, however, it can be helpful to divide the apical lower and main stem lower divisions

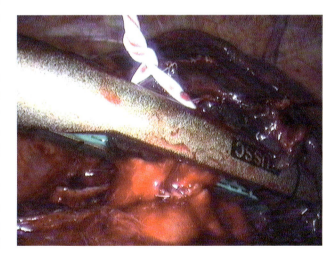

Figure 11.10 *Orientation of left upper lobe bronchus by sling. Note the 'crane' effect produced by twisting the endoforceps and so shortening the sling and elevating the bronchus, thereby providing better access to the bronchus.*

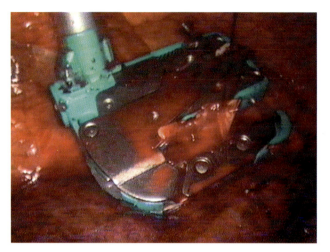

Figure 11.11 *Use of roticulating open stapler to restaple difficult bronchus.*

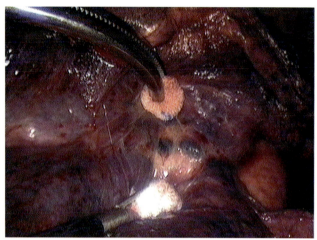

Figure 11.12 *Operative photograph of lymph nodes on sheath of pulmonary artery.*

separately so as to preserve the orifice of the middle lobe bronchus.

Rarely, the closure line may be inadequate or the tissues too thick to allow the use of an endostapler. In this instance, stay sutures should be inserted at either end of the bronchial stump, so that it can be elevated and reclosed with a conventional roticulated bronchial stapler introduced through the submammary incision (Fig. 11.11).

Dissection sequences

Lobectomy procedures

Left sided resection
If the fissure is complete, the sheath of the pulmonary artery is entered between the lobes so as to display the main artery and the apical lower and lingular branches.

When the fissure is incomplete, the pulmonary artery can usually be located by dissection within the fused fissure. The location of the artery within the fissure may be suggested initially by pulsation and confirmed by the presence of anthracotic nodes along the arterial sheath (Fig. 11.12) which is entered. The lung should then be retracted forwards, and the pleural reflection posterior to the lung root incised so that the artery can be identified and the sheath entered from the posterior, aspect of the lung root. A sling can then be passed between the two points of arterial access to elevate the fused posterior fissure which is then divided with an endostapler. The fused section of anterior fissure, is

divided when convenient or when the lobectomy has been completed.

Rarely, the fissure is completely fused with no fissural cleft. In this case, the lung is retracted forwards and the pulmonary artery is approached posteriorly. It may then be feasible to divide all the arterial branches passing to the lobe to be removed, after which the bronchus and vein can be divided. A sling can then be passed under the whole fused fissure which is divided with an endostapler. If this is not feasible, dissection should be continued within the sheath of the artery until it crosses the line of the fissure. A right-angled forceps can be pushed from the internal aspect of the fused fissure through to the external surface. The portion of fissure posterior to this breach can then be stapled, allowing better aspect to the artery and the hilum. The anterior portion of fused fissure is divided when convenient.

Left upper lobectomy. The lingular branches are divided and dissection continued up the pulmonary artery dividing each branch in turn. Considerable care is required when dealing with the apical and anterior mediastinal branches which are partially obscured by the bronchus and easy to injure. The bronchus is then cleared of surrounding tissue and divided. Finally the superior pulmonary vein is divided. The pulmonary ligament should be incised to free the lower lobe.

Left lower lobectomy. The apical lower and main stem lower arteries are taken separately. The pulmonary ligament is incised and the lower vein cleared and divided. The bronchus is then cleared of surrounding tissue and divided.

Right sided resection

For both right upper and lower lobectomy it is helpful to first enter the sheath of the pulmonary artery, after locating this by dissection in the confluence of the fissures.

When the fissure is incomplete posteriorly, the lung should be retracted anteriorly and the mediastinal pleura incised at the anterior border of the bronchus intermedius immediately below the upper lobe bronchus. A forceps can then be passed deep to the fused posterior fissure, lateral to the artery and anterior to the bronchus intermedius. A sling is passed in order to elevate the fused section of fissure which is divided.

If the oblique fissure is totally absent, or it is considered unsafe to directly dissect the artery at the confluence of the fissures, different strategies are needed. With an upper lobectomy, the lung should be retracted forwards and the upper lobe bronchus identified, cleared of surrounding tissue, and divided first. This exposes the pulmonary artery. With a lower lobectomy, the lung should be retracted anteriorly and somewhat superiorly so that the pulmonary ligament can be divided and the inferior vein identified. This is then divided, allowing the artery and bronchus to be approached from below.

After a right upper lobectomy or middle lobectomy the transverse fissure will have to be developed with an endostapler, taking care to preserve the relevant branch(es) of the superior pulmonary vein.

Right upper lobectomy. The posterior segmental artery is divided and the upper lobe bronchus cleared of surrounding tissue and divided. If the oblique fissure is totally absent, this order is reversed. The upper lobe is retracted forwards and the pulmonary artery cleaned to expose the apical and anterior segmental vessels, which are then divided separately or as a stem. The upper lobe branches of the superior pulmonary vein are cleared of surrounding tissue and the branch from the middle lobe identified. It is helpful to retract the lung posteriorly, and view the anterior aspect of the upper vein to allow that aspect to be cleaned and to verify the position of the middle lobe vein. The upper lobe veins are divided and the transverse fissure then completed.

Right lower lobectomy. If the posterior fissure is fused this is divided. The apical lower segmental artery and the main pulmonary arterial trunk are usually divided separately but it is sometimes feasible to divide the pulmonary trunk above the origin of the apical lower artery. The lower lobe is retracted anteriorly and the pulmonary ligament incised to expose the lower vein, which is cleared of surrounding tissue and divided. The lobe is retracted inferiorly and the anterior portion of the oblique fissure between the middle and lower lobes divided. The fissure is usually well developed and requires only sharp dissection, but if necessary an endostapler may be used. Finally, the lower lobe bronchus is divided, taking care to preserve the middle lobe origin. The author has occasionally found it helpful to confirm patency of the middle lobe bronchus by getting an assistant to view it with a fibre-optic bronchoscope when the lower lobe airway(s) are being stapled.

Middle lobectomy. After identifying the pulmonary artery just below the confluence of the fissures and entering its sheath, the lateral segmental artery is identified, cleaned and divided. The medial segmental artery is then cleaned, but it is usually easiest to divide the bronchus and then middle lobe vein before dividing this artery, to provide more room. The transverse fissure is completed.

Upper and middle lobectomy. If the fissures are reasonably well developed, the sheath of the pulmonary artery can be entered at the confluence of the fissures. The middle lobe hilar structures are divided and the fused portions of the oblique fissure separated. The upper lobar structures are then divided.

When the oblique fissure is virtually absent, the right upper lobe bronchus is divided and the lung reflected forwards. The arterial branches to the upper lobe and then the middle lobe are secured and the middle lobe bronchus divided prior to dividing the superior pulmonary vein. Finally, the fused oblique fissure is separated.

Middle and lower lobectomy. If possible, the sheath of the pulmonary artery is entered at the confluence of the fissures. The apical lower artery, the basal stem artery and the middle lobar branches may have to be separately divided, or the pulmonary artery sectioned obliquely, so as to include all the branches in one cut. This decision depends on the anatomy of the pulmonary artery. The posterior oblique fissure is completed and the bronchus intermedius divided. The inferior pulmonary vein and middle lobe vein are then divided and the transverse fissure is completed.

If the oblique fissure is completely fused, the inferior vein is divided and the lung retracted superiorly and anteriorly. This exposes the pulmonary artery and allows the apical lower and basal stem artery to be divided. The bronchus intermedius is divided and the middle lobar vessels dissected out and divided in turn from below. An opening is made in the area of the fused fissural confluence, having scrutinised the section of lung to be pierced from both sides to exclude any previously unnoticed vessels. This manoeuvre allows an endostapling device to be inserted so that the posterior fused oblique fissure and then the fused transverse fissure can be divided.

Closure

The bronchus stump should be tested under water and haemostasis of the resection area and incisions checked. Full inflation of the remaining lung can be confirmed thoracoscopically. The short submammary incision is closed in layers without pericostal sutures. The two inferior stab incisions are utilised as drain holes. As each of these holes is usually a little larger than a standard 32 FG drain, it is helpful to place one or two deep absorbable sutures to reduce the port size and so prevent air entering the chest. The thoracoscope incision is closed with absorbable sutures.

Pneumonectomy

Having verified that pneumonectomy is appropriate and feasible, the pulmonary ligament and the pleural reflection posterior to the hilum are incised. Vagal branches and bronchial arteries are divided peripheral to clips, and the major hilar structures cleared of surrounding connective tissue. It is helpful to divide the lower vein first as this improves mobility at the hilum, making it easier to orientate the structures for dissection and division. The main bronchus is then encircled with a sling and cleared of associated lymphatics. The subcarinal glands are block dissected or sampled as desired; the bronchus is then divided, taking care to ensure that clips placed on bronchial arteries do not come between the jaws of the stapler. The upper vein is divided and finally the main artery. It is imperative that the main artery is clamped centrally prior to division. A GIA staple is used to

section the artery peripheral to the clamp (Fig. 11.13a) and the closure line inspected prior to releasing the clamp (Fig. 11.13b).

About 5 cm of clear pulmonary artery are required to place the proximal clamp and endostapler safely. This can be difficult to achieve and it can be helpful to divide one or two early branches so as to create extra length before attempting to divide the pulmonary artery.

If the tumour does not allow an adequate length of extrapericardial vein for safe division, it is relatively simple to open the pericardium and divide the vessel at the intrapericardial level as would be performed at an open procedure (Fig. 11.14).

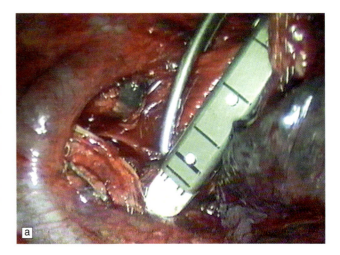

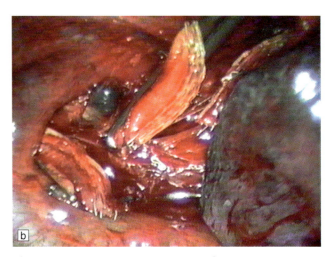

Figure 11.13 *(a) Operative photograph of right pulmonary artery with vascular clamp applied prior to division. (b) Operative photograph of clamped right pulmonary artery after stapler division of the vessel.*

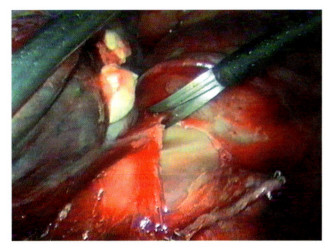

Figure 11.14 *Endoscopic intrapericardial dissection around the right upper pulmonary vein.*

When the lung has been removed mediastinal nodes can be dissected or sampled as preferred prior to testing the bronchus stump and ensuring haemostasis.

Closure is carried out in the same manner as after lobectomy.

Perioperative complications

The most significant potential perioperative complication during VATS pulmonary resection is major bleeding. This may result from inadvertent injury to a vessel or from failure of a stapling device used to divide and seal the vessel. Preparation for this event is the first line of management and should include the presence of an open thoracotomy tray at the operating table with a selection of vascular clamps, and a surgeon who is trained in general open thoracic surgery.[29]

If significant bleeding does occur, there are several immediate strategies available to control bleeding whilst the chest is opened:

- A swab mounted on sponge-holding forceps can be rapidly inserted through the submammary incision to compress the bleeding point. An assistant can then continue to apply pressure.
- It is sensible to open the jaws of a stapling device slowly and, if bleeding appears to be present, the jaws may be reclosed thereby controlling the bleeding.
- An obvious bleeding vessel of reasonable length can be clamped by passing a vascular clamp through the submammary incision. It is important, however, to beware of tearing an artery further.

Laceration of a bronchus may occur during dissection and occasionally there is inadequate closure of bronchial staples. The surgeon must then choose between several options. Application of a stapler to divide the bronchus may control a laceration but there is also the possibility of inserting an endoscopic suture. Failure of all or part of the staple line is best dealt with by restapling the bronchus, provided that adequate length is available. It may be helpful to place traction sutures at either end of the bronchus closure line to elevate the stump and facilitate the application of further staples or interrupted sutures. If the stapler failure is likely to be due to a thick bronchus, a roticulating stapler (as used in an open operation) may be employed since these are usually more robust than the endostapling devices.

Rarely, bleeding from one of the ports may be troublesome. In this instance the thoracoscope should be inserted through the port which provides the best view of the bleeding point and cautery or externally-placed sutures used to secure haemostasis. The cautery must be applied sparingly at port sites; excessive use can result in intercostal nerve damage.

Alternative techniques

Simultaneously stapled lobectomy

The simultaneously stapled (SS) lobectomy is a procedure devised by Lewis and associates[6,15,24] who utilise a single 60 mm conventional open stapler to close all the lobar hilar structure in one action. Their technique has evolved with time and this account is based on several of their descriptions. As with the endoscopic hilar dissection technique, visualisation is achieved entirely endoscopically and rib retraction is not used.

Positioning and access
Double lumen endobronchial intubation is used. The patient is placed in the lateral decubitus position and the table is arched so as to spread the interspaces. This process is augmented by placing an inflatable bag beneath the patient. Access is gained using four incisions (Fig. 11.15) in a 'grid iron' configuration. Two 2 cm incisions are made: one in the 6th or 7th intercostal space in the mid-axillary line for the thoracoscope (10 mm 0°), and one in the 4th intercostal space in the posterior axillary line for insertion of small

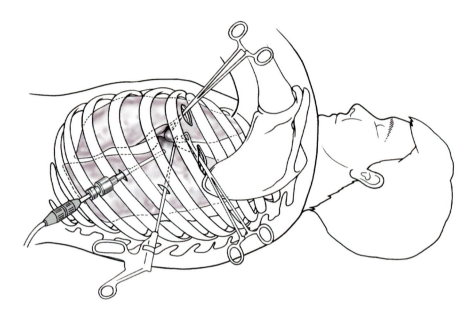

Figure 11.15 *The incisions used during SS lobectomy.*

instruments. A 5 cm access incision is created in the 3rd or 4th intercostal space in the anterior axillary line for larger instruments, digital palpation and delivery of the specimen.

Elements of technique

The mediastinal node stations are first explored and sampled and the hilar area then skeletonised with excision of hilar level nodes. The fissures relating to the lobe to be resected are separated by blunt dissection, cautery including an argon beam coagulator and linear endoscopic staplers (Ethicon: ELC35). The bronchus and vessels of the designated lobe are partially exposed and a rubber catheter is passed round the lobar pedicle and used to guide the lower jaw of a linear stapler (Ethicon: TL60) around the pedicle, which is secured by placing two double staple lines separated by 2 mm (Fig. 11.16). The degree of staple compression is varied to

Figure 11.16 *Mass hilar stapling as described by Dr Lewis.*

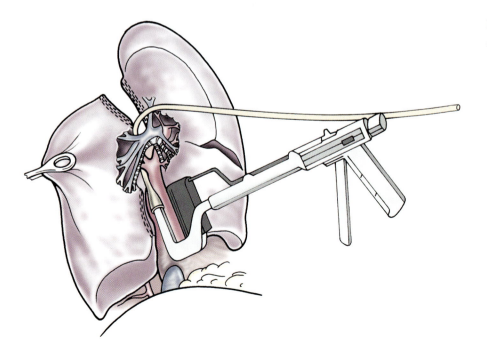

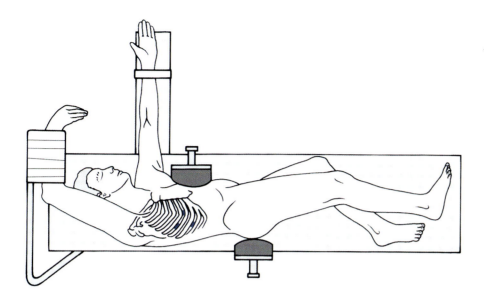

Figure 11.17 *Patient positioning for a mini-thoracotomy VATS lobectomy.*

produce a leg length of 1.5–2.5 mm (depending upon the thickness of the hilar structures). The lobe is then amputated and placed within a plastic bag. Having placed the specimen in the bag, large tumours are sectioned to facilitate delivery prior to delivery through the access incision. A single silastic 20 FG chest drain is inserted through a separate stab incision at the end of the procedure.

Video-assisted mini-thoracotomy

This technique utilises a mini-thoracotomy as the primary route for both visualisation and access. The concept, validation and documentation of this approach has largely been carried out by Giudicelli[8,13] from whose accounts this resumé is derived. This form of VATS resection has been described by other authors, notably Naruke.[25]

Positioning and access
The patient is placed in the lateral decubitus position and double lumen endobronchial intubation is required. The upper arm is suspended on a crossbar in order to expose the anterolateral chest (Fig. 11.17).

Elements of technique
The thoracoscope (10 mm 0°) is inserted through the 5th or 6th intercostal space in the anterior axillary line and a 10 cm intercostal incision is made in the mid-axillary line in the 5th interspace and opened with a small purpose-designed rib retractor (Karl Storz). The retractor is opened

to provide a 4 cm x 4 cm access opening. A standard lobectomy is then performed through this mini-thoracotomy incision using some specialised instruments (Karl Storz), particularly retractors, but predominantly normal instruments, ligatures and staplers. The bronchus is closed with a standard open surgical stapler (Autosuture; TA30). The specimen is delivered using a plastic sleeve to protect the wound. A full hilar and mediastinal lymph node dissection is performed. Visualisation is mainly obtained directly through the mini-thoracotomy and is necessarily restricted, but the view is supplemented by the videothoracoscope which also provides illumination of the operative field. At the end of the procedure, apical and basal chest drains are placed.

Results of VATS major pulmonary resection

The outcome of VATS pulmonary surgery in general has been reviewed in detail elsewhere.[37] Experience with VATS major pulmonary resection specifically is somewhat limited. To date, a reasonable estimate would suggest 2500 lobectomy cases have been performed worldwide but these are spread through many different units. Experience with VATS pneumonectomy is considerably less, and it is probable that under 100 pneumonectomy procedures have been performed thus far, which is not sufficient to allow statistically valid conclusions to be drawn. At this stage,

151

therefore, VATS pneumonectomy is best regarded as a procedure under evaluation.

The available published data can usefully be interpreted under several headings.

Pain

The most obvious potential benefit of VATS major pulmonary resection is the opportunity to reduce post-operative pain. Despite this, remarkably few authors have attempted to quantify their results with postoperative pain. Most have simply stated that, in their experience, post-operative pain was reduced, without justifying that assertion. Giudicelli[13] found a VATS approach to be associated with a significant (p < 0.006) reduction in post-operative pain at <1 week following surgery, in a non-randomised comparison between 44 mini-thoracotomy VATS cases and 23 open muscle-sparing thoracotomy cases. In the author's experience[18] (Table 11.4) comparison between 70 VATS lobectomy cases and a parallel audit group of 110 open standard thoracotomy lobectomy cases showed VATS lobectomy to be associated with a significant reduction in morphine consumption (p < 0.001). Also, in the VATS cases, there was a significant reduction in the need for post-

operative intercostal nerve blocks, and a significant increase in the number of recorded sleep episodes whilst the patient was in the HDU. Pain control in these patients was provided by intravenous morphine administered via a patient-controlled analgesia system. The only prospective randomised study reported to date[14] did not, remarkably, choose to look at in-hospital pain.

The issue of comparative levels of late pain between open and VATS surgery has been addressed by Landreneau and colleagues.[38] He utilised a questionnaire-based study to compare 165 patients undergoing a lateral thoracotomy (mostly muscle-sparing) with 178 patients who had undergone a VATS procedure. The majority of the VATS procedures were actually pulmonary wedge resections, but the study is relevant in that it confirmed a reduction in the perceived magnitude of pain in the VATS group for up to a year after surgery.

In a recent review of 83 VATS major pulmonary resections[18] the author has noted transient discomfort related to port sites at early postoperative review clinics in many VATS cases. This usually abates over several weeks. Only one patient has had persisting neuralgic symptoms sufficient to require specific drug therapy (although not

Table 11.4

Comparison between VATS and open thoracotomy lobectomy resection cases

	Open (n = 110)	VATS (n = 70)	P
Average age (years)	60.6	62.4	n.s.
Morphine usage*			
Total (mg)	83 (20–174)	57 (7–191)	<0.001
Rate (mg/hour)	2 (0.6–4.4)	1.5 (0.4–4.3)	<0.001
Extra (i.m. injections)*	2 (0–8)	1 (0–6)	<0.05
Intercostal nerve blocks (No./patient)*	0 (0–3)	0 (0–1)	<0.05
Sleep episodes (No./patient)*	1 (0–6)	2 (0–7)	<0.05

*Median values (ranges are given in parentheses).

Reproduced from *International Surgery* 1996: 81: 255–8.

sufficient to prevent him from crewing a transatlantic yacht!). This represents a possible incidence of 1.2% for late thoracotomy pain with VATS resection, and is comparable with that reported by McKenna[11] who described one patient with a late pain syndrome out of 45 VATS major resections (2.2%). These figures may be contrasted with the much greater incidence of persisting late pain (25+%) following open thoracotomy.[4]

Postoperative pain, both immediate and for up to a year after surgery is, therefore, definitely reduced with a VATS approach. Although the incidence of post-thoracotomy pain was thereafter reported by Landreneau and colleagues to be similar between VATS and open thoracotomy, the severity and need for treatment may not be as great with VATS surgery. It would seem likely also that technological advances leading to narrower stapler, instrument and telescope shafts, and the effects of improved VATS operative technique, may lead to a further reduction in intercostal nerve injury with a concomitant improvement in the results of VATS surgery.

Other morbidity

Giudicelli[13] in his comparison between muscle-sparing thoracotomy and his mini-thoracotomy VATS technique, reported that pain-related pulmonary complications were reduced in the VATS group (13.6% versus 21%) although this difference failed to achieve statistical significance. He was unable to demonstrate any difference in postoperative pulmonary function between the two groups; but it may be argued that this data is not representative of the possible benefit of a VATS approach as his technique requires the use of a rib retractor. Certainly, Waller,[39] in a randomised prospective study of patients undergoing VATS pleurectomy which was performed without rib spreading, found a significantly lesser reduction in FEV$_1$ (forced expiratory volume in one second) after a VATS approach than with an open approach.

Kirkby and colleagues[14] in their prospective study compared 30 patients undergoing standard lobectomy through a muscle-sparing thoracotomy with 25 patients undergoing VATS lobectomy by a hilar dissection type technique. They reported significantly less (p < 0.05) post-operative complications in the VATS group (six versus 16) than in the muscle sparing thoracotomy group. The author's experience would support the view that sputum retention

and pneumonia are relatively less frequent with VATS resection than with open resection. To date, the author has transferred three of 130 (2.3%) VATS major pulmonary resections to an ICU for observation, but ventilation was not required.

The incidence of cardiac dysrhythmia, principally atrial fibrillation, seems little different with either method of resection at 5–6%.[18]

Operative safety and peri-operative mortality

To date, only one intra-operative death occurring during a VATS major pulmonary resection has been described.[35] This was revealed in a survey of 1560 cases undertaken in 20 centres across the world and was due to myocardial infarction rather than operative mishap. Regardless of the operative approach used, however, the possibility of a major vascular accident occurring during a VATS major pulmonary resection is always present and requires a state of constant vigilance. The author advocates the use of centrally-placed vascular clamps prior to division of the pulmonary veins and the main or stem pulmonary arteries. Pre-planned strategies and routines must be in place to cope with the eventuality of a major bleed. It is obligatory that this form of surgery is only undertaken by surgeons and supporting teams with specific training in open thoracic surgery.[36]

None of the published accounts of endoscopic dissection[6,9–11,13,14] or the SS lobectomy technique[8,13,25] have reported an in-hospital mortality. Giudicelli[13] described a postoperative mortality of three out of 44 mini-thoracotomy technique cases (6.8%) but these were due to myocardial failure in two instances and a cytomegalovirus pneumonia in the third. In the author's continued experience,[20] currently totalling 150 VATS lobectomy cases, one postoperative in-patient death has occurred, due to a pulmonary embolism in a patient with a history of repeated emboli. Two further deaths have occurred after discharge and within 30 days. These deaths were from adrenal failure and pulmonary embolism, respectively. These results equate to an in-patient mortality of 1.3% and an overall 30-day mortality of 2%. It is not clear from the literature what the 30-day out-of-hospital death rate is for the other published series.

Overall, it would appear that VATS pulmonary resection is at least as safe as conventional open surgery.

Cost

Cost comparison between VATS and open major pulmonary resection is extremely difficult. This issue is complicated by several factors:

- Clinical practice differs greatly between the US where there are financial imperatives driving early discharge and Europe where there are often social considerations preventing it.
- Concentration on hospital costs may lead to inaccurate conclusions. Early discharge, for example, may simply represent transfer of cost from the surgical unit to a different stage in the health care chain.
- A method has not yet been determined to quantify the financial value of reduced pain and distress and earlier return to a good quality of life. These benefits cannot be offset against any increase in immediate cost associated with a new procedure.

In the author's experience, using the endoscopic hilar dissection technique, procedural costs are increased by about £1000–1200 in a VATS major pulmonary resection. Approximately 50% of this cost is spent on division of incomplete fissures by endostaplers. Operative time is increased by an average of about 60 minutes. Against this, the requirement for HDU care is reduced by about 16 hours, postoperative mobility is improved and discharge occurs about two days earlier than usual — typically on the fourth or fifth postoperative day. While it is difficult to cost the effects of these savings (48 hours of low-dependency care and 16 hours of high-dependency care), it would seem probable that the financial balance is neutral.

Giudicelli[13] identifies an additional 23 minutes of operating time for his mini-thoracotomy VATS approach but no additional disposables costs as endoscopic staplers were not used. This technique would appear inexpensive. The mean in-patient stay on the other hand for his VATS cases was 12 days, with a mean duration of chest tube drainage of eight days, suggesting that considerable in-patient time savings might have accrued from increasing his disposables spend in order to staple the fissures with endoscopic staplers at the time of the dissection. The procedure costs would have risen to nearer that of the endoscopic hilar dissection technique but much earlier discharge — surely a major potential benefits of a VATS approach — would have been possible.

Lewis and colleagues[40] compared their costs in detail for 15 patients undergoing standard open lobectomy (8) or

pneumonectomy (7), and 15 patients undergoing lobectomy (14) or pneumonectomy (1) using the SIS lobectomy technique. Remarkably, this detailed review of costs found that the VATS procedure was much less expensive, at an average cost of $8,660 compared with an average open procedure cost of $17,484. Length of stay was 3.3 days for the VATS cases and nine days for open cases while room and board charges were correspondingly less in the VATS group, producing a saving of $1,246. Open cases were routinely sent to an ICU whereas VATS cases were returned to 'floor' care thus producing an immediate saving of $4,800. Operating room costs and medical supplies costs were both slightly lower in the VATS group. This study is difficult to interpret for several reasons. Firstly, the groups are clearly not comparable with regard to the operations performed. Secondly, it must be open to debate whether open thoracotomy cases did really require ICU care. High dependency level care is accepted practice for open cases in the UK, at least. Thirdly, the author describes[15] the use of endostaplers to divide the fissures so it is difficult to understand why the disposable costs were actually less in the VATS group. Finally, it is not clear whether the patients undergoing early discharge do so to a zero-cost environment or whether they are transferred to hotel care or the supervision of a secondary health care provider. Despite these observations, it would seem that VATS SS lobectomy is definitely no more expensive than an open resection, has potential cost benefits and is associated with a major reduction in in-patient stay.

It is, unfortunately, difficult to view the whole cost of a patient's condition and treatment as the costs are often spread between different agencies, some are born by the patient and still more have not yet been assessed. Others which are intangibles such as distress, anxiety and pain may never truly be taken into account. It is, therefore, artificial to concentrate on in-patient costs when comparing procedures but there can be no doubt that hospital procedure cost is of the greatest importance in determining the likely uptake of any surgical procedure, simply because the healthcare purchaser will not wish to accept a higher total procedural cost. Operative disposables costs are certainly increased by the use of endostaplers, as is most evident with the endoscopic hilar dissection technique. Less advanced care requirements and shortened in-patient stay do, however, produce offsetting savings, as must reduced early and late clinic attendance and drug costs. The overall cost impact of VATS major pulmonary resection within the hospital setting is either neutral, as with total endoscopic hilar dissection, or favourable to the VATS procedure, as with the simultaneously stapled and mini-thoracotomy techniques. Viewed from a broader perspective which includes personal and social factors not usually considered, such as reduced pain, distress and earlier return to productive good quality life, VATS is likely to be cheaper than conventional surgery.

Physiological response to surgery

Surgery can have profound and often negative effects on cytokines and the immune system.[4,41] Comparative studies of laparoscopic versus open surgery have demonstrated that minimal access surgery is associated with reduced levels of stress hormones, C-reactive protein and interleukin-6[42,43] and less depression of the immune response based on T-cell proliferation 40 and neutrophil hypochlorous acid production.[45] These studies are of physiological interest but have been undertaken on relatively fit patients undergoing a modest surgical intervention (cholecystectomy) rather than major cancer resection.

Very little information is available regarding the comparative effects of VATS or open thoracotomy on stress response and immune function, despite the potential importance of this issue given that most patients undergo major pulmonary resection for malignant disease. The author has compared stress response and immune function in a randomised prospective study of VATS endoscopic hilar dissection lobectomy versus open lobectomy via a limited lateral thoracotomy. The data is currently in analysis but preliminary results confirm the VATS approach to be associated with a reduced stress response, as judged by decreased post-surgical C-reactive protein (Fig. 11.18) and interleukin-6[46] levels, and enhanced post-surgical cellular immune function with better preservation of neutrophil and monocyte function.[47]

Oncological validity of VATS major pulmonary resection for cancer

Most major pulmonary resections are undertaken for malignant disease. In this situation a VATS approach must provide equally effective management of malignant disease compared with open resection. Immunological considerations and the fact that tissue handling is necessarily

much reduced might suggest further potential advantages to a VATS resection but for present purposes this question may be judged by three issues:

● operative management of mediastinal lymph nodes
● long-term survival
● pattern of recurrent disease.

Operative management of mediastinal lymph nodes

Mediastinal nodes may be managed by sampling or 'radical' lymphadenectomy. While some surgeons believe that mediastinal lymph node block dissection is potentially curative, others would argue that excision of all mediastinal nodes serves only to increase the accuracy of surgical assessment of the extent of the cancer. Thus it is a matter of debate whether the advanced survival for early stage lung cancers reported by those groups performing adenectomy is any more than simply the result of accurate definition of the stage of the cancer — the so-called 'staging effect'.

The adequacy of the total lymph node harvest during endoscopic hilar dissection VATS lobectomy with mediastinal dissection has been studied by McKenna[11] who reported a yield of up to 26 nodes (range 15–26). Kirkby and colleagues[14] in their prospective randomised comparison between hilar dissection VATS and open lobectomy, both with mediastinal sampling, found equivalent sample rates (nine nodal sites) with either technique. Lewis and colleagues have described sampling as his technique for

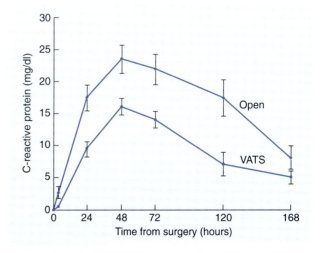

Figure 11.18 *C-reactive protein levels post open and VATS lobectomy.*

SS lobectomy[24] with a sample rate of 7–18 nodes. Other authors have described full gland dissection with the endoscopic hilar dissection approach[5,7,17] or the mini-thoracotomy approach.[8,13] The author practices a hybrid solution. VATS resection is selected on the basis of a negative CT and, in every case, negative mediastinoscopy. Hilar level clearance is carried out and then mediastinal gland sampling performed unless large mediastinal nodes are encountered when a mediastinal dissection is performed.

Long-term survival

Most surgical teams have deliberately selected presumed Stage I (T1 or 2, N0) or early Stage II (T1 or 2, N1) lesions for a VATS approach. As with other aspects of VATS surgery for major pulmonary resection, published information is limited and, given the very small number of pneumonectomies performed, is essentially restricted to lobectomy cases. Kirkby and colleagues[14] reported on early follow-up at a mean of 13 months. One patient in their entire randomized study had developed recurrent disease and had died at 15 months. Lewis,[24] in the most recent update of his experience, describes 90 patients with primary lung cancer (40 Stage I, 45 Stage II, two stage IIIa and three Stage IV). Follow-up averaged 26.5 months with six lung cancer deaths at between six and 18 months post-operatively. Four of these patients were node negative. Naruke,[25] using his variation of Giudicelli's mini-thoracotomy technique, describes 46 patients (43 stage I, one Stage II and two Stage III) with predominantly mediastinal node sampling and modest follow-up ranging between six and 36 months. In this group of patients, he has had no recurrence with Stage I disease and a 95% survival for the group as a whole. The absolute recurrence rate is unclear.

The author reported one bronchogenic carcinoma-related death amongst 49 patients with non-small cell lung cancer (NSCLC) at mean follow-up of 16.5 months.[18] More recent experience demonstrates three lung cancer related deaths at nine, 17 and 37 months post-operatively, occurring among 72 Stage I NSCLC patients. Average follow-up was 27 months, extending to a maximum of 58 months. This represented an at-risk period of 1914 patient months and a predicted survival free of cancer-related death for Stage I of 89.7% at 4.5 years. This figure may be compared with the 80% and 63% survivals at five years for T1N0 and T2N0

NSCLC patients, respectively, reported by Williams and colleagues.[48]

Patterns of recurrent disease

Inadequate local clearance might logically be expected to result in a high rate of local recurrence. Lewis[24] does not report how many of his patients were alive with recurrence but does comment that each of the dead patients had first presented with distant metastases. In addition to the three dead patients in the author's Stage I group, there is one other patient with recurrent disease, and all four patients had systemic metastatic recurrence. VATS lobectomy was performed on 16 other NSCLC patients (nine had Stage II and seven Stage III). Recurrent disease has occurred in seven of these: systemic in five and local in two (one N1, the other N2). Thus in the entire NSCLC series of 88 patients, 10 have had recurrent disease which has been local in only two cases (22.2%).

As with open surgery, therefore, either lymph node sampling or block dissection can be performed. The final choice is, as it should be, a matter of surgical preference (Table 11.5) rather than a function of whether or not a VATS approach is used. The available evidence supports the view that survival after VATS lobectomy is at least equal to that achieved with open surgery and that the pattern of recurrent disease after VATS resection does not suggest inadequate local clearance.

Summary

VATS major pulmonary resection is safe, associated with reduced postoperative pain and should not compromise the standard surgical principles governing the resection of malignant disease. It provides an opportunity for pre-resectional inspection of the thoracic cavity, which can extend surgery to poorer risk patients and can help to reduce the open and closed thoracotomy rate. Although the procedure may be more expensive, the overall cost of care is probably unchanged or even reduced due to quicker discharge, better post-surgical condition and reduced late pain. There are potential benefits to immune function which may be important in cancer patients. Long-term survival and patterns of bronchogenic carcinoma recurrence suggest that this form of resection is at least equally as effective as a conventional open thoracotomy approach.

Surgeon	Technique	Experience	Mediastinoscopy	Op. node strategy
Gossot (France)	EHD	53	–	Sampling
Giudicelli (France)	MT	70	–	Radical dissection
Hazelrigg (USA)	EHD	43	–	Sampling
Iwasaki (Japan)	MT	128	–	Radical dissection
Lewis (USA)	SS	231	–	Sampling
Loscertales (Spain)	EHD	51	–	Radical dissection
Mackinlay (Argentina)	MT	67	–	Radical dissection
McKenna (USA)	EHD	170	–	Radical dissection
Naruke (Japan)	MT	45	–	Radical dissection
Roviaro (Italy)	EHD	147	–	Radical dissection
Sayer (UK)	EHD	63	Routine	Sampling
Stamatis (Germany)	EHD	40	Routine	Radical dissection
Walker (UK)	EHD	135	Routine	Sampling (rarely, dissection)
Yim (Hong Kong)	MT	76	Occasional	Sampling

Table 11.5

Management of mediastinal lymph nodes during VATS lobectomy among centres with operative experience >20 cases

MT = minithoracotomy; EHD = endoscopic hilar dissection; SS = simultaneously stapled.
(With grateful thanks to Dr Thomas Mackinlay for permission to quote aspects of data gathered from American and Asian surgeons and presented at the IV International Symposium on Thoracoscopy and Video-Assisted Thoracic Surgery, Sao Paulo, Brazil, May 1997).

Major pulmonary resection by VATS — safe practice points

- Do not embark on this form of surgery without a trained thoracic surgical team:
  - experienced thoracic surgeon (endoscopic and open surgical skills, extended knowledge of pulmonary resection)
  - anaesthetic support (double lumen endobronchial intubation)
  - alert and fully trained nursing team (awareness of endoscopic surgery, response to emergency conversion).

- Select early clinical Stage I NSCLC lesions or benign disease
- Exclude patients with obvious adhesions
- Ensure that a full thoracotomy tray is open by the operating table at the time of surgery
- Ensure that a large venous catheter is placed in case of intraoperative haemorrhage
- Define the location of lesion
- Obtain proximal control of large vessels prior to division
- Deliver the operative specimen inside a plastic bag
- Convert to open thoracotomy if the anatomy is obscure or the operative situation is difficult.

References

1 Conacher ID. Pain relief after thoracotomy. *Br J Anaesth* 1990; **65**: 806–12.

2 Hazelrigg SR, Landreneau RJ, Boley TM *et al*. The effect of muscle-sparing versus standard posterolateral thoracotomy on pulmonary function, muscle strength and post-operative pain. *J Thorac Cardiovasc Surg* 1991; **101**: 394–401.

3 Leaver HA, Craig SR, Yap PL, Williams JR, Walker WS. Arachidonic acid metabolism and activation of monocyte and neutrophil reactive oxygen in lung cancer patients undergoing pulmonary resection. *Biologicals* 1997: in press.

4 Dajczman E, Gordon A, Kreisman H, Wolkove N. Long term post thoracotomy pain. *Chest* 1991; **99**: 270–4.

5 Roviaro GC, Rebuffat C, Varoli F *et al*. Videoendoscopic pulmonary lobectomy for cancer. *Surg Laparosc Endosc* 1992; **2**: 244–7.

6 Lewis RJ, Sisler GE, Caccavale RJ. Imaged thoracic lobectomy: should it be done? *Ann Thorac Surg* 1992; **54**: 80–3.

7 Roviaro GC, Varoli F, Rebuffat C *et al*. Major pulmonary resections: pneumonectomies and lobectomies. *Ann Thorac Surg* 1993; **56**: 779–83.

8 Giudicelli R, Thomas P, Lonjon T *et al*. Major pulmonary resection by video-assisted minithoracotomy. *Eur J Cardiothorac Surg* 1994; **8**: 254–8.

9 Kirkby TJ, Mack MJ, Landreneau RJ, Rice TW. Initial experience with video-assisted thoracoscopic lobectomy. *Ann Thorac Surg* 1993; **56**: 1248–53.

10 Walker WS, Carnochan FM, Pugh GC. Thoracoscopic pulmonary lobectomy: early operative experience and preliminary clinical results. *J Thorac Cardiovasc Surg* 1993; **106**: 111–17.

11 McKenna RJ. Lobectomy by video-assisted thoracic surgery with mediastinal node sampling *J Thorac Cardiovasc Surg* 1994; **107**: 879–82.

12 Walker WS, Carnochan FM, Mattar S. Video-assisted thoracoscopic pneumonectomy. *Br J Surg* 1994; **81**: 81–2.

13 Giudicelli R, Thomas P, Lonjon T *et al*. Video-assisted minthoracotomy versus muscle sparing thoracotomy for preforming lobectomy. *Ann Thorac Surg* 1994; **58**: 712–18.

14 Kirkby TJ, Mack MJ, Landreneau RJ *et al*. Lobectomy — video-assisted thoracic surgery versus muscle-sparing thoracotomy. A randomized trial. *J Thorac Cardiovasc Surg* 1995; **109**: 997–1002.

15 Lewis RJ. Simultaneously stapled lobectomy: a safe technique for video-assisted thoracic surgery. *J Thorac Cardiovasc Surg* 1995; **109**: 619–25.

16 Lewis RJ, Caccavale RJ, Sisler GE *et al*. VATS-SS Lobectomy: A kinder, gentler, more cost-effective lobectomy? *Chest* 1995; **108**(Suppl): 143S (abstr).

17 Roviaro G, Varoli F, Rebuffat C *et al*. Videothoracoscopic staging and treatment of lung cancer. *Ann Thorac Surg* 1995; **59**: 971–4.

18 Walker WS, Pugh GC, Craig SR, Carnochan FM. Continued experience with thoracoscopic major pulmonary resection. *Int Surg* 1996; **81**: 255–8.

19 Walker WS. Video-assisted thoracic surgery: pulmonary lobectomy. *Semin Laparosc Surg* 1996; **3**: 233–44.

20 Walker WS. Video-assisted thoracic surgery (VATS) lobectomy: the Edinburgh experience. *Seminars in Thoracic and Cardiovascular Surgery* 1998; **10**: 291–299.

21 Yim APC, Liv H-P. Thoracoscopic major lung resection-indications, technique and early results: experience from two centres in Asia. *Surgical Laparoscopy and Endoscopy* 1997; **7**: 241–4.

22 Craig SR, Walker WS. Initial experience of video-assisted thoracoscopic pneumonectomy. *Thorax* 1995; **50**: 392–5.

23 Kerr KM, Lamb D, Wathen CG, Walker WS, Douglas NJ. Pathological assessment of mediastinal lymph nodes in lung cancer: implications for non-invasive mediastinal staging. *Thorax* 1992; **47**: 337–41.

24 Lewis RJ, Caccavale RJ, Sisler GE, Bocage J-P, Mackenzie JW. 100 video assisted thoracic surgical non-rib spread simultaneously stapled lobectomies. *Ann Thorac Surg*: in press.

25 Naruke T. Thoracoscopic surgery for small, non small-cell lung cancer. Is video-assisted lobectomy an adequate treatment? *Journal de Pneumologia* 23: **S17**, 1997 (abstr.).

26 Leaver HA, Craig SR, Yap PL *et al*. Phagocyte activation after minimally invasive and conventional pulmonary lobectomy. *Eur J Clin Invest* 1996; **26**: Suppl.1. A37, 210 (abst).

27 Lenglinger FX, Schwartz CD, Artmann W. Localization of pulmonary nodules before thoracoscopic surgery: value of percutaneous staining with methylene blue. *Am J Roentgenol* 1994; **163**: 297–300.

28 Mack MJ, Shennib H, Landreneau RJ, Hazelrigg SR. Techniques for localization of pulmonary nodules for thoracoscopic resection. *J Thorac Cardiovasc Surg* 1993; **106**: 550–3.

29 Shaw RM, Spirn PW, Salazar AM *et al*. Localization of peripheral pulmonary nodules for thoracoscopic excision: value of CT-guided wire placement. *Am J Roentgenol* 1993; **161**: 279–83.

30 Shennib H, Bret P. Intraoperative transthoracic ultrasonographic localization of occult lung lesions. *Ann Thorac Surg* 1993; **55**: 767–9.

31 Fry WA, Siddiqui A, Pensler JM *et al*. Thoracoscopic implantation of cancer with a fatal outcome. *Ann Thorac Surg* 1995; **59**: 542–9.

32 Craig SR, Walker WS. Potential complications of vascular stapling in thoracoscopic surgery. *Ann Thorac Surg* 1995; **59**: 736–8.

33 Shields TW. Surgical anatomy of the lungs. In: Shields TW, ed. *General Thoracic Surgery*. 3rd Edition. Philadelphia, London: Lea & Febiger, 1989: pp 62–7.

34 Cooper JD. Technique to reduce air leaks after resection of emphysematous lung. *Ann Thorac Surg* 1994; **57**: 1038–9.

35 Mackinlay TA. 'VATS lobectomy: an international survey'. Presented at the IVth International Symposium on Thoracoscopy and Video-Assisted Thoracic Surgery, Sao Paulo, May 1997.

36 Statement of the AATS/STS Joint Committee on Thoracoscopy and Video Assisted Thoracic Surgery. *J Thorac Cardiovasc Surg* 1992; **104**: 1.

37 Walker WS, Craig SR. Video-assisted thoracoscopic pulmonary surgery: current status and potential evolution. *Eur J Cardiothorac Surg* 1996; **10**: 161–7.

38 Landreneau RJ, Mack MJ, Hazelrigg SR *et al.* Prevalence of chronic pain after pulmonary resection by thoracotomy or video-assisted thoracic surgery. *J Thorac Cardiovasc Surg* 1995; **107**: 1079–86.

39 Waller DA, Forty J, Morrit G. Video-assisted thoracoscopic surgery versus thoracotomy for spontaneous pneumothorax. *Ann Thorac Surg* 1994; **58**: 372–7.

40 Lewis RJ, Caccavale RJ, Sisler GE *et al.* Is video-assisted thoracic surgery cost effective? *New Jersey Medicine* 1996; **93**: 35–41.

41 Salo M. Effects of anaesthesia and surgery on the immune response. *Acta Anaes Scand* 1992; **36**: 201–20.

42 Mealy K, Gallagher H, Barry M *et al.* Physiological and metabolic responses to open and laparoscopic cholecystectomy. *Br J Surg* 1992; **79**: 1061–4.

43 Roumen RM, Meurs PA, Kuypers H, Kraak WA, Sauerwein RW. Serum interleukin-6 and C-reactive protein responses in patients after laparoscopic or conventional cholecystectomy. *Eur J Surg* 1992; **158**: 541–4.

44 Grifith J, Everitt N, Curley P, McMahon M. Laparoscopic versus 'open' cholecystectomy: reduced influence upon immune function and the acute phase response. *Surg Endosc* 1993; **7**: 123 (abstr).

45 Carey PD, Wakefield CH, Thayeb A *et al.* Effects of minimally invasive surgery on hypochlorous acid production by neutrophils. *Br J Surg* 1994; **81**: 557–60.

46 SR Craig, WS Walker. Unpublished data: in preparation for submission.

47 Leaver HA, Craig SR, Yap PL, Walker WS. Phagocyte activation after minimally invasive and conventional pulmonary lobectomy. *Eur J Clin Invest* 1996; **26**(Suppl.1): 210 (abstr).

48 Williams DE, Pairolero PC, Davis CS *et al.* Survival of patients surgically treated for Stage I lung cancer. *J Thorac Cardiovasc Surg* 1981; **82**: 70–6.

Endoscopic oesophageal myotomy

A. Cuschieri

12

Introduction

Despite alternative management options, myotomy remains the definitive treatment for specific oesophageal motility disorders. Until fairly recently, surgical myotomy had one significant disadvantage, i.e. it entailed a major surgical intervention: laparotomy or posterolateral thoracotomy. Largely for this reason, and despite unequivocal evidence from prospective randomised studies of the long-term superiority of myotomy in terms of relief of dysphagia and return of propulsive oesophageal contractions over balloon dilatation,[1,2] most gastroenterologists favoured the much less invasive balloon dilatation as the first line treatment.[3–5] Surgical myotomy was reserved for failures after dilatation.

The advent of minimal access surgery (MAS) and, in particular, of endoscopic myotomy[6–16] has changed the situation. The MAS approach, laparoscopic or thoracoscopic, is particularly suited to functional operations such as myotomy where the ratio of procedure-related trauma to access trauma is low so that the major traumatic insult to the patient is the thoracotomy or laparotomy needed to access the relevant segments of the oesophagus.[17] There is now sufficient reported experience from a variety of centres worldwide[6–16] to establish the safety and efficacy of endoscopic myotomy with evidence of clear benefit to patients over the conventional open surgical approach. These benefits include enhanced patient acceptability, diminished disruption of the normal oesophageal attachments, reduced hospital stay and a drastic curtailment of the period of short-term disability with early return to full activity and work. There are, however, a number of unresolved surgical issues, including the optimal endoscopic approach and the need for an antireflux component and its nature.

Oesophageal motility disorders and investigations

Oesophageal motility disorders may be primary or secondary to neurological or systemic disease, for example, pseudobulbar palsy, dermatomyositis and myasthenia gravis. Primary oesophageal motility disorders may affect the upper sphincter (defective oropharyngeal transfer), the body of the oesophagus (impaired propulsion) or the lower oesophageal sphincter (impaired relaxation or incompetence). In practice, it is customary to consider abnormalities within the body of the oesophagus and lower sphincter together, as abnormalities in these regions frequently coexist in the common specific motility disorders of the oesophagus and they have distinctive contrast radiological and manometric features. The manometric details of the common specific motility disorders of the body and/or the lower oesophageal sphincter are shown in Table 12.1. Myotomy is usually considered for achalasia and diffuse oesophageal spasm (DES) and much less commonly for Nutcracker oesophagus (symptomatic hypertensive oesophageal peristalsis).

Contrast radiological findings are important in achalasia and DES. In early achalasia, there is mild dilatation of the oesophagus and a contracted lower oesophageal high-pressure zone accounting for the classical 'bird beak' deformity (Fig. 12.1). With long-standing disease, increasing dilatation and lengthening ensues with the development of the sigmoid mega-oesophagus (Fig. 12.2). The contrast radiological appearance of DES is also often characteristic

Table 12.1

Manometric features of the specific oesophageal motility disorders

Disorder	Manometric features
Achalasia	Aperistalsis in oesophageal body Elevated LES pressure ($\geq$26 mmHg) Incomplete relaxation of the LES Increased intraoesophageal baseline pressure relative to gastric
Diffuse oesophageal spasm	Simultaneous non-peristaltic contractions Multiple peaks of increased amplitude and duration Spontaneous contractions Periods of normal peristalsis
Nutcracker oesophagus	Hypertensive peristaltic contractions ($\geq$180 mmHg in distal oesophagus) of increased duration (>5.5 s) Normal peristaltic sequence

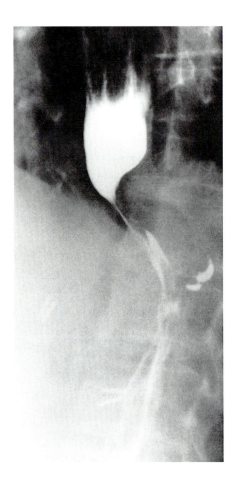

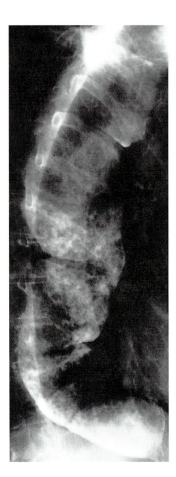

Figure 12.1 *(Left) Early achalasia: 'bird beak' deformity.*

Figure 12.2 *Late achalasia: sigmoid mega-oesophagus.*

with a typical 'corkscrew' appearance (Fig. 12.3). The oesophagogram of patients with Nutcracker disease is usually normal. It should be stressed that exclusive reliance on contrast radiology for the diagnosis of specific motility disorders of the oesophagus is unsafe since the radiological findings may be atypical and, more importantly, 'typical' radiological appearances may be encountered in organic disease including oesophageal cancer. Thus, upper gastrointestinal endoscopy is essential in the investigation of all patients with oesophageal symptoms. Radionuclide studies provide useful quantitative information on oesophageal transit. With the solid egg-white labelled bolus test[18,19] in addition to time–activity curves, the pattern of oesophageal transit in the various segments can be demonstrated by the row summation technique utilising an on-line computer. The normal total oesophageal transit time with this test is 8–10 seconds. It is elevated in all specific and non-specific motility disorders indicating that the radio-labelled egg-white bolus is a useful non-invasive screening test but cannot be regarded as a definitive or specific investigation.

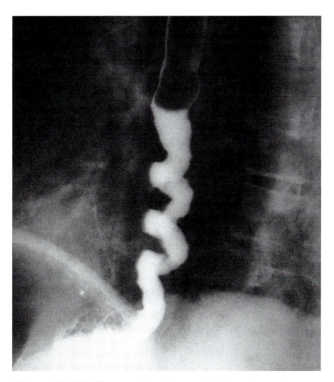

Figure 12.3 *Diffuse oesophageal spasm: 'corkscrew' oesophagus. (Reproduced with permisson from The Slide Atlas of Gastroenterology, London: Gower Medical Publishing)*

Symptoms necessitating treatment

The most common symptom is dysphagia. This may or may not be accompanied by retrosternal tightness amounting at times to episodes of severe non-cardiac chest pain which closely simulate anginal attacks. Other oesophageal symptoms include regurgitation, choking and aspiration. It is typical of the dysphagia to affect both solids and liquids and to vary in intensity with periods of remission. The trend is, however, towards deterioration with increasing difficulty in swallowing.

Dysphagia is the symptom that responds best to myotomy, although in the author's experience palliation of non-cardiac chest pain can be achieved in patients with DES and Nutcracker oesophagus.

Treatment options

Conservative management

Medical therapy for the relief of dysphagia and non-cardiac chest pain by antispasmodics including calcium-blocking agents is rarely successful except as a short-term measure whilst waiting for definitive treatment. Recently, endoscopic injection of botulinum toxin has been shown to be effective in the relief of dysphagia caused by achalasia[20] but data on long-term relief and on the need for repeat injections are not available. At best, this treatment option has to be regarded as promising.

Endoscopic balloon dilatation

The standard conservative management consists of either pneumatic dilatation or surgical myotomy. Prior to the advent of endoscopic surgery most gastroenterologists resorted to balloon dilatation in the first instance. Although the results of dilatation are good in 70% of cases,[1,2,21–24] there are problems. In particular, the relief of dysphagia is often not permanent, necessitating repeat dilatation, and the incidence of reflux following forceful dilatation is high. Repeat dilatations enhance the risk of perforation and render the subsequent myotomy more difficult as the loose submucosal plane is lost as a result of repeated disruption of the mucosal integrity by the forceful dilatations. Thus the current policy of reserving surgical myotomy for treatment failures is no longer sustainable as a definitive endoscopic procedure can be performed with minimum disruption to the patient and rapid return to full activity or work.

Open surgical myotomy

Cardiomyotomy for achalasia and a tailored long myotomy for DES and Nutcracker oesophagus are the standard procedures. Prior to the advent of MAS, cardiomyotomy was performed either abdominally through an upper midline laparotomy or transthoracically through the left chest. Both were major operations and abdominal cardiomyotomy was attended by a 13–15% incidence of reflux.[25] Many surgeons undertaking the latter approach have favoured an additional antireflux procedure.[26–28] In clinical trials, open cardiomyotomy has been demonstrated to be superior to balloon dilatation in terms of long-term relief of dysphagia and in the improvement of the propulsive peristaltic activity in the body of the oesophagus.[1,2] The benefits of long oesophageal myotomy, which is always performed through the left chest, are not as well documented and the evidence for relief of non-cardiac chest pain by this operation remains to be established.

Endoscopic myotomy

In the author's opinion, this is now the best treatment option and is indicated in all patients except those who are unfit for surgery and general anaesthesia in whom balloon dilatation is performed. The myotomy is carried out endoscopically with minimum disruption to the oesophageal attachments and its extent is tailored to the length of the manometrically defined abnormality. There are, however, a number of unsettled issues concerning cardiomyotomy. These relate to the nature of the endoscopic approach (laparoscopic or thoracoscopic) and to the need or otherwise for an antireflux procedure. The increased incidence of oesophago-gastric (O-G) reflux after open abdominal cardiomyotomy is due to the mobilisation of the O-G junction with disruption of the normal oesophageal attachments including the phreno-oesophageal membrane. It is also related to the length of the myotomy.[29] Laparoscopic cardiomyotomy can and should be performed with limited mobilisation. If this technique is followed,[8,10] the postoperative incidence of reflux is small. In the author's experience with 26 patients who have undergone laparoscopic cardiomyotomy for achalasia, postoperative reflux was documented in two (7%). There are two reasons for avoiding an antireflux procedure during endoscopic cardiomyotomy. The first concerns the pump failure due to the absence of propulsive peristaltic activity in the body of the oesophagus which invariably accompanies the cardiospasm. Secondly, should reflux develop after surgery, a laparoscopic antireflux procedure can be undertaken. Our experience indicates that the need for this arises very infrequently and this experience is confirmed by a recently reported study.[16] If an antireflux procedure is considered necessary, either at the time of cardiomyotomy or subsequently, it should not consist of a total wrap. Currently, most surgeons favour a partial anterior fundoplication of the Dor type.

The author's practice consists of the following:

- Laparoscopic cardiomyotomy with minimal mobilisation of the O-G junction and without an antireflux procedure for achalasia.
- Thoracoscopic long myotomy for DES and Nutcracker oesophagus.

Endoscopic approaches

The approach depends on the intended procedure. Cardiomyotomy can be performed either via the left thoracoscopic approach with the patient in the classical posterolateral position or by the laparoscopic route with the patient supine and in a steep head-up tilt. Long oesophageal myotomy is undertaken by the thoracoscopic route, left or right with the patient in the classical posterolateral position or in the posterior prone jackknife position.

Instrumentation for endoscopic myotomy

In addition to the standard instrumentation and equipment, a 30° forward oblique 10 mm telescope is necessary both for thoracoscopic myotomies and for laparoscopic cardiomyotomy. For chest work, the coaxial distal curved instruments introduced through metal flexible cannulae* are recommended.[30] A good liver retractor is essential for laparoscopic cardiomyotomy. A flexible endoscope and a colleague who is experienced in flexible endoscopy should be available during the conduct of thoracoscopic myotomies.

---

* Storz, Tuttlingen, Germany

Technique of thoracoscopic long myotomy

Approaches and patient positioning

Thoracoscopic long myotomy can be performed either through a left posterolateral or through a right prone posterior approach. The latter is favoured by the author because it gives better access to the oesophagus and often avoids single lung ventilation. Irrespective of the approach, the operation is performed under general anaesthesia with endobronchial intubation in order to allow bronchial occlusion and lung collapse on the operative side. Before positioning, a flexible endoscope is passed as far as the O-G junction.

Operative procedure

Standard left posterolateral. The position of the patient and the port sites are shown in Fig. 12.4. The operating table must be split to widen the intercostal spaces and the left upper arm held forward on its support away from the chest and in the adducted position. The optical port is introduced first. This is placed in the 5th interspace along the posterior axillary line. The author recommends the use of a Visiport§ for safe entry into the pleural cavity. The two operating flexible ports are then introduced on either side of the telescope cannula and the assistant's cannula is introduced last.

Despite bronchial occlusion, complete collapse of the lung may be hastened by insufflation of CO_2 using a standard laparoscopic insufflator set at a pressure of 6–8 mmHg.

Technique. The first step of the procedure consists of division of the inferior pulmonary ligament. This usually contains small vessels which require electrocoagulation. The ligament is divided completely in order to expose the inferior pulmonary vein. At this stage the endoscope light is switched on and the tip of the instrument bent forward to lift the oesophagus out of the aorto-vertebral gutter. The light is switched off and the endoscope held in the position which gives maximal exposure of the oesophagus. This may have to be altered as the operation progresses. The pleura covering the oesophagus is divided with care to avoid damage to the vagal fibres. Some small anterior oesophageal vessels may require electrocoagulation. The extent of the myotomy is determined by the preoperative manometric findings but for DES it usually extends from the diaphragm to the aortic arch. The myotomy is usually restricted to the lower third in patients with Nutcracker oesophagus.

There are several techniques which are used for executing the myotomy:
- the tenting electrosurgical hook method
- the use of the endoscopic pericardiectomy scissors
- the distraction–splitting technique.[10]

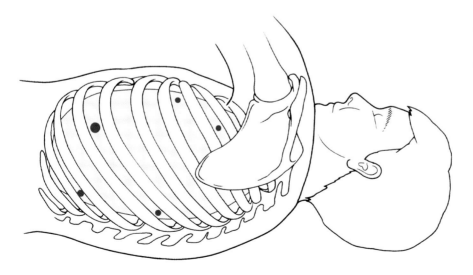

Figure 12.4 *Position of the patient and port sites for long oesophageal myotomy using the left posterolateral thoracoscopic approach.*

§ USSC, Norwalk, USA

The tenting electrosurgical technique is intrinsically unsound, as collateral damage may extend to the mucosal layer despite adequate tenting of the muscle layers unless the quasi-bipolar cutting technology is used. The safest method is the distraction–splitting technique. It is easiest to start at the middle of the proposed myotomy and then work up and down until the desired limits of the myotomy are reached (Fig. 12.5). The surface longitudinal muscle of the oesophagus is coagulated along the proposed line of the intended myotomy. Next, the coagulated muscle is split with the coaxial curve scissors and one of the edges grasped and lifted (Fig. 12.6a). The deeper muscular layer is then seen and cut by the scissors until the white mucosal tube is identified (Fig. 12.6b). At this stage, the two edges are grasped on either side and gently distracted (Fig. 12.6c) to achieve extension of the myotomy. The process is continued by 'walking along the muscle edges' with the two grasping forceps and then distracting them to achieve the desired length of myotomized oesophagus in either direction. Some of the deeper circular fibres are not split by this technique. These residual bands are cut with the curved coaxial scissors. If bleeding is encountered during the myotomy, simple pressure with adjacent tissue followed by irrigation always results in haemostasis and the need for electrocoagulation seldom arises. During suction, it is important that the tip of the sucker is kept well away from the mucosal tube as otherwise this will be breached by being sucked into the tip of the sucker.

At the end of the operation, the endoscope is retracted proximal to the myotomy and then air insufflation used to distend the myotomised region, thereby confirming mucosal integrity. A basal chest drain is inserted before the lung is expanded.

Posterior prone approach through the right chest. This gives better access to the entire thoracic oesophagus and single lung anaesthesia is often unnecessary since lung compression with CO_2 suffices to displace the lung away from the operative field. In addition, proximal extension of the myotomy to the upper third poses no problems in those patients where the DES affects the entire oesophagus.

The positioning of the patient and port sites is shown in Figure 12.7. The author favours the Visiport for insertion of the optical cannula which is sited in the first easily palpable intercostal space below and in line with the inferior angle of the right scapula. With the right posterior approach, the myotomy is situated at the back of the oesophagus and division of the inferior pulmonary ligament is unnecessary. Following division of the mediastinal pleura over the oesophagus, the myotomy is performed using the identical distraction–splitting technique described above. Again an underwater seal basal drain is inserted at the end of the procedure.

Technique of thoracoscopic cardiomyotomy

Although the author's initial experience of endoscopic cardiomyotomy was with the thoracoscopic approach, his preference is now to undertake this operation laparoscopically. Nonetheless, thoracoscopic cardiomyotomy is still favoured by some surgeons, especially in the USA.[9,11]

Advantages and disadvantages

Undoubtedly, the thoracoscopic access is good and the mobilisation is kept to a minimum. However, this approach has the following limitations:

- it requires the services of a good flexible endoscopist
- suturing of the mucosa if this is breached during the myotomy can be difficult because of the transmitted aortic and cardiac pulsations and may necessitate conversion
- an additional antireflux procedure, if considered necessary, usually requires the addition of a mini-thoracotomy.

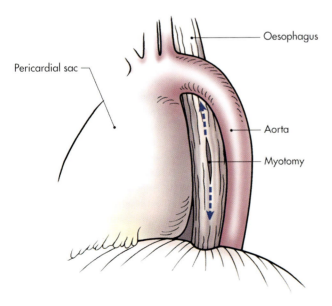

Figure 12.5 *It is easiest to start at the middle of the proposed myotomy and then work up and down until the desired limits of the myotomy are reached.*

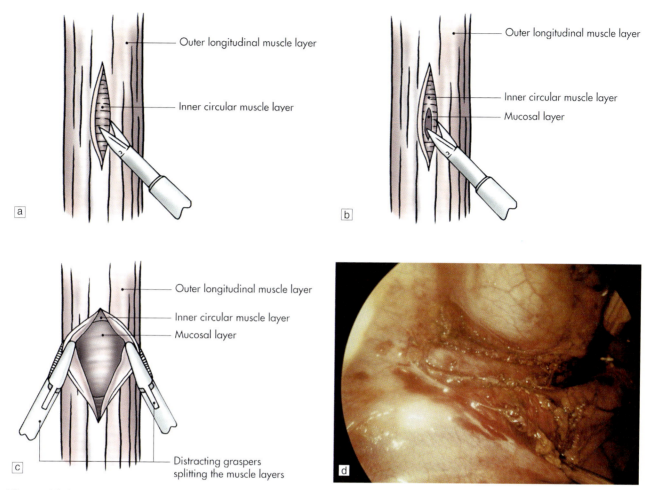

Figure 12.6 *Distraction–splitting technique. (a) The coagulated muscle is split with the coaxial curved scissors and one of the edges grasped and lifted; (b) the deeper muscular layer is cut by the scissors until the white mucosal tube is identified; (c) the two edges are grasped on either side and gently distracted to achieve extension of the myotomy; (d) completed long myotomy with distraction–splitting technique.*

Approaches and patient positioning

Thoracoscopic cardiomyotomy is conducted with the patient in the classical left posterolateral position (left chest uppermost). Prior to positioning of the patient, a flexible endoscope is inserted. The procedure entails close cooperation between the flexible endoscopist and the endoscopic surgeon. The endoscope is used to lift the oesophagus out of the aorto-vertebral gutter (Fig. 12.8) which greatly facilitates the procedure and minimises the dissection required. In addition, the endoscopist determines for the surgeon the distal limit of the myotomy in order to ensure that the division of the muscle layers extends beyond the O-G junction. This is essential for a good functional result.

The positioning and port sites are identical to those described for thoracoscopic long myotomy.

Procedure

The technique of the myotomy is important and it is best to start proximally at the junction of the dilated with the contracted segment and then proceed distally towards the oesophageal hiatus and then beyond the O-G junction to reach the proximal stomach. Guidance by the endoscopist on the distal limit of the cardiomyotomy is essential for a good result. An underwater seal chest drain is left at the end of the operation.

167

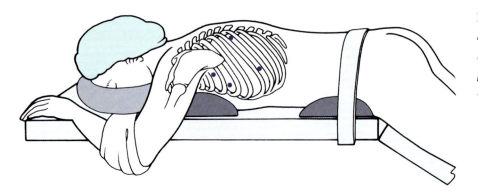

Figure 12.7 *Position of the patient and port sites for long oesophageal myotomy using the right posterior prone jack-knife thoracoscopic approach.*

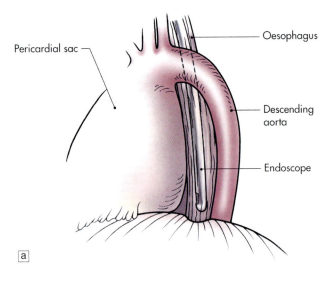

Pericardial sac

Oesophagus

Descending aorta

Endoscope

a

Technique of laparoscopic cardiomyotomy

Dissection is confined to the anterior surface of the O-G junction and lower oesophagus, with the myotomy being performed to the left of the anterior vagus and extending from the dilated segment proximally to about 1 cm below the O-G junction. A Dor type antireflux procedure is added only in the following situations:

- in patients with a concomitant hiatal hernia
- when the mucosa is breached during the myotomy as a buttress to the repair.

Approach and patient positioning
The patient is placed in the supine position with a steep head-up tilt. A Salem sump nasogastric tube is passed to ensure complete and sustained deflation of the stomach during the operation. The position of the port sites is shown in Figure 12.9. The passage of a flexible endoscope is unnecessary.

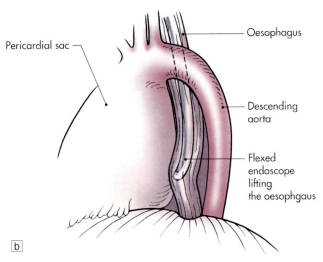

Pericardial sac

Oesophagus

Descending aorta

Flexed endoscope lifting the oesophgaus

b

Figure 12.8 *The endoscope is used to lift the oesophagus out of the aorto-vertebral gutter.*

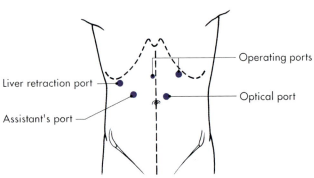

Operating ports

Liver retraction port

Optical port

Assistant's port

Figure 12.9 *Position of the port sites for laparoscopic cardiomyotomy.*

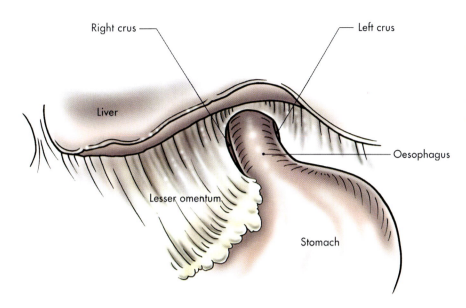

Right crus — Left crus

Liver

Oesophagus

Lesser omentum

Stomach

Procedure

The left lobe of the liver is retracted upwards. A good atraumatic laparoscopic retractor is essential for this purpose. The anterior wall of the fundus of the stomach is grasped by the assistant and pulled downwards and to the right. The dissection is limited to the anterior aspect of the oesophagus and O-G junction. It starts on the left side with division of the peritoneum over the left crus and this is extended along the superior margin of the hiatus across the right crus to the transparent section of the lesser omentum (Fig. 12.10). The caudate lobe of the liver is visualised once the proximal part of the lesser omentum is divided. The fat pad overlying the right crus is then detached in a distal direction until the whole length of the right crus is exposed. At this stage the right crus is gently retracted away from the oesophagus which is cleared anteriorly with care to preserve the anterior vagus nerve and the phreno-oesophageal membrane which is gently teased upwards inside the hiatal canal. The anterior margin of the hiatal canal is lifted up and the oesophagus mobilized anteriorly until the dilated segment is reached (usually within 2 cm of the margin of the hiatus).

The removal of the fat pad overlying the O-G junction is the most difficult part of the operation and has to be undertaken with care to avoid bleeding and damage to the anterior vagal fibres. This fat pad is best excised using coagulation with an insulated duckbill forceps and curved coaxial scissors. Underneath the fat pad a branch of the left gastric artery crosses the O-G junction and has to be secured (by clips) prior to division.

The myotomy is performed to the left of the anterior vagus nerve and starts in the middle of the abdominal oesophagus (Fig. 12.11). Again the distraction–splitting technique is favoured by the author. The myotomy is first extended proximally and then distally to cross the O-G junction to the adjacent stomach for a distance of about 1cm. The total length of the cardiomyotomy is usually about 4 cm (Fig. 12.12). The myotomy becomes more

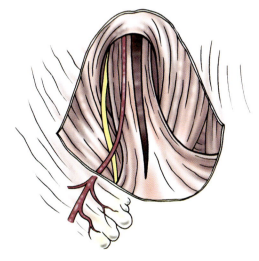

Figure 12.11 *The myotomy is performed to the left of the anterior vagus nerve and starts in the middle of the abdominal oesophagus.*

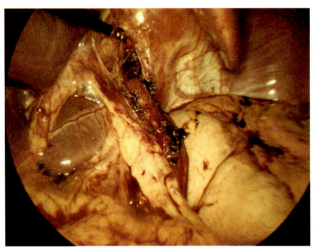

Figure 12.12 *The total length of the cardiomyotomy is usually about 4 cm.*

difficult as the stomach is approached since the submucosal plane is less well defined. Careful scissors division of the muscle bands is needed here. Laparoscopic cardiomyotomy can be difficult in patients who have previously undergone balloon dilatations as the loose submucosal plane is lost; and the risk of perforation of the mucosal coat is higher. If the mucosal tube is breached, conversion is unnecessary provided the surgeon is experienced in endoscopic suturing as the defect can be repaired with 4/0 Polysorb or Vicryl.

On completion of the cardiomyotomy, the nasogastric tube is withdrawn proximal to the myotomy and air injected into the oesophagus to distend the myotomised segment and identify any mucosal leaks.

Dor anterior fundoplication. This is performed selectively. It requires some mobilisation of the fundus by division of the gastrophrenic peritoneum and underlying fascial attachments. The mobilised fundus is brought over the O-G junction and sutures in the following fashion and order:

- to the left edge of the myotomy (Fig. 12.13a)
- to the right edge of the myotomy (Fig. 12.13b)
- to the right crus (Fig. 12.13c).

The completed appearance of the fundoplication is shown in Figure 12.13d.

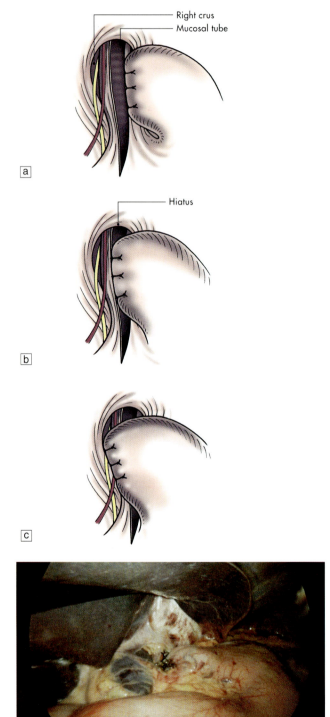

Figure 12.13 *Dor anterior fundoplication. (a) Suture of fundus to the left edge of the myotomy; (b) fundus to the right edge of the myotomy; (c) fundus to the right crus; (d) completed Dor anterior fundoplication.*

Postoperative management of patients undergoing oesophageal myotomy

In thoracoscopically conducted cases, the chest drain is usually removed within 12–24 hours depending on the chest X-ray findings.

Oral fluids are started the next day in patients in whom the mucosal tube was intact at the time of the myotomy (oesophageal insufflation test) without recourse to gastrografin contrast studies. The patients then rapidly progress to solid diet and are usually discharged on the second or third postoperative day. If the mucosa has been perforated during surgery, the patient is kept nil-by-mouth for five days and a gastrografin study is then performed. Fluids are started if this radiological assessment confirms mucosal integrity. These patients are put on antibiotics (usually a cephalosporin) for five days.

Results of oesophageal myotomy

The author has found the results for endoscopic cardiomyotomy to be very good with 22 out of 26 patients having no complications following a single intervention. One patient with long-standing achalasia and a sigmoid mega-oesophagus required repeat intervention (thoracoscopic and laparoscopic) to achieve complete relief of the dysphagia. There were three perforations: all occurred in patients who had undergone previous pneumatic dilatation. Two of these were sutured endoscopically but one was converted. Dysphagia persisted but was improved in this patient. To date, with a maximal follow-up period of six years (median 32 months), reflux symptoms have developed in three patients with documentation of gastro-oesophageal reflux by pH monitoring in two.

The results of long myotomy in 17 patients have been mixed. Dysphagia was relieved or improved in all the patients and non-cardiac chest pain was relieved in 10 (60%). Three patients in this group have developed gastro-oesophageal reflux (18%).

Conclusions

The author's experience and that reported in the literature with endoscopic cardiomyotomy indicates that this procedure should now be regarded as the definitive first-line treatment for patients with achalasia. It should replace pneumatic dilatation except in poor risk patients and in centres where the necessary endoscopic surgical expertise is not available. In general, the laparoscopic approach is favoured over the thoracoscopic route for cardiomyotomy. The need for an anti-antireflux procedure remains an unsettled issue and will be determined only by long-term follow-up from centres who do not add an antireflux component routinely, and by randomised clinical trials. The latter are, however, difficult to conduct in view of the low incidence of the disease in Western countries.

The thoracoscopic approach is best reserved for long myotomy and has the benefit of avoiding a posterolateral thoracotomy. Overall, the results are not as good as those following cardiomyotomy for achalasia. Long myotomy for non-cardiac chest pain cannot be regarded as a routine procedure until sufficient experience has been gained with adequate follow-up to document sustained relief of pain in a significant percentage of these patients.

References

1. Csendes A, Velasco N, Bragetto I, Henriquez A. A prospective randomized study comparing forceful dilatation and esophagomyotomy in patients with achalasia of the esophagus. *Gastroenterology* 1981; **80**: 789–95.
2. Csendes A, Braghetto I, Henriquez A *et al*. Late results of a prospective randomised study comparing forceful dilatation and esophagomyotomy in patients with achalasia. *Gut* 1989; **30**: 299–304.
3. Fellows IW, Ogilvie AL, Atkinson M. Pneumatic dilatation in achalasia. *Gut* 1983; **24**: 1020–3.
4. Levine ML, Moskowitz GW, Dorf BS, Bank S. Pneumatic dilation in patients with achalasia with a modified Gruntzig dilator (Levine) under direct endoscopic control: results after 5 years. *Am J Gastroenterol* 1991; **86**: 1581–4.
5. Kadakia SC, Wong RK. Graded pneumatic dilation using Rigiflex achalasia dilators in patients with primary esophageal achalasia. *Am J Gastroenterol* 1993; **88**: 34–8.
6. Shimi S, Nathanson LK, Cuschieri A. Laparoscopic cardiomyotomy for achalasia. *J Roy Coll Surg Edinb* 1991; **36**: 152–4.
7. Cuschieri A. Treatment of oesophageal disease: medical, surgical or endoscopic? *Curr Surg Pract* 1991; **3**: 187–9.
8. Shimi SM, Nathanson LK, Cuschieri A. Thoracoscopic long myotomy for nutcracker oesophagus: initial experience of a new surgical approach. *Br J Surg* 1992; **79**: 533–6.
9. Pellegrini C, Wetter LA, Patti M *et al*. Thoracoscopic esophagomyotomy. Initial experience with a new approach for the treatment of achalasia. *Ann Surg* 1992; **216**: 291–6.
10. Cuschieri A. Endoscopic oesophageal myotomy for specific motility disorders and non-cardiac chest pain. *End Surg* 1993; **1**: 280–5.
11. Pellegrini C, Leichter R, Patti M *et al*. Thoracoscopic esophageal myotomy in the treatment of achalasia. *Ann Thorac Surg* 1992; **56**: 680–2.
12. Buess G, Cuschieri A, Manncke K *et al*. Technique and preliminary results of laparoscopic cardiomyotomy. *End Surg* 1993; **1**: 76–81.

13 Ancona E, Peracchia A, Zaninotto G, Rossi M *et al*. Heller laparoscopic cardiomyotomy with antireflux anterior fundoplication (Dor) in the treatment of esophageal achalasia. *Surg Endosc* 1993; **7**: 459–61.

14 Anselmino M, Hinder RA, Filipi CJ, Wilson P. Laparoscopic Heller cardiomyotomy and thoracoscopic esophageal long myotomy for the treatment of primary esophageal motor disorders. *Surg Laparosc Endosc* 1993; **3**: 437–41.

15 Cuschieri A. Endoscopic surgery for oesophageal disorders. *Cur Surg Pract* 1994; **6**: 31–8.

16 Robertson GSM, Lloyd DM, Wicks ACB, De Caestecker J, Veitch PS. Laparoscopic Heller's cardiomyotomy without an antireflux procedure. *Br J Surg* 1995; **82**: 957–9.

17 Cuschieri A. Wither minimal access surgery: tribulations and expectations. *Am J Surg* 1995; **169**: 9–19.

18 Cranford CA Jr, Sutton D, Sadek SA, Kennedy N, Cuschieri A. New physiological method of evaluating oesophageal transit. *Br J Surg* 1987; **74**: 411–15.

19 Eriksen CA, Sadek SA, Cranford C, Sutton D, Kennedy N, Cuschieri A. Solid bolus oesophageal transit in patients with reflux oesophagitis. *Br J Surg* 1989; **73**: 496.

20 Pasricha PJ, Ravich WJ, Hendrix TR *et al*. Intrasphincteric botulinum toxin for the treatment of achalasia. *N Engl J Med* 1995; **332**: 774–8.

21 Ferguson MK. Achalasia: current evaluation and therapy. *Ann Thorac Surg* 1991; **52**: 336–42.

22 Vantrappen G, Janssens J. To dilate or to operate? That is the question. *Gut* 1983; **24**: 1013–19.

23 Vantrappen G, Hellemans J. Treatment of achalasia and related motor disorders. *Gastroenterology* 1980; **79**: 144–54.

24 Reynolds JC, Parkman HP. Achalasia. *Gastroenterol Clin North Am* 1989; **18**: 223–55.

25 Andreollo NA, Earlam RJ. Heller's myotomy for achalasia: is an added anti-reflux procedure necessary? *Br J Surg* 1987; **74**: 765–9.

26 Bonavina L, Nosadinia A, Bardini R *et al*. Primary treatment of esophageal achalasia: long-term results of myotomy and Dor fundoplication. *Arch Surg* 1992; **127**: 222–6.

27 Paricio P, Martinez de Haro L, Ortiz A *et al*. Achalasia of the cardia: Long-term results of oesophagomyotomy and posterior partial fundoplication. *Br J Surg* 1990; **77**: 1371–4.

28 Donahue PE, Schlesinger PK, Sluss KF *et al*. Esophagocardiomyotomy – Floppy Nissen fundoplication effectively treats achalasia without causing esophageal obstruction. *Surgery* 1994; **116**: 719–25.

29 Ellis FH Jr, Kiser JC, Schlegel JF *et al*. Esophagomyotomy for esophageal achalasia: experimental. Clinical and manometric aspects. *Ann Surg* 1967; **166**: 640–56.

30 Cuschieri A, Shimi S, Banting G, Vander Velpen G, Dunkley P. Coaxial curved instruments for minimal access surgery. *End Surg* 1993; **1**: 303–5.

Minimally invasive surgical treatment of gastroesophageal reflux disease

13

E.S. Kassis and J.D. Luketich

Gastroesophageal reflux disease

Epidemiology

Gastroesophageal reflux disease (GERD) is common and has been estimated to affect 5–10% of the adult population.[1] In Western countries, occasional heartburn is experienced by 20–40% of the population but oesophagitis and other complications such as ulceration, stricture, or Barrett's are estimated to be present in less than 10% of this group.[2,3] The incidence of GERD is increased by age, smoking, weight, and pregnancy[4] and men are affected more commonly than women. Although GERD is a condition associated with significant morbidity and decreased quality of life, the annual mortality rate is very low at only 1 death per 100,000 patients annually.[2]

Pathophysiology

The antireflux barrier in humans can be thought of as consisting of three components. The oesophageal body acts as a propulsive pump, the lower oesophageal sphincter (LES) functions as a one-way valve, and the stomach serves as a reservoir (Fig. 13.1).[5] Normal function at the gastroesophageal junction is complex with many anatomical and physiological factors affecting the coordination of swallowing and the prevention of reflux. These functions depend on adequate oesophageal motility coordinated with

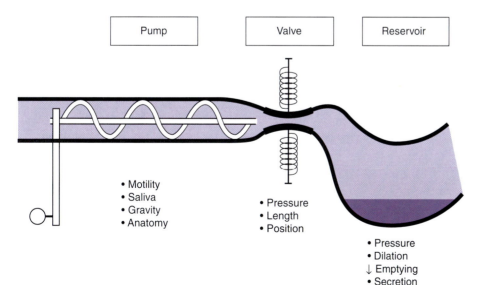

Pump | Valve | Reservoir

- Motility
- Saliva
- Gravity
- Anatomy

- Pressure
- Length
- Position

- Pressure
- Dilation
- ↓ Emptying
- Secretion

Figure 13.1 *The three components of the antireflux barrier. The oesophagus acts as a propulsive pump, the stomach serves as a reservoir, and the lower oesophageal sphincter functions as a one-way valve.*

relaxation and contraction of the LES. Changes in intragastric pressure and normal stomach emptying also play crucial roles in the correct synchronisation of these functions. A disturbance of any of these components may lead to reflux.[6]

The most common mechanism of pathological reflux is a defective LES, accounting for 50–70% of cases. The competency of the LES depends on the sphincter pressure, overall LES length, and the length of oesophagus exposed to the positive pressure environment of the abdomen. A greater length of abdominal oesophagus increases the effectiveness of this barrier mechanism. When LES tone is decreased, regurgitation of gastric contents into the oesophagus may occur.

A second pathophysiological mechanism leading to GERD involves the inefficient clearance of refluxate by the oesophagus. Oesophageal clearance depends on gravity, oesophageal motor function, salivation, and anchoring of the distal oesophagus in the abdomen. Reflux symptoms due to primary oesophageal disorders include oesophageal dysmotility, oesophageal spasm and achalasia. The third general cause of reflux involves disorders of the stomach. In the normal state, intragastric pressure rarely exceeds LES tone, and reflux does not occur to any clinically significant degree. In certain pathological conditions, the intragastric pressure may exceed normal LES tone resulting in reflux. This situation may occur in patients with other disease processes, such as diabetes mellitus, which affect gastric emptying.

Hiatal hernia is a common co-existing finding in the setting of clinically significant reflux. However, many patients with GERD do not have a hiatal hernia and many patients with hiatal hernia do not reflux significantly. Thus, this association is present but not consistent. In addition there are many drugs, hormones and foods that promote reflux by diminishing the tone of the LES. Although many acid suppressing agents often ameliorate the symptoms of GERD, gastric acid hypersecretion is an uncommon aetiological factor.

Diagnosis

The clinical presentation of GERD can mimic many other disease processes.[7,8] Although there are some classic features, such as heartburn, there are a variety of other signs and symptoms that must be kept in mind in order for the proper diagnosis to be made. For example, dysphagia, odynophagia, and chest pain are common complaints in patients with GERD. In 25% of patients pulmonary manifestations are present including chronic cough, chronic bronchitis, pulmonary fibrosis, recurrent pneumonia, and asthma. Gastrointestinal symptoms such as bloating, early satiety, belching, nausea, and acute and chronic blood loss may be present. Other symptoms of GERD include regurgitation of gastric contents into the mouth, water brash, globus, hoarseness, and hiccups.

Despite its prevalence, GERD is a challenging diagnostic problem. Since oesophageal, gastric, pulmonary, and cardiac disorders may all present in a similar manner, it is difficult to differentiate between them based on symptomatology alone. Therefore, objective methods must be employed to confirm the diagnosis of GERD.

The most commonly employed diagnostic tests are:

- oesophageal manometry
- 24-hour pH monitoring
- endoscopy
- barium swallow with fluoroscopy.

Oesophageal pH monitoring

Oesophageal pH monitoring allows for the recording of the pH changes under physiological conditions over a 24-hour period. This study allows for the quantitation of the actual time that the oesophagus is exposed to gastric contents, measurement of the oesophageal ability to clear the refluxate, and a correlation of reflux with the patient's symptoms. This study has the highest sensitivity and specificity in the detection of reflux, but is not able to determine the cause. An acid reflux episode is defined each time the pH falls to four or less. Using 24-hour pH monitoring, oesophageal exposure to gastric acid can be compared to a number of normal parameters (Table 13.1).[5,8,9] In analysing these six components from patients with typical symptoms of GERD it was found that not all of these parameters are abnormal in each case. These parameters can be combined to form a composite score to assess disease severity.[5]

Oesophageal manometric analysis

Oesophageal manometric analysis evaluates pressure, overall length, and abdominal length of the LES and allows comparison to normal values (Table 13.2).[10,11] A defect in any one of these parameters decreases the effectiveness of

pH <4	Normal value
Episodes per 24 hours	<50
Fraction of total time	<4.2%
Fraction of upright time	<6.3%
Fraction of supine time	<1.22%
Episodes greater than 5 minutes	≤3
Duration of longest episode	<9.2 minutes

Table 13.1

Parameters measured by 24-hour oesophageal pH monitoring

Adapted from Bremner RM, Bremner CG, DeMeester TR. Gastroesophageal reflux: the use of pH monitoring. *Current Problems in Surgery* 1995; **6**: 429–568.

Parameter	Mean value (5th/95th percentile)
Pressure (mmHg)	13.8 (8/26.5)
Overall length (cm)	3.7 (2.6/5.4)
Abdominal length (cm)	2.2 (1.1/3.4)
Intra-abdominal SVV* (mmHg . mm)	3,613 (684/12,918)
Total SVV* (mmHg . mm)	5,723 (1,212/16,780)

Table 13.2

Normal LES parameters

*Sphincter vector volume.

Adapted from DeMeester TR, Constantini M. Function Tests. In: Pearson FG, Deslauriers J, Ginsberg RJ *et al.* (eds) *Esophageal Surgery*. New York, Churchill Livingstone, 1995; pp 119–50.

the LES mechanism and increases the risk of reflux. In addition, manometric analysis can assess the propulsive force of the oesophageal body.[12] Antireflux procedures are designed to restore normal LES length and resting pressure. Abnormal motility of the oesophageal body can lead to dysphagia following anti-reflux surgery and should be considered preoperatively.

Endoscopy

Endoscopy with biopsies is important to identify complications of GERD such as oesophagitis, stricture, and/or Barrett's. These endoscopic signs are useful in assessing the severity of disease, but are unable to provide information on the mechanism of reflux.

Barium swallow

Barium swallow with fluoroscopy will show spontaneous reflux in only 40% of patients with classic GERD symptoms. In the majority of these patients who show spontaneous reflux, the diagnosis of increased acid exposure is confirmed on 24-hour pH studies. Therefore, the absence of radiological evidence of reflux does not indicate absence of disease.

Surgical management of GERD

Recently, interest in antireflux surgery for long-term treatment of GERD has been increasing. Several reasons account for this renewed interest. Surgery has been demonstrated in a prospective randomised trial to be superior to medical treatment in providing symptomatic relief and healing of oesophagitis[13] and the advent of a minimally invasive approach to antireflux surgery has made this option more attractive to both patient and physician. Also, concerns regarding the side effects associated with long-term use of acid suppressing agents, such as omeprazole, are leading to an increased recognition of the surgical alternative[14] and cost analyses have demonstrated that surgery is less expensive than chronic medical therapy in younger patient populations.[15] In addition, it has be

recognised that the majority of patients with GERD have an ineffective lower oesophageal sphincter (LES).[3,8] Medical management such as omeprazole, H2 blockers, and prokinetic agents commonly used in medical therapy do not address the issue of a mechanically deficient LES. Surgical therapy, on the other hand, corrects the antireflux mechanism and re-establishes the barrier to reflux.

Patient selection for antireflux surgery

Antireflux surgical therapy is indicated only for those with clinically significant GERD and an incompetent LES. Therefore, when confronted with a patient with symptoms of GERD it is important to determine the underlying pathophysiology. Inappropriate patient selection is one of the most common reasons for the failure of antireflux surgery.[16]

Most patients with symptoms of GERD will respond to medical intervention and will not require further testing. Indications for the surgical evaluation include persistent or recurrent symptoms and/or complications after 8–12 weeks of acid suppression therapy (Fig. 13.2).[6] Objective tests should be obtained including 24-hour pH testing,

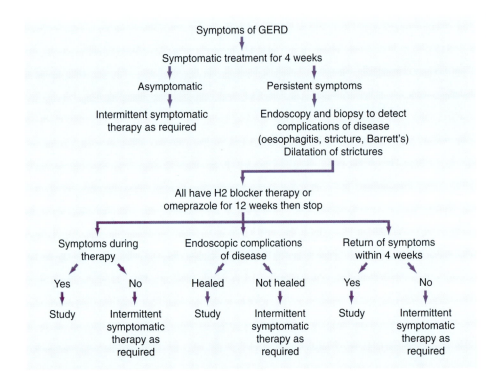

Figure 13.2 *Algorithm used in the evaluation of patients with symptoms of gastroesophageal reflux disease.*

manometry, barium oesophagram, and upper endoscopy. We perform 24-hour pH monitoring off medications in order to document increased exposure to gastric acid and formulate a DeMeester composite score.[5] If this demonstrates symptomatic acid reflux, manometry is obtained. Since the goal of antireflux surgery is to establish a barrier to reflux, a defective LES should be present in any patient undergoing surgical intervention (Table 13.3).[6] Next, oesophago-gastroduodenoscopy is performed to evaluate the extent of oesophagitis and to search for complications of GERD such as stricture or Barrett's. In our practice, a barium video oesophagram is also obtained to rule out other oesophageal pathology.

These tests allow the surgeon to establish the degree of acid reflux, amount of mucosal damage, LES incompetence and the functional status of the oesophageal body and stomach. This information is used to decide if an antireflux procedure should be considered and if necessary, what type. In addition, underlying disorders mimicking GERD such as achalasia, scleroderma, and motility abnormalities of the oesophageal body can be ruled out which influence treatment decisions.

Surgical techniques

The ultimate goal of antireflux surgery is to increase LES tone to promote a more effective barrier to reflux. A successful operation accomplishes this goal by: fixation of the LES in the abdomen to expose it to the positive intra-abdominal pressure, narrowing the oesophageal hiatus by approximating the diaphragmatic crura to keep the fundoplication in the abdomen, lengthening the intra-abdominal LES, and reduction of a hiatal hernia.[17]

Laparoscopic Nissen fundoplication

Historical background

In 1956, Rudolph Nissen described a fundoplication procedure for the surgical management of GERD.[18] This technique involved encircling the lower oesophageal sphincter with a 360° wrap of the gastric fundus and has become the most common surgical procedure for the treatment of GERD (Fig. 13.3). Many modifications of this procedure have occurred since its conception. The degree of fundal wrap was decreased by both Dor (Fig. 13.4) and Toupet (Fig. 13.5) in order to decrease the rate of post-operative complications, such as gasbloat syndrome, and dysphagia associated with the original procedure.[19,20] For similar reasons, Donahue[21] and DeMeester[22] have recommended performing a loose and shorter wrap, respectively. Other important modifications included the narrowing of the oesophageal hiatus posterior to the oesophagus and division of the short gastric vessels to enable better mobilisation of the gastric fundus. The Nissen procedure has become widely accepted for the surgical management of GERD. In 1991, Dallemagne[23] demonstrated the feasibility of a laparoscopic approach to the Nissen procedure.

Technique of laparoscopic Nissen fundoplication

The laparoscopic fundoplication has been described by a number of surgeons.[3,17,24] In most descriptions, the patient is placed in the lithotomy position in steep reverse Trendelenburg. Initially, most surgeons positioned themselves between the patient's legs. Recently, good success has been reported with the surgeon in the traditional right-sided position and the patient supine.

Table 13.3

Criteria defining an abnormal lower oesophageal sphincter (LES)

Parameter	Normal value
Mean LES pressure	<6 mmHg
Mean length of the abdominal LES	<1 cm
Mean overall sphincter length	<2 cm

Adapted from Stein HJ, DeMeester TR. Who benefits from antireflux surgery? *World Journal of Surgery* 1992; **16**: 313–319.

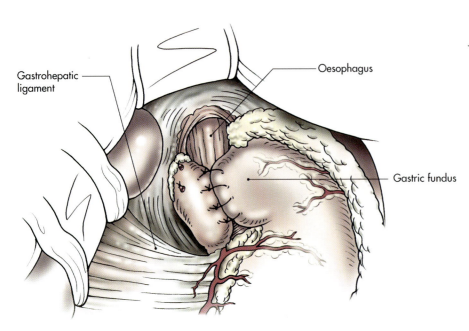

Figure 13.3 *Completed Nissen fundoplication demonstrating the 360° wrap of the gastric fundus around the esophagus.*

Gastrohepatic ligament

Oesophagus

Gastric fundus

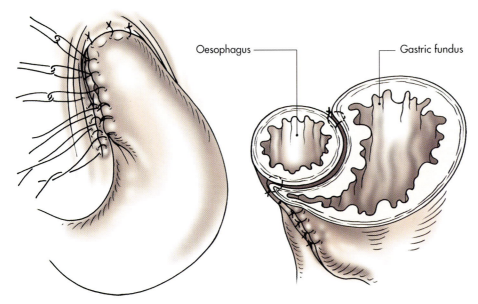

Figure 13.4 *The Dor (anterior) partial fundoplication.*

Oesophagus

Gastric fundus

Once patient position and pneumoperitoneum have been established we place five trocars in the abdominal cavity. One 10 mm port is placed in the midline, approximately midway between the xiphoid and the umbilicus. The 30° endoscope is inserted in the supra-umbilical port. Two 5 mm ports, are placed along the right costal margin (Fig. 13.6). Another port is placed along the subcostal margin in the left midclavicular line (Fig. 13.7). The lower right costal margin port is used for the liver retractor. We use the Diamond-Flex Retractor System* (Fig. 13.8). The upper right costal port is used for the operating surgeon's grasper. Another 10 mm

---

*   Deknatel Snowden Pencer, Tucker Georgia

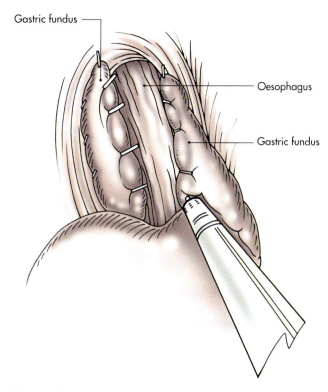

Figure 13.5 *The Toupet (posterior) partial fundoplication.*

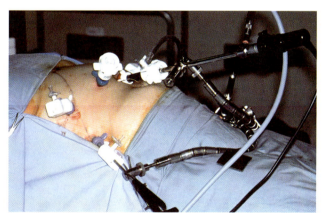

Figure 13.6 *Right-sided port placement for the laparoscopic Nissen fundoplication.*

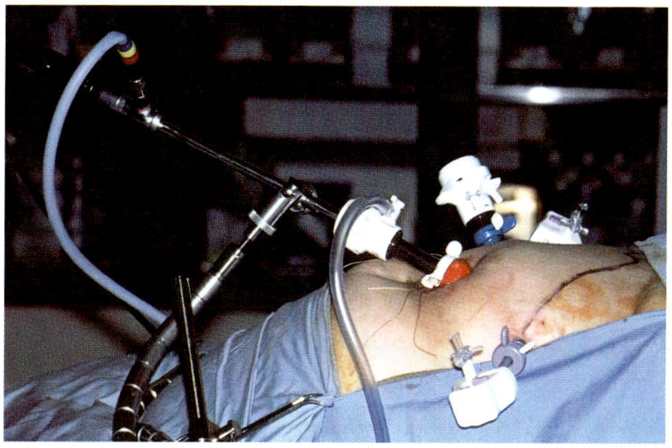

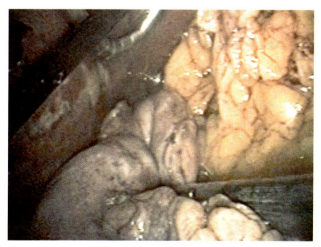

Figure 13.7 *Left sided port placement for the laparoscopic Nissen fundoplication.*

Figure 13.8 *Operative photograph of liver retraction using the Diamond-Flex Retractor System (Deknatel Snowden Pencer Worldwide, Tucker, Georgia).*

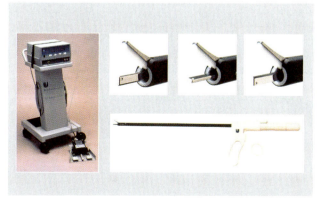

Figure 13.9 *The Harmonic Scalpel System (Ethicon Endo-Surgery, Cincinnati, Ohio).*

port is placed between the camera port and the upper right costal margin port to allow for insertion of a dissecting instrument. We have found the endoshear of the Harmonic Scalpel† (Fig. 13.9) both useful in para-oesophageal dissection

†   Ethicon Endo-Surgery, Cincinnati, Ohio

and short gastric division. The left subcostal margin port allows for retraction of the stomach by the first assistant.

Following port placement and liver retraction the first step in the Nissen is division of the gastrohepatic ligament and identification of the right crus (Fig. 13.10). Next, we dissect the right diaphragmatic crus from the oesophagus. The anterior vagus is left in contact with the oesophagus. Dissection of the right crus should continue until the point where the left and right crura meet posterior to the oesophagus. The left crus is now dissected off of the oesophagus. The oesophagus is then retracted upward using an atraumatic grasper. This greatly increases access to the area posterior to the oesophagus. Posterior dissection of the oesophagus continues until a window is formed viewing the diaphragm. Once the window has been established the crura are rejoined with one or two non-absorbable sutures placed in the crura posterior to the oesophagus with a 54–60F bougie in place (Fig. 13.11).

The fundus is mobilised by division of the most superior three to four short gastric vessels. This dissection must be continued to the posterior aspect of the stomach in order to achieve maximal mobilisation so that a loose, floppy fundoplication may be performed. The harmonic scalpel greatly facilitates mobilisation of the oesophagus and division of the short gastric vessels (Fig. 13.12).

Once the fundus has been mobilised it is pulled through the window posterior to the oesophagus using an atraumatic grasper. The fundus is pulled posteriorly and then anteriorly around the oesophagus with a 54F bougie in place to prevent excessive narrowing of the oesophagus. The fundoplication is then performed sutured with non-absorbable suture (Fig. 13.13) and the bougie removed. A nasogastric tube is placed and air is removed from the stomach. The trocars are then removed and sites closed with absorbable suture. The nasogastric tube is removed in the operating room.

Results

Many centres have reported results of the laparoscopic Nissen procedure.[25–31] The short-term results of these series have demonstrated that the laparoscopic approach has a success rate of approximately 90%. This is comparable to the success rate of the open procedure. The operative mortality of the laparoscopic procedure is consistently reported to be less than 1% and is zero in most series. Operative time varies between centres, from 109–186 minutes, and is somewhat longer than the time needed to complete the open procedure. Hospital stay is reduced to less than 72 hours in most series. In our series, 90% are discharged within 48 hours of surgery.[31]

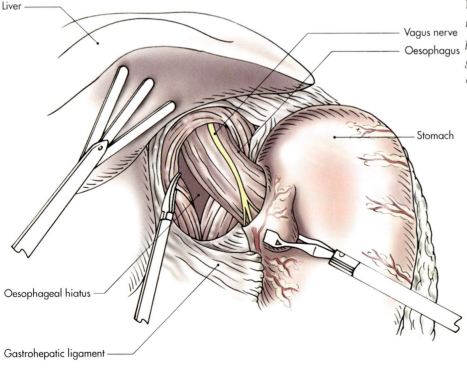

Figure 13.10 *The initial step in the laparoscopic Nissen fundoplication is division of the gastrohepatic ligament to expose the oesophageal hiatus.*

Liver

Vagus nerve

Oesophagus

Stomach

Oesophageal hiatus

Gastrohepatic ligament

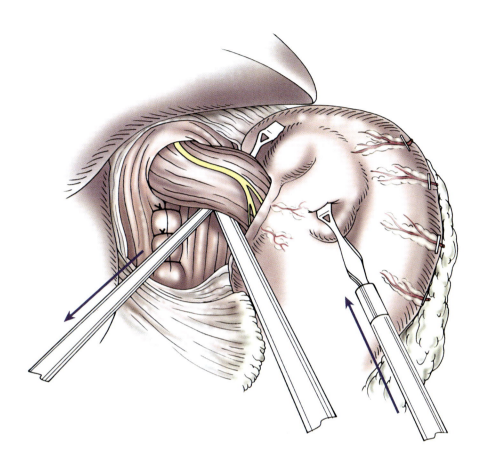

Figure 13.11 *Diagram demonstrating the creation of a window posterior to the oesophagus and crural closure.*

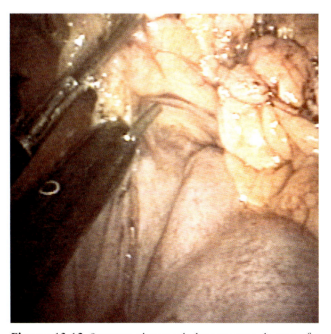

Figure 13.12 *Operative photograph demonstrating division of a short gastric vessel using the Harmonic Scalpel.*

Early postoperative gastrointestinal complaints are common following the laparoscopic procedure. Common complaints include dysphagia (often requiring dilation), heartburn, epigastric pain, bloating, nausea, diarrhoea, early satiety, and the inability to vomit or belch. These complaints have been reported to occur in upwards of 50% of patients undergoing the procedure. Although common, these complaints resolve within 4–6 weeks and long-term complaints are relatively uncommon. Studies analysing the long-term results of the laparoscopic technique are underway.

Operative complications seen in the laparoscopic procedure have varied between 5–25%. The lowest operative complication rates occur in those studies with the highest number of patients. This exemplifies the long learning curve before the technique is mastered. Therefore, the technique should only be undertaken by surgeons who have considerable experience in advanced laparoscopic technique. Complications have included oesophageal,

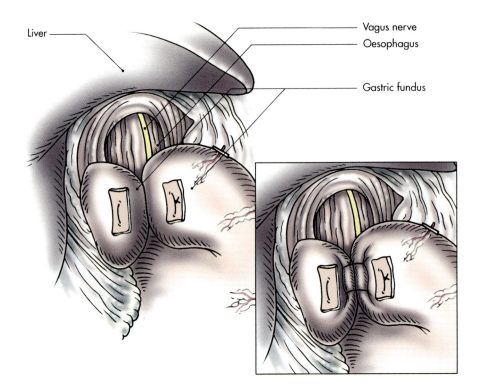

Liver

Vagus nerve

Oesophagus

Gastric fundus

Figure 13.13 *The fundus is wrapped around the oesophagus then sutured in place.*

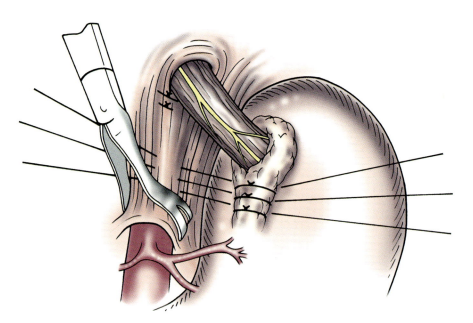

Figure 13.14 *The diaphragm has been closed loosely around the oesophagus and sutures have been placed in the anterior and posterior phrenoesophageal bundles. Sutures are then taken through these bundles and are carried through the pre-aortic fascia. The lower two sutures are tied and a pressure measurement is taken before tying the top knot.*

gastric, small bowel and pleural perforations, haemorrhage, hepatic lacerations, and pneumothoraces. In approximately 6% of procedures reported, complications necessitated conversion to an open fundoplication.

The major benefits of the laparoscopic procedure over the open procedure deal primarily with patient comfort and hospital costs. Low published a study where cost and outcome data were compared between the open and laparoscopic procedure.[32] The hospital stay for the patients undergoing laparoscopic Nissen was on average three days shorter than patients undergoing the open procedure. Laparoscopic patients returned to work greater than four days earlier than the open patients. Importantly, patients in each group did not differ with regard to complication rates, return-to-work statistics and quality-of-life assessments at three months. Therefore patients are leaving the hospital and resuming normal activities earlier without any ill effect when compared to the open procedure. Recently, we have initiated a protocol for same-day discharge for low-risk patients after laparoscopic Nissen fundoplication.[33]

Laparoscopic Toupet fundoplication

Historical background

Toupet[20] devised a modification of the traditional operation in an attempt to ameliorate the postoperative gastrointestinal complaints of dysphagia and bloating in patients undergoing the Nissen procedure. This modification of the Nissen fundoplication involves a reduction on the degree of the fundal wrap to 180–200° (see Fig. 13.5) rather than the 360° originally described. The fundus is only wrapped along the posterior aspect of the oesophagus. There have been reports that the Toupet procedure is associated with fewer postoperative digestive complications.[34]

Results

Tucker[35] and McKernan[36] have recently published data comparing the effectiveness of the Toupet fundoplication versus the Nissen fundoplication. The success of these two procedures in achieving symptomatic relief and patient satisfaction were similar. The distinction between these procedures was in relation to the postoperative complaints. In the study by Tucker, nearly 50% of the patients undergoing the Nissen procedure complained of post-operative dysphagia or bloating. None of the patients who underwent the Toupet procedure had these complaints. McKernan reported that the average time until patients were able to swallow normally was greater than two weeks longer for the patients in the Nissen group. Although these studies are small and more data is clearly needed, it seems that the Toupet procedure has the potential to be as effective as the Nissen with a lower rate of postoperative side-effects.

Laparoscopic Hill repair

Historical background

In 1967, Lucius D. Hill described a surgical approach for the treatment of GERD. The goal of this procedure is to restore the normal functioning of the gastroesophageal junction.

This is accomplished via posterior fixation of the gastroesophageal junction to the pre-aortic fascia, and restoration of the gastroesophageal valve mechanism.[37] In 1978, Hill described the use of intra-operative manometry with a modified nasogastric tube so that the surgeon can calibrate the LES pressure intra-operatively.[38]

Hill has recently developed a laparoscopic approach to the procedure that he developed nearly 30 years ago. The goals of the laparoscopic approach are the same as the open and include posterior fixation of the gastroesophageal junction, intraoperative calibration of the LES, and recreation of a normal gastroesophageal valve mechanism (Figs. 13.14–13.16). The initial report on 51 patients was published in 1994.[39]

Results

Early reports on the effectiveness of the laparoscopic Hill repair have been published.[39,40,41] Hill reported that in over 2,000 patients undergoing the open Hill repair greater than 90% reported a good or excellent result. Early results with the laparoscopic approach indicate that it is as effective as the open approach. The operative mortality is very low, and operative time varies between 139–244 minutes. Operative complications were exceedingly rare. There was only one reported operative complication among 81 patients in the Aye and Snow reports. The hospital stay averaged less than three days.

Early postoperative gastrointestinal complaints are frequent with dysphagia being the most common. This dysphagia often requires dilation. There were few long-term complications or side-effects.

Belsey Mark IV repair

Historical background

In 1961, Ronald Belsey[42] published the results of 71 patients treated with the Mark IV procedure for gastroesophageal reflux. In 1967, Skinner and Belsey[43] reported on over 1,000 patients for oesophageal reflux and hiatal hernia. The goal of this procedure is to restore four to five cm of oesophagus to the abdomen and to fix it in place. There were various techniques for maintaining this segment.[44] The first of these involved shortening of the crura to augment Allison's pinchcock action. The second technique involved creating an exaggerated angle of His and suture of the fundus to the undersurface of the

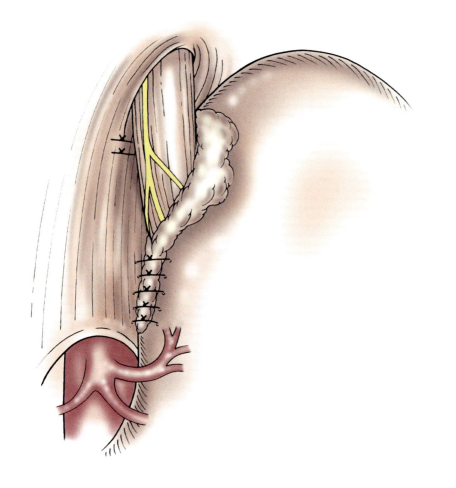

Figure 13.15 *All attachment sutures have been tied.*

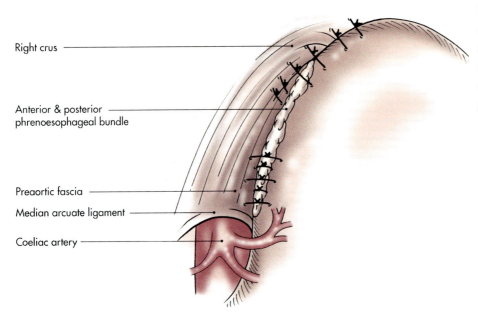

Right crus

Anterior & posterior
phrenoesophageal bundle

Preaortic fascia

Median arcuate ligament

Coeliac artery

Figure 13.16 *Additional sutures have been placed between the fundus and the diaphragm in order to close the opening into the posterior mediastinum and reinforce the gastroesophageal valve.*

diaphragm. The third attempt used a 270° fundoplication surrounding four to five cm of oesophagus. These techniques were known as the Belsey Mark I, II, and III respectively. The Mark III procedure was the most effective in securing the lower segment of the oesophagus. The Belsey Mark III was further modified by reducing the number of fundoplicating sutures from three to two to simplify the training of residents. In 1952 the Belsey Mark IV was adopted (Fig. 13.17). The procedure has four elements, namely exposure, mobilisation, crus approximation, and fundoplication.

Long-term results of the Belsey Mark IV have been reported by many groups.[45–47] These studies have reported good to excellent results in 78 to 84% of patients undergoing this procedure by conventional (open) means.

Preliminary results of the thoracoscopic Belsey Mark IV repair
In 1997, we reported our first series of 11 patients treated with a video-thoracoscopic (VATS) Belsey Mark IV antireflux procedure.[49] All patients had severe gastroesophageal reflux. The primary indication for the Belsey Mark IV surgery was oesophageal dysmotility. Four 10 mm ports were inserted over the left hemithorax and were used for the thoracoscopic procedure.

In three patients, a conversion to mini-thoracotomy (8 mm incision) was required — two for repair of a gastric perforation and one for dense adhesions. The remaining seven patients were completed thoracoscopically. The average operating time was 3.9 hours. Postoperative barium swallow showed no leaks, and a typical Mark IV appearance. Hospital stay averaged 4.6 days overall and less than three days for the last five patients. All patients are off antacids, and asymptomatic at a mean follow-up of three months. The results of this series demonstrate that the thoracoscopic technique is feasible with good short-term results. Subsequent follow-up of 15 patients at a median interval of 19 months[50] showed that two-thirds were asymptomatic. Three required further laparoscopic Nissen wrap for persistent reflux. One was maintained on H_2 anatagonist therapy and one with concurrent achalasia underwent oesophagectomy. Champion has recently presented his series of 17 patients undergoing thoracoscopic Belsey Mark IV.[48] His preliminary results showed good relief of symptoms and minimal morbidity.

Long-term follow-up is necessary to adequately gauge the effectiveness of this procedure in comparison to the open approach.

Conclusion

Gastroesophageal reflux disease is a chronic condition affecting 5–10% of the population. The diagnosis of GERD

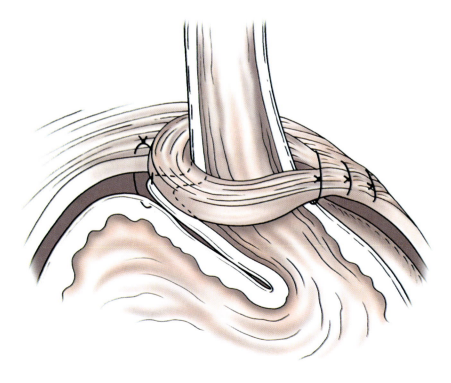

Figure 13.17 *Saggital section of a completed Belsey Mark IV. This figure depicts a 3–4 cm length of abdominal oesophagus and a 240° wrap of stomach around the oesophagus.*

is a challenging one to the physician because of the wide variety of presentations associated with this disease. In addition to patient history, the diagnosis relies heavily on the use of objective tests to determine the presence of pathological reflux. Surgical management of GERD is aimed at restoring the antireflux barrier. Because surgery repairs a defective antireflux mechanism it is important that a defective mechanism be noted.

There are a variety of antireflux surgical options. Many of these procedures are now routinely approached laparoscopically. The success rates of these minimally invasive approaches appear to be as effective as their respective open procedures. Patient comfort, pain management, hospital stay, and return to work have all improved dramatically with the minimally invasive approach.

References

1 Petersen H. The prevalence of gastroesophageal reflux disease. *Scandinavian Journal of Gastroenterology*-Supplement; **211**: 5–6.

2 Spechler SJ. Epidemiology and natural history of gastroesophageal reflux disease (review). *Digestion* 1992 51-supplement; **1**: 24–9.

3 Hinder RA, Filipi CJ. The laparoscopic management of gastroesophageal reflux disease. *Advances in Surgery*; **28**: 41–58.

4 Isolauri J, Laippala P. Prevalence of symptoms suggestive of gastroesophageal reflux disease in the adult population. *Annals of Medicine* 1995 Feb; **27**(1): 67–70.

5 Bremner RM, Bremner CG, DeMeester TR. Gastroesophageal reflux: the use of pH monitoring. *Current Problems in Surgery* 1995; **6**: 429–568.

6 Stein HJ, DeMeester TR. Who benefits from antireflux surgery? *World Journal of Surgery* 1992; **16**: 313–19.

7 Traube M. The spectrum of symptoms and presentations of gastroesophageal reflux disease. *Gastroenterology clinics of North America* 1990; **19**(3): 609–16.

8 Peters JH, DeMeester TR. Gastroesophageal reflux. *Surgical Clinics of North America* 1993; **73**(6): 1119–44.

9 DeMeester TR, Wang CI, Wernly JA *et al*. Technique, indications, and clinical use of 24 hour esophageal monitoring. *J Thoracic and Cardiovascular Surgery* 1980; **79**: 656–70.

10 DeMeester TR, Constantini M. Function tests. In: Pearson FG, Deslauriers J, Ginsberg RJ *et al*. (eds) Esophageal Surgery. New York, Churchill Livingstone, 1995; 119–150.

11 Zaninolto, DeMeester TR, Schweizer W *et al*. The lower esophageal sphincter in health and disease. *Am J Surg* 1988; **155**: 104–11.

12 Kahrilas PJ, Dodds WJ, Hogan WJ. Effect of peristaltic dysfunction on esophageal volume clearance. *Gastroenterology* 1988; **94**: 73–80.

13 Spechler SJ and the Department of Veterans Affairs Gastroesophageal Reflux Study Group. Comparison of medical and surgical treatments for gastroesophageal reflux in Veterans. *NEJM* 1992; **326**: 786–92.

14 Anonymous. Omeprazole. *Med Lett Ther* 1990; **32**: 19–21.

15 Coley CM, Barry MJ, Spechler SJ *et al*. Initial medical versus surgical therapy for complicated or chronic gastroesophageal reflux disease. *Gastroenterology* 1993; **104**: A5 (Abstract).

16 Stein HJ, Feussner H, Siewart JR. Failure of antireflux surgery: causes and management. *American Journal of Surgery*; **171**(1): 36–9. Discussion, 39–40 1996 Jan.

17 Condon RE, Hinder RA. Laparoscopic Nissen fundoplication. *Current Techniques in General Surgery*; Volume 2 Issue 4 1993.

18 Nissen R. Eine einfache operation zur beinflussung der reflux esophagitis. *Schweiz Med Wochenschhr* 1956; **86**: 590–92.

19 Dor J, Humbert P, Dor V, Figarella J. L'intérêt de la technique du Nissen modifée la prevention aprés cardiomyotomie extra muquese de Heller. *Mem Acad Chir* 1962; **88**: 877.

20 Toupet A. Technique d'oesophagogastroplastie avec phrenogastroplexie appliquée dans la crure radical les hernia hiatales et comme complement de l'operation de Heller dans les cardiospasmus. *Mem Acad Chir* 1963; **89**: 374.

21 Donahue PE, Samelson S, Nyhus LM, Bombeck CT. The floppy Nissen fundoplication: effective long-term control of pathologic reflux. *Arch Surg* 1985; **120**: 663.

22 DeMeester TR, Bonavina L, Albertucci M. Nissen fundoplication for gastroesophageal reflux disease: evaluation of primary repair in 100 consecutive patients. *Annals of Surgery* 1986; **204**: 9.

23 Dallemagne B, Weerts JM, Jehacs C *et al*. Laparoscopic Nissen fundoplication: preliminary report. *Surgical Laparoscopic Endoscopy* 1991; **1**: 138–43.

24 Hinder RA, Filipi CJ. The technique of laparoscopic Nissen fundoplication. *Surg Lap Endo* 1992; **2**: 265.

25 Ferguson CM, Rattner DW. Initial experience with laparoscopic Nissen fundoplication. *The American Surgeon* 1995; **61**: 21–3.

26 Cadiére GB, Houben JJ, Bruyns J *et al*. Laparoscopic Nissen fundoplication: technique and preliminary results. *Brit J Surg* 1994; **81**: 400–3.

27 Bittner HB, Meyers WC, Brazer SR, Pappas TN. Laparoscopic Nissen fundoplication: operative results and short-term follow up. *The American Journal of Surgery*; **167**: 193–98. Discussion 199–200.

28 Pitcher DE, Curet MJ, Martin DT et al. Successful management of severe gastroesophageal reflux disease with laparoscopic Nissen fundoplication. *The American Journal of Surgery*; **168**: 547–53. Discussion 553–554.

29 Hinder RA, Filipi CJ, Wetscher G et al. Laparoscopic Nissen fundoplication is an effective treatment for gastroesophageal reflux disease. *Annals of Surgery*; **220**(4): 472–83.

30 Jameison GG, Watson DI, Britten-Jones R *et al*. Laparoscopic Nissen fundoplication. *Annals of Surgery* 1994; **220**(2): 137–45.

31 Naunheim KS, Landreneau RJ, Andrus CH *et al*. Laparoscopic fundoplication: a natural extension for the thoracic surgeon. Accepted for presentation at the 1996 Annual Meeting of The Southern Thoracic Surgical Association.

32 Low DE. Examination of outcome and cost data of open and laparoscopic antireflux operations at Virginia Mason Medical Center in Seattle. *Surgical Endoscopy* 1995; **9**(12): 1326–8.

33 Schauer PR, Luketich JD, Dunkleman M *et al*. Outpatient laparoscopic Nissen fundoplication is safe and cost effective in selected patients. Submitted for presentation at the 1997 Annual Meeting of the Society of American Gastrointestinal Endoscopic Surgeons.

34 Thor KBA, Silander T. A long-term randomized prospective trial of the Nissen procedure versus a modified Toupet technique. *Annals of Surgery* 1989; **210**: 719–24.

35 Tucker JG, Ramshaw BJ, Newman CL et al. Laparoscopic fundoplication in treatment of severe gastroesophageal disease: preliminary results of a prospective trial. *Southern Medical Journal* 1996; **89**(1): 60–4.

36 McKernan JB. Laparoscopic repair of gastroesophageal reflux: Toupet partial fundoplication versus Nissen fundoplication. *Surgical Endoscopy* 1994; **8**: 851–6.

37 Hill LD. Progress in the surgical management of hiatal hernia. *World Journal of Surgery* 1977; **1**: 425.

38 Hill LD. Intraoperative measurements of LES pressure. *Journal of Thoracic and Cardiovascular Surgery* 1978; **75**: 3.

39 Hill LD, Kraemer SJM, Aye RM, Kozarek RA, Snopkowski P. Laparoscopic Hill repair. *Contemporary Surgery*; 1994; **44**(1): 13–20.

40 Aye RW, Hill LD, Kraemer SJM, Snopkowski P. Early results with the laparoscopic Hill repair. *American Journal of Surgery* 1993; **167**: 542–6.

41 Snow LL, Weinstein LS, Hannon JK. Laparoscopic construction of gastroesophageal anatomy for treatment of reflux disease. *Surgical Endoscopy* 1995; **9**: 774–80.

42 Hiebert CA, Belsey R. Incompetency of the gastric cardia without radiologic evidence of hiatal hernia. *J Thoracic and Cardiovasc Surg* 1961; **53**: 33.

43 Skinner DB, Belsey R. Surgical management of esophageal reflux and hiatus hernia: long-term results in 1,030 patients. *J Thoracic and Cardiovasc Surg* 1967; **53**: 33.

44 Belsey RHR. History of antireflux surgery. In: Pearson FG, Deslauriers J, Ginsberg RJ *et al.* (eds) *Esophageal Surgery*. New York, Churchill Livingstone, 1995; pp 209–13.

45 Lerut T, Coosemans, Christaens R, Gruwez JA. The Belsey Mark IV antireflux procedure: reflections on indications and long-term results. *Acta Gastro-enterologica Belgica* 1990; **13**: 585.

46 Hiebert GA, O'Meara CS. The Belsey operation for hiatal hernia: a twenty year experience. *Am J Surg* 1979; **137**: 532.

47 Orringer MB, Belsey R, Skinner DB. Long-term results of the Mark IV operation for hiatal hernia and analyses of recurrences and their treatment. *J Thorac and Cardiovasc Surgery* 1972; **63**: 25.

48 Champion JK, McKernan JB. Thoracoscopic Belsey fundoplication for complicated gastroesophageal disease. Presented at The Minimally Invasive Thoracic Surgery Interest Group, First International Symposium. Boston, Massachusetts, September 1996.

49 Luketich JD, Hutson B, Ninan M *et al.* Videothoracoscopic Belsey Mark IV antireflux procedure. Presentation at the 1997 Annual Meeting of the Society of American Gastrointestinal Endoscopic Surgeons.

50 Nguyen NT, Schauer PR, Hutson W *et al.* Preliminary results of thoracoscopic Belsey Mark IV antireflux procedure. *Surg Lap Endosc* 1998; **8**: 185–8.

Oesophagectomy

O.J. McAnena

14

Introduction

The five-year overall survival rate for carcinoma of the oesophagus is less than 5%.[1,2] Although conventional oesophageal resection achieves some cures, it may be associated with a morbidity rate of up to 45% in patients who are often elderly and infirm.[3,4] Mortality rates vary quite widely between different centres, but range from 0–28% with a median around 10–12%.[3,4] Other options such as radiotherapy, chemotherapy, intubation and laser re-cannulisation, provide palliation in some patients but may have complications which result in a poorer palliative outcome than surgery,[5] and which may even be lethal.

Surgical strategies

The complexities of surgical resection for oesophageal carcinoma are exacerbated by the anatomical difficulties in access. Several quite different approaches are currently used in conventional oesophagectomy (Table 14.1).[6,7,8]

While blunt (trans-hiatal) oesophagectomy appears to decrease the risk of postoperative pulmonary dysfunction,[9] it is a blind procedure which is associated with well-defined perioperative risks. These include haemorrhage (particularly from azygos vein trauma), chylous leak from thoracic duct injury[10] and an increased incidence of tumour rupture and bronchial injury compared with an open thorax procedure.[11] Formal lymph node dissection is not possible using the trans-

Technique	Typical incisions	Anastomosis
Three-stage (McKeown)	Upper midline abdominal Right posterolateral Thoracotomy cervical	Cervical
Two-stage (Ivor Lewis)	Upper midline abdominal Right posterolateral Thoracotomy	Intrathoracic
Thoraco-abdominal	Oblique left thoracolaparotomy	Intrathoracic
Trans-hiatal	Upper midline abdominal Cervical	Cervical

Table 14.1

Access routes and anastomotic sites for conventional open oesophagectomy techniques

hiatal route and there is evidence to suggest improved long-term survival if this is undertaken by open thoracotomy.[12] Open thoracotomy is required for nodal dissection which contributes to postoperative pulmonary dysfunction and can lead to morbidity from thoracic wound pain. Formal thoracotomy restricts postoperative respiratory excursion, provoking atelectasis and chest infection. Moreover, a multi-cavity approach and the necessity to re-position, prolongs the operating time and magnifies the physiological insult. Avoidance of formal thoracotomy by the abdomino-cervical approach may allow more rapid oesophagectomy without increasing the risk of postoperative death, and appears to give a quality of palliation at least equivalent to that of conventional trans-thoracic oesophageal excision.[13]

Against this background, a minimal access approach to oesophagectomy utilising video endoscopic surgical techniques is an attractive option. In theory, at least, the deficiencies of trans-hiatal oesophagectomy are overcome as the surgical resection is performed under direct vision and the potential exists to perform a full lymph node dissection whilst avoiding the perceived insult of a thoracic incision and exposure of the thoracic cavity.[14]

An alternate minimal access strategy for oesophagectomy — endoscopic mediastinal dissection — has been described by Buess[15] who has reported an experience of over 35 cases. This technique is, however, suited only to T1 lesions. The majority of tumours will, therefore, require a trans-thoracic endoscopic approach as will be described in detail for our own technique.

Patient selection

Careful patient selection is important for successful application of videothoracoscopic techniques to oesophagectomy as this form of oesophageal dissection is technically demanding. In the initial phase of surgical experience it is preferable to have the optimum opportunity to appreciate the technique by operating on a lower-third oesophageal carcinoma as tumours in the upper- and middle-thirds are even more demanding. The ideal applications are, therefore, the management of benign disease such as a lye stricture and early malignant lesions of the oesophagogastric junction and lower-third of the oesophagus.

Pre-operative evaluation will depend on the underlying diagnosis, but for malignant cases should include the standard investigations of endoscopy and biopsy, barium swallow and meal, liver ultrasound, oesophageal ultrasound bronchoscopy (for middle- and upper-third tumours) and computerised tomographic scanning of the thorax and upper abdomen. Pre-operative plain chest films, pulmonary function tests, arterial blood gas estimation and cardiological assessment are routine. Intravenous digoxin may be considered in the peri-operative period to decrease the effect of postoperative supraventricular dysrhythmias. As with any such major surgery, an experienced anaesthetist is mandatory.

Thoracoscopic oesophagectomy

Anaesthesia, positioning and patient preparation

The standard surgical procedure is as follows. Anaesthesia by double-lumen endobronchial tube is required. Monitoring is effected by bladder catheterisation, right internal jugular CVP catheter, a left radial arterial line and continuous intra-operative pulse oximetry measurement. The patient is positioned, prepared and draped as for a standard right thoracotomy (Fig. 14.1). A flexible gastroscope is advanced before draping the patient.

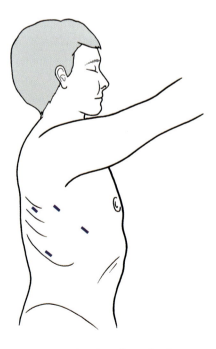

Figure 14.1 *Patient is placed in the right thoracotomy position. The gastroscope is inserted prior to draping.*

Port placement

A 10 mm trocar is sited in the fifth interspace in the anterior axillary line and the thoracoscope is advanced through this port into the chest cavity. The remaining ports are then placed such that:

- the ports are as far away from each other as possible,
- instruments can be moved in all directions freely, and
- the trocar sites allow repositioning of the telescope wherever they are placed.

These considerations usually require a 12 mm trocar placed in the 9th interspace in the posterior axillary line, a 10 mm trocar sited just below, and 1 cm anterior to the inferior angle of the scapula and an additional trocar is placed later on in the procedure in the sixth or seventh interspace in the anterior axillary line (Fig. 14.2).

Operating team positions

The operating surgeon stands initially on the patient's left hand side with the operating monitor placed opposite, to the left of the operating assistant's shoulder. The assistant's monitor is placed to the right of the operating surgeon (Fig. 14.3). The nurse stands to the left of the operating surgeon. A second assistant, who is experienced in gastroscopy, sits with the anaesthetist at the head of the table.

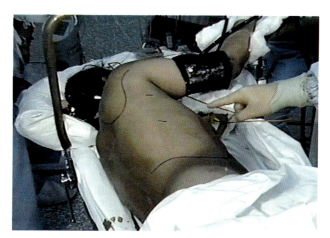

Figure 14.2 *Port placement.*

General considerations

Prior to insertion of the ports, the right lung is deflated by the anaesthetist. In the initial stages, despite effective single lung anaesthesia, there may be residual air trapping in the right lung which will require to be controlled by pressure from a lung retractor for a period of time. This can last up to 30 minutes before lung collapse on the right side is complete. Carbon dioxide insufflation can be utilised, but great caution should be exercised. Use of an automatic insufflator set at 5 mm of mercury pressure will decrease the risk of creating a tension pneumothorax. Occasionally, it

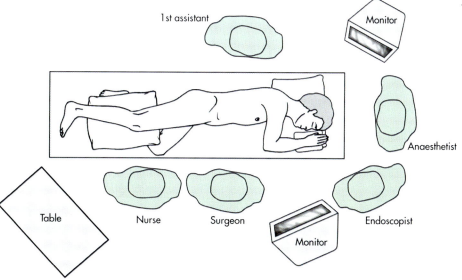

Figure 14.3 *Operator positions.*

may be necessary to use up to 1 litre of carbon dioxide insufflation in the early stages to aid in right lung compression. Some authors have suggested that placing the patient in a more prone position for oesophageal dissection may have technical advantages and by reducing post-operative respiratory complications.[16]

During the course of the procedure, the operating surgeon transfers to the opposite side of the table. This facilitates dissection of the upper third of the oesophagus. Advancement of the gastroscope confirms the exact position of the oesophagus in the posterior mediastinum. The tumour is visualised to detect any unforeseen invasion of adjacent structures that may have been missed on pre-operative imaging. Thoracoscopy in addition will facilitate identification of pleural metastatic deposits that may have gone unrecognised on pre-operative staging. Once deemed resectable, the dissection is initiated away from the primary tumour. The initial steps are designed to encircle the oesophagus. The parietal pleura is divided by sharp dissection (Fig. 14.4). Either diathermy or ultrasonic dissection is utilised. It has been the author's preference to use a Harmonic* scalpel. This device coagulates by ultrasonic energy and reduces the risk of adjacent organ damage because tissue temperatures do not usually exceed 90 degrees centigrade. It also avoids build-up of smoke in the

thoracic cavity and creates minimal nerve stimulation. An adequate suction irrigation system is mandatory. Even small amounts of blood in the operating field will absorb light and diminish the picture quality significantly.

Operative technique

Dissection for lower third tumours begins just below the azygos vein, advancing caudally to the inferior pulmonary ligament. The pleura overlying the azygos is then carefully mobilised and divided cephalad to the thoracic inlet. Careful scissors dissection close to the under surface of the azygos vein is the key to its mobilisation. Care is taken to avoid small tributaries that occasionally enter on its under surface and need to be clipped. The azygos vein is then divided using an endostapler, Vascular‡ endoscopic stapler (Fig. 14.5(a)–(f)). The oesophagus is then mobilised over a distance of 3–4 cm by a combination of distraction of the oesophageal wall with the endoscope within the oesophagus and sharp dissection. Arterial vessels from the anterior wall of the thoracic aorta or intercostal arteries are readily identified, clipped and divided. Eventually the posterior and left walls of the oesophagus free to allow passage of a shaped memory instrument, Roticulating Endo-Grasp,‡ under the oesophagus (Fig. 14.6(a) and (b)). The instrument is manipulated carefully to avoid injury to the oesophageal wall. Once a shaped memory instrument is in

Figure 14.4 *Gastroscope in oesophageal lumen. Pleura is divided over azygos vein by sharp dissection.*

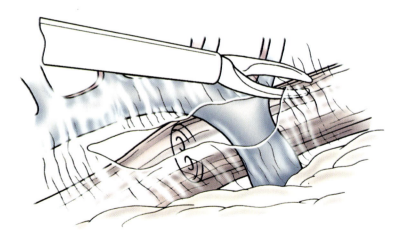

*   Ultracision, Providence, Rhode Island, USA
‡   US Surgical Corp, CT

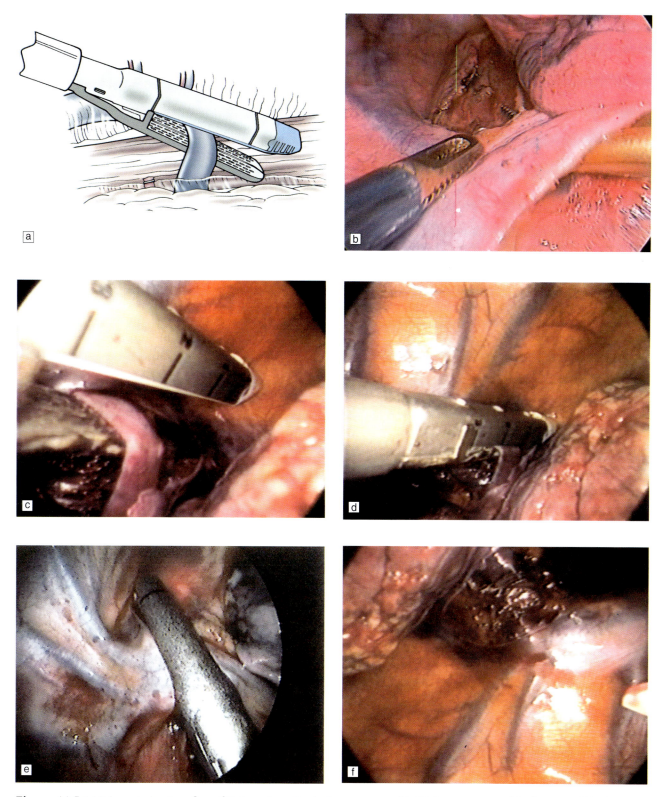

Figure 14.5 *(a) Schematic drawing of use of Endostapler to divide the azygos vein. (b)–(d) Operative views of the dissection of (b) the azygos arch and (c) and (d) the placement of the stapler. (e) Occasionally, use of an angled videothoracoscope may be helpful in showing the position of the stapler across the vein more clearly. (f) Appearance of the stapled stump of the azygos vein. (b) and (e) are courtesy of Dr. D Gossot.*

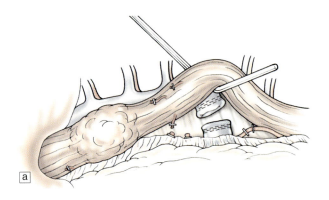

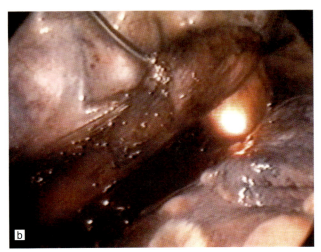

Figure 14.6 *(a) Diagrammatic and (b) operative views of the use of a shaped memory instrument to elevate the oesophagus during dissection.*

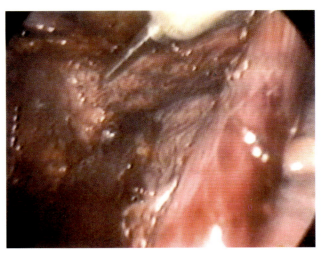

Figure 14.7 *Harmonic scalpel in use for peri-oesophageal dissection.*

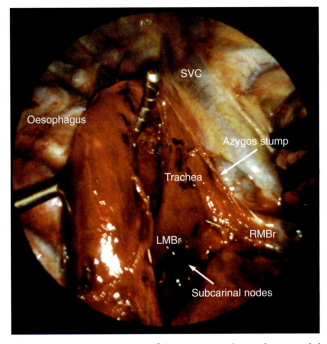

Figure 14.8 *Operative view of the upper oesophagus during nodal dissection. The oesophagus has been elevated and the upper mediastinum and posterior tracheal wall has been cleared of surrounding tissue. Partially mobilised subcarinal glands remain to be excised. (Courtesy of Dr D Gossot).*

position, traction and angulation of the introducer proximally will facilitate oesophageal dissection under direct vision. Dissection between the oesophagus and trachea is performed by sharp scissors, without diathermy or by Harmonic scalpel dissection (Fig. 14.7). Diathermy at this point may cause heat injury to the membranous trachea with disastrous consequences.[17]

With increasing experience, a complete lymphadenectomy encompassing the right para-oesophageal, bilateral middle and lower para-oesophageal, right paratracheal, sub-carinal, posterior mediastinal and bilateral pulmonary nodes can potentially be performed in a manner similar to that at open thoracotomy. This type of dissection is extensive, difficult and time consuming. One cannot expect to be able to perform this without considerable experience in the technique (Fig. 14.8).

Dissection can be performed cephalad to behind the thyroid gland and caudad to the diaphragmatic hiatus. For large, bulky tumours the dissection is more difficult and demanding, and may require resection of some of the contralateral mediastinal pleura. Once haemostasis has been achieved, a 24 or 28 French thoracostomy tube is advanced through the most inferior and anterior port before lung inflation, under direct vision. The skin incisions are then closed.

The patient is then placed in the supine position and the abdominal phase of the procedure is performed through either a bilateral subcostal or an upper midline incision. Gastric mobilisation is performed in the usual manner. We usually perform the neck dissection on the left side, carefully identifying and preserving the left recurrent laryngeal nerve. The specimen is delivered into the abdomen and divided at the gastric cardia. A greater curvature gastric tube is constructed and brought through the posterior mediastinal tunnel. Oesophago-gastrostomy is then performed in the neck. We prefer to use 3.0. polyglycolic acid for the anastomosis and routinely place a jejunostomy feeding tube.

All patients are transferred to the Intensive Care Unit post-operatively and depending on their overall condition, they may remain routinely ventilated overnight or longer. Jejunostomy feeding is initiated within 36 hours of surgery.

Post-operative considerations

Thoracoscopically-assisted oesophagectomy has the theoretical appeal of allowing oesophageal dissection under direct vision whilst avoiding the need for thoracotomy. This conceptually overcomes the adverse problems of open thoracotomy in a thoracolaparotomy, three-stage or Ivor Lewis oesophagectomy and the blunt nature of a trans-hiatal oesophageal dissection. Experience with thoracoscopic oesophagectomy is internationally limited. The available data (Tables 14.2, 14.3) would suggest that a thoracoscopic approach to dissection of the oesophagus is both feasible and

Table 14.2

Reported series of VATS oesophagectomy

Report (year)	Collard[16] (1993)	Gossot[17] (1993)	Descottes[18] (1993)	Azagra[19] (1993)	Cuschieri[20] (1994)	McAnena[14] (1994)	Mitchell[21] (1994)	Perachia[22] (1995)	Law[23] (1997)
Patients	15	15	19	8	26	9	8	18	22
Conversions	3	3	5	0	1	1	0	0	4
Severe respiratory complication	2	2	3	7	3	3	2	2	3
Blood loss (ml)	–	200	–	600	Nil Measured*	>600	1500	210	450
Thoracoscopy time (mins.)	150–360	–	–	180	–	128	150	114	110
Lymph node harvest (no.)	21–15	–	–	–	–	9–26	11	12	7
Operative mortality	1	0	0	0	0	0	0	1	1

Adapted from Peracchia A, Rosati R, Fumagalli U, Bona S, Chella B. Thoracoscopic dissection of the esophagus for cancer. *Int Surg* 1997; **82**: 1–4

* Excludes one patient with massive blood loss from aortic injury

Table 14.3

Combined data from collected oesophagectomy series in Table 14.2*

Total number of collected patients	140
Rate of conversion to open thoracotomy	12%
Incidence of severe respiratory complications	19%
Average blood loss during thoracoscopic phase	486 ml
Average duration of thoracoscopic phase	151 minutes
Average number of lymph nodes harvested	16
Operative mortality	2.1%

*Derived and averaged from available reported data — some inaccuracy will result from the effect of missing data.

safe with low conversion and operative mortality rates. Lymph node harvest is similar to that achieved at open dissection suggesting that oncological principles can be respected for appropriate early tumours. In our experience, however,[14] the mean time for thoracoscopic oesophageal mobilisation has ranged from 100 to 160 minutes and the mean total operating procedure time has ranged from 250 to 360 minutes. Prolonged right lung collapse increases the risk of postoperative pulmonary complications, and we have indeed noted that virtually all patients who have had such prolonged single lung ventilation will demonstrate, on the immediate postoperative chest X-ray after re-expansion of the lung, evidence of persistent segmental collapse. (Our single most significant complication has been pulmonary, in that all patients developed some degree of right lung consolidation. Some required bronchoscopy to assist removal of right bronchial secretions and most required assisted ventilation for at least 72 hours. None however needed formal tracheotomy). Cuschieri[20] has described the use of a prone position in an attempt to avoid prolonged single lung ventilation (see Chapter 12, Figure 12.7), and has stated that there were no significant pulmonary complications with this approach although only six patients had undergone prone surgery at the time of his report. Our impression, however, which is shared by Peracchia[22] from his review of the literature, is that the perceived potential

for improved postoperative pulmonary function and diminished pulmonary complications which could potentially have been provided by a thoracoscopic approach to oesophageal dissection, has not been realised.

Other techniques

Trans-mediastinal endoscopic oesophageal dissection

This technique involves oesophageal endo-dissection which allows for mediastinal dissection of the thoracic oesophagus by the use of a mediastinoscope, video endoscopy and dedicated instruments. Structures such as the trachea, both main bronchi, the vagal trunks, the parietal pleura and mediastinal lymph nodes can be regularly identified. Bumm and Siewert[24] found that endo-dissection is helpful intra-operatively because mediastinal dissection can be performed simultaneously with the abdominal approach: the main anatomic structures as well as tumour staging information can be determined even before the hiatus is opened by the abdominal team. Major intra-operative complications are rare (5.3%), and can usually be managed without thoracotomy.[18] The comparative data from a previous prospective study performed revealed that the main clinical advantage of endo-dissection over conventional trans-hiatal oesophagectomy was a low rate of postoperative pulmonary complications and recurrent laryngeal nerve palsy. The author feels that this is a technical improvement, but it does not solve the problem of the limited dissection of trans-hiatal oesophagectomy, because a systemic lymphadenectomy cannot be performed. In order to utilise this technique, it would be advisable to attend a course or proctorship with the surgeons who practise this very specialised procedure.

Thoracoscopic oesophagectomy with intrathoracic stapled anastomosis

The techniques are experimental at present and involve either a trans-oral or trans-hiatal approach.[25] For the trans-oral technique the stapler is inserted from above. The anvil, which is connected to a wire, is drawn into the abdomen together with the distal oesophagus. Retracting the wire pulls both the anvil and the stomach up into the thorax after the insertion of the anvil. The second technique requires a special attachment to introduce the anvil trans-hiatally into the thorax and into the oesophageal stump. The gastric tube is pushed into the thorax by the stapler gun, which is inserted into the stomach through an antrostomy. The insertion of the anvil into the oesophageal stump can also be achieved with the support of a flexible endoscope including a polyp snare.

Combined thoracoscopic and laparoscopic oesophagectomy

Bessell *et al.*[26] have described a combined thoracoscopic and laparoscopic approach with oesophago-gastric reconstruction in the chest. These surgeons have utilised this technique in an experimental setting. A three-step operation has been performed consisting of thoracoscopic oesophageal dissection, laparoscopic gastric mobilisation, and thoracoscopic oesophago-gastric anastomosis using a circular endoluminal stapler. Conversion to open surgery was required only once during a gastric dissection, and all anastomoses were safely constructed thoracoscopically. The question of intrathoracic anastomosis is a matter for considerable debate and individual surgeon preference. One is always fearful of the breakdown of an intra-mediastinal anastomosis. However, an Ivor Lewis type laparoscopic dissection of the stomach and thoracoscopic dissection of the lower-third of the oesophagus would appear feasible.

Discussion

The prognosis for patients with oesophageal carcinoma remains very poor. Therapy for dysphagia from tumour obstruction varies through dilatation, laser therapy, electro-coagulation and intubation, to various forms of surgery. When resection is performed with curative intent, it gives the best results for dysphagia and is the only hope of cure. The present options for surgery carry certain advantages and disadvantages. Trans-hiatal oesophagectomy is believed to carry a lower incidence of postoperative pulmonary complications compared to either the three-stage or thoraco-abdominal approaches, which necessitate an open thoracotomy. Because it is a blind procedure, there is significantly greater risk of haemorrhage from bleeding oesophageal vessels, or from the azygos vein tributaries which may require emergency thoracotomy. Bronchial rupture may occur, particularly for middle-third carcinomas and the incidence of thoracic duct injury seems higher than with open surgery. Lymph node dissection, which may improve survival in some cases, is not an option with trans-hiatal resection.

Thoracotomy incisions facilitate dissection under direct vision and allow for lymph node dissection. The risks of haemorrhage, chylothorax, bronchial rupture, or tumour rupture are diminished, but the risk of postoperative pulmonary complications is believed to increase. Thoracotomy incisions induce considerable pain and may result in long-term discomfort. Both the two- and three-stage procedures involve significant post-operation morbidity which is undesirable, particularly in patients with poor long-term outlook, and who from the outset are frequently elderly and debilitated.

Right thoracoscopic-assisted oesophagectomy is conceptually appealing in that a thoracotomy incision is avoided and dissection and haemostasis are performed under direct vision. Although we have not pursued a policy of formal mediastinal lymph node dissection, we believe that with increasing experience it is feasible through this approach. In this respect it is superior to the mediastinoscopic approach developed by Buess *et al.*[27] Because the mediastinoscopic instrument is straight, the olive at the end of the operating mediastinoscope impinges on the aorta when the lower third of the thoracic oesophagus is reached, rendering this part of the dissection difficult unless the instrument is held in the correct alignment by the abdominal surgeon. This mediastinoscopic technique has the advantage of allowing the surgeon to perform the entire operation without changing the position of the patient on the operating table.[27]

Careful selection is important as patients with small, mobile tumours appear to be more suitable for VATS oesophagectomy. With bigger tumours, the loss of surgical planes complicates thoracoscopic dissection and requires increasing expertise.

The size of the thoracic cavity varies from patient to patient. In trocar placement it is better to err on the side of separating trocar positions as far away as possible, especially in the smaller patient. This reduces the technical problem of 'crossing swords' (instruments), during dissection. The port positions described are guidelines and, as in laparoscopic surgery, are not absolute.

Simultaneous use of the gastroscope within the oesophagus improves visualisation and facilitates elevation of the oesophagus from its mediastinal bed. This is helpful when encircling the oesophagus, which can be difficult. This manoeuvre must be done carefully and patiently in order to avoid the risk of oesophageal perforation. The oesophagus should be encircled well away from the tumour so as to avoid disturbing the tumour and because this makes subsequent dissection of the tumour easier. We have found that dividing the azygos vein in the early stages of the dissection helps encirclement of the oesophagus. The use of the gastroscope as an aid in improving illumination and distracting the oesophageal wall from within is a very helpful measure. Illumination is essential to dissection and increasing familiarity with the use of the Harmonic* scalpel, has decreased the need for frequent suction–irrigation, which unnecessarily prolongs the procedure. Heat transmission from monopolar diathermy can be more extensive than intended and is particularly dangerous when dissecting the upper third of the oesophagus close to the thin membranous trachea.

Prolonged deflation of the right lung certainly contributes to the frequency of postoperative lung complications. Hopefully this can be overcome by decreasing the time for dissection of the oesophagus. Perhaps the surgical approach using the prone position, as recommended by Cuschieri[16], may go some way towards improving the problem. Alternatively, intermittent re-inflation may decrease the postoperative pulmonary complications that we have experienced.

Thoracoscopic oesophagectomy holds some potential for future management of oesophageal problems. However, surgeons who undertake this form of surgery must have training and capability to proceed immediately to standard open thoracotomy if necessary. Prior laboratory experience is helpful. It has been the author's experience that the pig model is not particularly helpful in learning oesophageal dissection techniques thoracoscopically. Canine models appear to more resemble the human dissection.

Present data suggest that hospital stay is not shortened. As experience increases, intra-operative measures may be adopted to help overcome the postoperative problems. Until these are resolved, or contrary data is presented from other centres, the use of thoracoscopic oesophagectomy cannot be universally recommended. A VATS approach may, however, be of some limited value in the staging and assessment of oesophageal carcinoma. In this context it has been shown to offer significant accuracy (88%) in determining intrathoracic lymph node status, and overall staging is particularly effective when combined with laparoscopic sample of the coeliac nodes.[28,29] This technique may prove to be useful in the evaluation of patients with regard to entry into study protocols, although the primary decision regarding whether or not to operate is likely to continue to be made on the basis of conventional techniques.

---

* Ultracision, Providence, Rhode Island, USA

VATS oesophagectomy — summary points

- Intractable benign strictures or very early stage cancers are appropriate cases
- An endoscope placed within the oesophageal lumen prior to surgery can be used to elevate the oesophagus intraoperatively in order to facilitate dissection
- The azygos arch should be divided in order to provide good access to the oesophagus
- Considerable care is required during dissection of the upper third because of the risk of posterior tracheal, vascular or neural injury
- Full mediastinal lymphadenectomy is feasible but difficult
- Collected experience suggests that the procedure is infrequent but safe with a reported operative mortality of 2% and conversion rate of 12%
- Postoperative pulmonary complications are common, prevent early discharge and limit the potential advantages of the procedure.

References

1 Earlam R, Cunha-Melo JR. Oesophageal squamous cell carcinoma: 1. A critical review of surgery. Br J Surg 1980; 67: 381–90.
2 Silverberg E. Cancer statistics 1979. Cancer J Clin 1979; 29: 20.
3 Mitchell RL. Abdominal and right thoracotomy approach as standard procedure for oesophago-gastrectomy with low morbidity. J Thorac Cardiovasc Surg 1987; 93: 205–11.
4 Lam KH, Cheung HC, Wong J, Ong GB. The present state of surgical treatment of carcinoma of the oesophagus. J R Coll Surg Edinb 1982; 27: 315–26.
5 Skinner DB. En bloc resection for neoplasms of the oesophagus and cardia. J Thorac Cardiovasc Surg 1983; 85: 59–71.
6 McKeown KC. The surgical treatment of carcinoma of the oesophagus. A review of the results in 478 cases. J R Coll Surg Edinb 1985; 30: 1–14.
7 Orringer MB. Trans-thoracic versus trans-hiatal oesophagectomy: what different does it make? Ann Thorac Surg 1987; 44: 116–8.
8 Tanner NC. The present position of carcinoma of the oesophagus. Postgrad Med J 1947; 23: 109–39.
9 Muller JM, Erasmi H, Stelzner M, Zieren U et al. Surgical therapy of oesophageal carcinoma. Br J Surg 1990; 77: A45–57.
10 Fok M, Siu KF, Wong J. A comparison of transhiatal and trans thoracic resection for carcinoma of the thoracic oesophagus. Am J Surg 1989; 158: 414–9.
11 Bolger C, Walsh TN, Tanner WA et al. Chylothorax after oesophagectomy. Br J Surg 1991; 78: 587–9.
12 Khoury GA. Oesophageal surgery under Akiyama. Lancet 1989; i: 91–2.
13 Gotley DC, Beard J, Kruper MJ et al. Abdomino-cervical trans-hiatal oesophagectomy in the management of oesophageal carcinoma. Br J Surg 1990; 77: 815–19.
14 McAnena OJ, Rogers J, Williams NS. Right thoracoscopically assisted oesophagectomy for cancer. Br J Surg 1994; 81: 236–8.
15 Manncke K, Raestrup H, Walter D et al. Technique of endoscopic mediastinal dissection of the oesophagus. Endoscopic Surgery and Allied Technologies 1994; 2: 10–15.
16 McAnena OJ, Willson PD. Diathermy in laparoscopic surgery. Br J Surg 1993; 80: 1094–96.
16 Collard JM, Lengele B, One JB, Kestens PJ. En bloc and standard esophagectomies by thoracoscopy. Ann Thorac Surg 1993; 56: 675–9.
17 Gossot D, Fourquier P, Celerier M. Thoracoscopic esophagectomy: technique and initital results. Ann Thorac Surg 1993; 56: 667–70.
18 Descottes B, Valleix D, Sodji M et al. Oesophagectomie sous thoracoscopie. Proceedings XVI Journées Niçoises Pathologie et Chirurgie Digestives – Video Laparoscopie. Nice 11–12 Feb 1993.
19 Azagra JS, Ceuterick M, Goergen M et al. Thoracoscopic in oesophagectomy for oesophageal cancer. Br J Surg 1993; 80: 320–1.
20 Cuschieri A. Thoracoscopic subtotal oesophagectomy. Endoscopic Surgery and Allied Technologies 1994; 2: 21–25.
21 Mitchell I, Corless DJ, Deligiannis E, Wastell C. Thoracoscopy oesophagectomy. Minimally Invasive Therapy 1994; 3: 307–10
22 Peracchia A, Rosati R, Fumagalli U et al. Thoracoscopic dissection of the esophagus for cancer. Int Surg 1997; 82: 1–4
23 Law S, Fok M, Chu KM, Wong J. Thoracoscopic esophagectomy for esophageal cancer. Surgery 1997; 122: 8–14
24 Bumm R, Siewert JR. Results of tran-mediastinal endoscopic oesophageal dissection. Endoscopic Surgery and Allied Technologies 1994; 2: 16–20.
25 Manncke K, Raestrup H, Kanehira E et al. Thoracoscopic oesophagectomy with intra-thoracal stapled anastomosis. Endoscopic Surgery and Allied Technologies 1994; 2: 37–41.
26 Bessell JR, Maddern GJ, Manncke K et al. Combined thoracoscopic and laparoscopic oesophagectomy and oesophago-gastric reconstruction. Endoscopic Surgery and Allied Technologies 1994; 2: 32–6.
27 Buess G, Kipfmuller K, Nahrun M, Melzer A. Endoskopischemikrochirurgische dissektion des osophagus. I; Buess G, Ed. Endoskopie. Koln: Arzte-Verlag, 1990: 358–75.
28 Krasna MJ, Reed CE, Jaklitsch MT et al. Thoracoscopic staging of esophageal cancer: a prospective, multicentre trial. Ann Thorac Surg 1995; 60: 1337–40.
29 Krasna MJ, Advances in staging of esophageal carcinoma. Chest 1998; 113(1 Suppl): 107S–111S.

Pericardiectomy

S.R. Hazelrigg and M.J. McGee

15

Introduction

Thoracoscopy or video-assisted thoracic surgery (VATS) provides excellent visualisation of the intrathoracic and mediastinal structures. The pericardium is well seen from either thoracic cavity, and the consequent feasibility of VATS pericardiectomy raises questions as to when this surgical route should now be preferred to more traditional approaches. This chapter will attempt to describe the surgical technique of VATS pericardiectomy and outline the potential pitfalls and advantages in order to define the role of this procedure.

History and function

The pericardium has been recognised as an anatomical structure since the time of Hippocrates (460 BC). Lower is credited with the first account of pericardial disease in humans and Riolan, in 1649, suggested pericardiectomy for effusive pericarditis. The physiological consequences of constrictive pericarditis or a large pericardial effusion have been well described, including Kussmaul's (1873) description of paradoxical pulses and elevated venous pressure with inspiration.

The pericardium is a fibrous sac with a smooth serous lining that allows the heart to move in a frictionless manner. There have been several suggested functions for the pericardium. These include preventing the rapid over-dilation of the cardiac chambers especially the right heart; preventing cardiac torsion and impairment of vena caval inflow, and acting as a barrier to infection. The congenital absence, or surgical removal of the pericardium is, however, accompanied by little if any clinical consequences.

Pericardial disease

Several disorders may affect the pericardium but most produce clinical symptoms because of inflammation, the production of a pericardial fluid or by the development of constriction. The inflammatory process may be induced by infection (viral, bacterial, fungal, etc.), myocardial infarction, trauma, or systemic disorders such as connective tissue disease. There are unusual causes such as cholesterol pericarditis which may be seen in association with hypothyroidism. Pericarditis may produce symptoms such as pain and fever as well as the occasional complaints of shortness of breath and dry cough. Symptoms may be improved by sitting and leaning forward. Examination may reveal dysrhythmias and a friction rub. Leukocytosis with a lymphocyte predominance has been described as the classic presentation. Other clinical findings may include ST segment elevation on the electrocardiogram without evidence of infarction. Fluid in the pericardial space may accompany the inflammation and result in an enlarged cardiac silhouette on chest X-rays (Fig. 15.1).

Pericarditis is usually a self-limiting problem although it may recur. It is caused by a diverse group of aetiologic agents including viruses such as Coxsackie and influenza. Treatment of simple non-specific pericarditis generally includes anti-inflammatory agents, but steroids have been used for non responders with success.

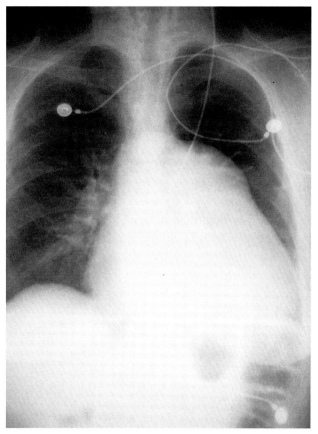

Figure 15.1 *Enlarged cardiac silhouette from a pericardial effusion.*

Surgical consideration for pericardial disease

Pericardial constriction

Invasive intervention in pericardial disease is generally considered because of the development of a pericardial effusion or constriction. Constriction may develop months to years after pericarditis as the fibrous, thickened pericardium constricts around the heart limiting diastolic filling. Constrictive pericarditis eventually reduces cardiac output and results in end organ dysfunction such as renal and hepatic insufficiency. The development of right-sided failure becomes evident by jugular venous distention, hepatomegaly, hepatojugular reflex and ascites. Although peripheral oedema may be present this may be less noticeable than the ascites. Pulsus paradoxus develops when the pulse pressure decreases on inspiration.

Constrictive pericarditis can be a challenging diagnosis to establish and may be confused with myocarditis. Cardiac catheterisation has been the most discriminating test and

demonstrates a diastolic pressure trace in the right ventricle which rises rapidly and then plateaus $\sqrt{}$ with a small "α" wave. There is equalisation of diastolic pressures. Left ventricular end diastolic pressure approximates that of the right but is not as elevated to the extent seen in myopathies and myocarditis.

Pericardiectomy relieves the constrictive process and traditionally has been performed via a median sternotomy or a left thoracotomy. After finding the appropriate plane of dissection above the pericardium, the left ventricle is freed followed by the right so as to prevent the development of pulmonary oedema during surgery. The use of cardiopulmonary bypass is possible but the necessary anticoagulation increases bleeding. Thoracoscopic pericardiectomy, although possible, does not seem appropriate for cases with constriction. The dissection is often difficult and small bleeding sources may require frequent sutures. At present, pericardiectomy for constriction seems too technically demanding to be performed as a VATS procedure.

Pericardial effusion

Pericardial effusive disease is the main area where VATS has been advocated. Pericardial effusions may be due to infectious causes that produce an acute suppurative pericarditis or more commonly may be secondary to an inflammatory process or malignancy (Table 15.1).[1–5]

The group of idiopathic effusions are presumably viral in origin but without culture confirmation. Cardiac surgical procedures may produce delayed effusions causing clinical symptoms several days to weeks later.

Surgical intervention for cardiac effusions may be primarily diagnostic or therapeutic. Options for drainage include:

- simple pericardial aspiration
- placement of pericardial drainage catheters
- pericardial window formation
- partial or complete pericardiectomy.

The simplest procedure is pericardiocentesis. This may be done blindly or with radiologic or echocardiographic guidance. This approach is attractive for a malignant effusion when sclerosant agents may be instilled to prevent recurrent effusion. Recurrence rates of around 10% have been

Table 15.1

Common causes of pericardial effusion

- Malignancy (lung, breast, lymphoma)

- Infection

- Uraemia

- Radiation

- Collagen vascular diseases

- Trauma

- Idiopathic

- Cardiac surgery

reported[6] but may be as high as 83%.[7] For patients with a short expected survival time, this approach may be preferable. Complications may include laceration of the heart and bleeding leading to an urgent surgical repair procedure or death.[8,9]

The therapeutic goals for pericardial effusions are to relieve the effusion, make a definitive diagnosis, and prevent recurrent fluid or the development of constriction. This should be accompanied by the lowest possible morbidity and mortality. Surgical approaches include: subxiphoid, median sternotomy, thoracotomy, and VATS. A median sternotomy has definite advantages for constrictive pericarditis although it is less useful for purely effusive disorders. It allows complete pericardial resection with less pulmonary morbidity than with a thoracotomy. The subxiphoid route has been popular because it is simple and may be performed under local anaesthesia. However, it allows only limited exposure and results in a restricted pericardial excision. Direct comparisons between subxiphoid and thoracotomy pericardiectomy have documented fewer pulmonary complications with the subxiphoid route[5] but recurrence rates after the subxiphoid approach have varied between 2.5–18% depending upon the reporting centre and the mixture of aetiologic agents.[1–3,5,10,11] There has been some evidence suggesting that a larger pericardial resection correlates with fewer recurrent effusions.[1,3]

Thoracotomy affords good exposure of the pericardium for a wide resection but its main drawback in the management of pericardial effusions relates to the morbidity of the incision — primarily pulmonary complications and pain.[12]

Video-assisted pericardiectomy is attractive because it allows exposure and pericardial resection comparable to that of a formal thoracotomy while avoiding the morbidity of this larger incision.[13–15] Pericardiectomy performed thoracoscopically is fairly straightforward. The main issue has been the relative merits of this procedure compared with the subxiphoid route. Video-assisted surgery requires a double lumen endotracheal tube and general anaesthesia.[16] More complicated anaesthetic management may be a significant consideration in the very ill patient. Clearly one can resect a larger amount of pericardium by the VATS technique than the subxiphoid route, but does this impact upon recurrence rates and the development of constriction?

Techniques of video-assisted pericardiectomy

Anaesthetic considerations

Although theoretically one can perform VATS pericardiectomy with an induced pneumothorax or with a single lumen endotracheal tube and CO_2 insufflation, the authors have found the most satisfactory method to be general anaesthesia with a double lumen endotracheal tube and single lung ventilation. This approach affords excellent exposure with which to work.[12,17,18] Patients with a haemodynamically significant effusion may require pericardiocentesis to prevent hypertension with anaesthetic induction. In the authors' experience this is rarely required for patients who are not hypotensive preoperatively.

Positioning and port placement

Pericardiectomy may be performed from either pleural cavity. With a large effusion, much of the left pleural space may be taken up by the pericardium leaving little room to operate. The right pleural cavity provides good exposure to a large portion of the pericardium and often allows more working space. In addition, pericardial fat is more prevalent on the left side of the pericardium. Often, however, the side from which the pericardium is approached is dictated by the presence of other pathological processes such as pleural effusions or lung abnormalities that require biopsy.

The patient is positioned in the full lateral position with a slight tilt backwards to allow gravity to assist in lung retraction (Fig. 15.2). If the pericardium is approached from the left chest, the initial trocar site should be posterior to the mid axillary line to prevent injury to the cardiac structures. The first trocar is generally placed in the seventh or eighth intercostal space. The thoracoscope is then introduced into the chest to allow subsequent trocars to be placed under direct vision. For most procedures, a total of three access sites is required for pericardiectomy. On occasion, a fourth site is required to retract the lung (Fig. 15.3).

Surgical technique

After placement of the trocars, a careful examination of the chest cavity is undertaken. Pericardiectomy will be performed by grasping the pericardium and incising it anterior to the phrenic nerve (Fig. 15.4). A very distended pericardium may be difficult to grasp and aspiration of some of the pericardial fluid under direct vision is helpful. After aspirating fluid the pericardium becomes redundant and is easily grasped and incised. Another option with a distended pericardium is to use a sharp hook to tent the pericardium up and incise it. Pericardiectomy is generally performed with endoscopic scissors. Care is taken to prevent injury to the phrenic nerve and its surrounding vascular pedicle. The authors usually excise as much pericardium anterior of the phrenic nerve as possible (Fig. 15.5). Pericardium posterior to the phrenic nerve may also be excised, but this has

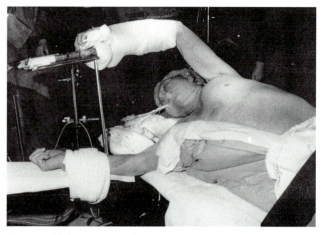

Figure 15.2 *Positioning for a VATS pericardiectomy.*

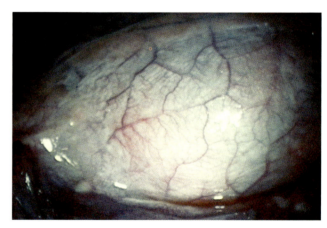

Figure 15.3 *View of the pericardium from the left pleural cavity at thoracoscopy.*

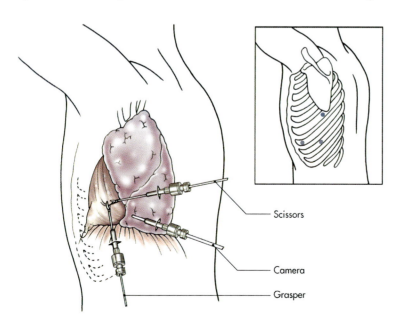

— Scissors

— Camera

— Grasper

Figure 15.4 *The typical trocar sites for performance of thoracoscopic pericardiectomy. The initial trocar should be placed posterior to the posterior axillary line when done from the left pleural cavity to avoid injury to cardiac structures. (Reprinted with permission from Ann Thor Surg 1993; 56: 792–5, Hazelrigg, et al. Thoracoscopic Pericardiectomy for Effusive Pericardial Disease).*

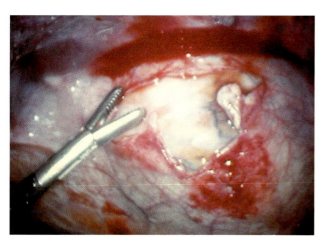

Figure 15.5 *VATS pericardiectomy in progress from left pleural cavity.*

generally been reserved for effusions that have posterior locations (Fig. 15.6).

If the pericardium is thickened and inflamed the endoscopic stapler may be used with a vascular insert to excise the pericardium and prevent bleeding. Electrocautery is routinely used for pericardial bleeding. Care should be taken with unipolar cautery to avoid contact with the heart as this can induce arrhythmias. Bipolar cautery may make this less likely, as may an Argon Beam Coagulator. The operative team should be prepared to manage cardiac dysrhythmias should they arise.

Postoperative management

After partial pericardiectomy a drainage tube is directed into the pericardial space and not removed until drainage is minimal i.e. less than 150 cc/24 hours. The lung is then re-expanded.

Postoperative care may be routine and the preoperative condition of the patient will dictate the level of required postoperative nursing care. Postoperative pain control is largely accomplished with non-steroidal anti-inflammatory agents.

Results of thoracoscopic pericardiectomy

The authors reported upon their first 35 VATS pericardiectomies all performed for effusive pericardial disease.[12] Eighteen effusions were due to malignancy and 17 were benign aetiologies (Table 15.2). Fourteen patients simultaneously had a pulmonary or pleural abnormality. These included two pleural masses, two pulmonary nodules, and 12 pleural effusions.

The side from which the VATS pericardiectomy was performed was often dictated by these pulmonary and pleural abnormalities. Eight pericardiectomies were performed for the right side. There were no intraoperative complications and during follow-up (mean of nine months) there were no recurrent effusions or constrictive changes.

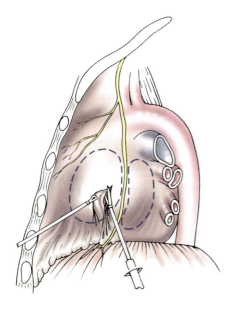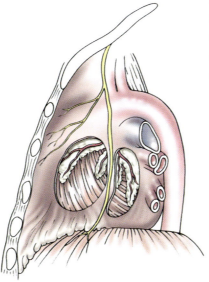

Figure 15.6 *Pericardium may be resected both anterior and posterior to the phrenic nerve for loculated effusions or when a larger resection is desired.*

Table 15.2

Aetiology of effusions

Malignant (*n*=18)

Lung	8
Breast	6
Lymphoma	3
Cervical	1

Benign (*n*=17)

Idiopathic	10
Uraemic	2
Post-cardiac surgery	5

The pulmonary abnormalities were addressed simultaneously with the pericardiectomy. Both pleural-based lesions were malignant implants and one lung nodule was a metastatic breast lesion while the other was benign. Nine of the coexisting pleural effusions were malignant and they were treated with instillation of talc.

Postoperative complications were uncommon: two cases of dysrhythmia and two cases of pneumonia. The average duration of chest tubes was 2.5 days for benign effusions and three days for malignant. The hospital stay averaged 4.6 days for benign effusions but in the malignant group there was a large range of hospital stay (7–36 days) due to the need for further testing, treatment, and generally poor health status.

In the group of benign effusions there were five patients who had undergone open heart surgery 3–4 weeks prior to presenting with evidence of a pericardial fluid collection. One patient was a transplant patient and the others were on anticoagulants. Often, these effusions were more loculated and portions of the pericardium posterior to the phrenic nerve were resected in addition to the anterior pericardium. The VATS approach was felt to be an advantage because it allowed complete drainage of the fluid without the need to re-open the sternotomy incision with its attendant potential infections and sternal healing problems.

Since the publication of these results the authors have continued to perform VATS pericardiectomy but have done so more selectively. In their opinion, it is a valuable approach for benign effusions because a large amount of pericardium can be removed without the morbidity of an open thoracotomy. Certainly a larger pericardial resection can be performed at thoracoscopy than by a subxiphoid route and this will lessen the chance of recurrent effusions or development of constriction over time.

Patients with malignant effusions, especially those with short expected remaining life spans should be managed in the simplest and safest fashion. Patients with lung cancer and a pericardial effusion had an average postoperative life span of less than 3 months,[12] so the amount of pericardium resected in this group of patients is less important as development of late constriction is not an issue. For malignant effusions catheter drainage or a subxiphoid pericardiectomy seem most logical. The subxiphoid approach can be performed with a local or general anaesthetic. A recent report suggested a 2.5% recurrence rate of effusions with a subxiphoid drainage with few complications.[11]

It has been suggested by several authors that prolonged pericardial drainage is of paramount importance as this allows obliteration of the pericardial space.[10,11] Sugimoto and colleagues[10] demonstrated this in four patients at autopsy. Failure to obliterate the pericardial space may indeed be the predominate factor in recurrent effusions, while the amount of pericardium resected may be more important when looking at the development of late constriction.

Patients with coexistent pleural and pulmonary lesions are often managed thoracoscopically. This allows direct visualisation and treatment of these abnormalities at the same time that the pericardiectomy is performed.

The group of patients who present with delayed tamponade after median sternotomy and open heart procedures are still approached by us thoracoscopically to avoid reopening the sternotomy incision.

Pericardial disease due to radiation-induced pericarditis and purulent pericarditis in children have been two groups in which a complete pericardiectomy has been advocated.[5,19] Whether a VATS pericardiectomy would be adequate has not been addressed.

The authors have recently performed several pericardial resections using the subxiphoid route and a modified mediastinoscope (Fig. 15.7). This may allow a wider resection while avoiding the problems of single lung ventilation. A 5 mm scope fits through a separate channel on

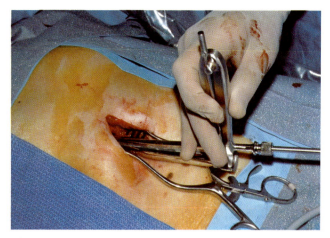

Figure 15.7 *Subxiphoid approach with a modified mediastinoscope that allows a 5 mm rigid thoracoscope to be inserted. This approach may allow a wider pericardial resection than the traditional subxiphoid pericardiectomy.*

the mediastinoscope. Resection is possible either by dissecting the retrosternal space or by operating from inside the pericardial space. Early experience using this modified mediastinoscope has been favourable and the authors have been able to perform the procedure under local anaesthesia in several cases.

Conclusions

VATS allows excellent vision of the pericardium through a relatively non-invasive approach. Pericardiectomy similar to that performed at thoracotomy is possible while avoiding the peri-operative morbidity of the open approach. The subxiphoid route offers the advantages of a simpler anaesthetic management and the option of being performed under local anaesthesia. Low recurrence rates for the subxiphoid route have been reported[11] making this seem an attractive surgical choice. There have however been reports of higher recurrence rates[13] after the subxiphoid approach and the amount of resected pericardium may be of importance with respect to the likelihood of recurrent problems.

Given this present information, the authors have approached pericardiectomy on an individual basis. An open approach (sternotomy or thoracotomy) is used for constrictive pericarditis. The subxiphoid route is used for malignant effusions especially if a short remaining life span is

suggested. The video-assisted route is used for suspected benign aetiologies, those with other intrathoracic pathology that can be addressed simultaneously, those presenting weeks after cardiac surgery with effusions and for those in whom a subxiphoid route would be contra-indicated (e.g. substernal colon). Video-assisted pericardiectomy is a safe and effective procedure which may at times offer advantages over other surgical routes. At present, the main advantage of the subxiphoid route is the lack of requirement for single lung ventilation. It may be that the combination of the subxiphoid route with endoscopic instrumentation will prove to be the best of both routes.

References

1 Piehler JM, Pluth JR, Schaff HV *et al.* Surgical management of effusive pericardial disease. *J Thorac Cardiovasc Surg* 1985; **90**: 506–16.

2 Gregory JR, McMutrey MJ, Mountain CF. A surgical approach to the treatment of pericardial effusion in cancer patients. *Am J Clin Oncol* 1985; **8**: 319.

3 Santos GH, Frater RWM. The subxiphoid approach in the treatment of pericardial effusion. *Ann Thorac Surg* 1977; **23**: 467–70.

4 Spodick DH. The normal and diseased pericardium, current concepts of pericardial physiology, diagnosis and treatment. *J Am Coll Cardiol* 1983; **1**: 240–51.

5 Naunheim KS, Kesler KA, Fiore AC *et al.* Pericardial drainage: subxiphoid vs transthoracic approach. *Eur J Cardiothorac Surg* 1991; **5**: 99–104.

6 Celermajer DS, Beyer MJ, Bailey BP, Tattersall MH. Pericardiocentesis for symptomatic malignant pericardial effusions: a study of 36 patients. *Med J Aust* 1990; **154**: 19–22.

7 Markiewicz W, Borovik R, Ecker S. Cardiac tamponade in medical patients: treatment and prognosis in the echocardiographic era. *Am Heart J* 1986; **111**: 1138–42.

8 Duvernoy O, Borowiee J, Helmins G, Erikson U. Complications of percutaneous pericardiocentesis under fluoroscopic guidance. *Acta Radiol* 1992; **33**: 309–13.

9 Wong B, Murphy J, Chang CJ, Hassenein K, Dunn M. The risk of pericardiocentesis. *Am J Cardiol* 1979; **44**: 1110–14.

10 Sugimoto JT, Little AG, Ferguson MK *et al.* Pericardial window: mechanisms of efficacy. *Ann Thorac Surg* 1990; **50**: 442–5.

11 Moores DWO, Allen KB, Faber LP *et al.* Subxiphoid pericardial drainage for pericardial tamponade. *J Thorac Cardiovasc Surg* 1995; **109**: 546–52.

12 Hazelrigg SR, Landreneau RJ, Boley TM *et al.* The effect of muscle-sparing versus standard posterolateral thoracotomy on pulmonary function, muscle strength, and postoperative pain. *J Thorac Cardiovasc Surg* 1991; 394–401.

13 Hazelrigg SR, Mack MJ, Landreneau RJ *et al.* Thoracoscopic pericardiectomy for effusive pericardial disease. *Ann Thorac Surg* 1993; 792–5.

14 Landreneau RJ, Hazelrigg SR, Mack MJ *et al.* Postoperative pain-related morbidity: video-assisted thoracic surgery versus thoracotomy. *Ann Thorac Surg* 1993; **56**: 1285–9.

15 Landreneau RJ, Mack MJ, Hazelrigg SR *et al.* Prevalence of chronic pain following pulmonary resection by thoracotomy or video-assisted thoracic surgery. *J Thorac Cardiovasc Surg* 1994; **107**: 1079–86.

16 Landreneau RJ, Mack MJ, Keenan RJ *et al.* Strategic planning for video-assisted thoracic surgery. *Ann Thorac Surg* 1993; **56**: 615–19.

17 Landreneau RJ, Mack MJ, Hazelrigg SR *et al*. Video-assisted thoracic surgery: basic technical concepts and intercostal approach strategies. *Ann Thorac Surg* 1992; **54**: 800-7.

18 Mack MJ, Landreneau RJ, Hazelrigg SR, Acuff T. Video thoracoscopic management of benign and malignant pericardial effusions. *Chest* 1993; **103**: 390S–93S.

19 Morgan RJ, Stephenson LW, Woolf PK, Edie RN, Edmunds LH Jr. Surgical treatment of purulent pericarditis in children. *J Thorac Cardiovasc Surg* 1983; **85**: 527–31.

Interruption of the patent ductus arteriosus in children

16

F. Laborde, T. Folliguet, E. Le Bret, A. Batisse, E. Dacruz, D. Carbognani, J. Pétri and A. Dibie

Introduction

A large patent ductus arteriosus (PDA) creates a significant left-to-right shunt which may cause refractory congestive cardiac failure in the neonatal period and may require emergency closure. Even in an asymptomatic PDA, however, closure is necessary in view of the continuing haemodynamic and pulmonary consequences of the persistent shunt and because of the small but definite risk of bacterial endocarditis developing within the ductus. A new technique for video endoscopic closure of the PDA using two titanium clips is described in this chapter. This technique results in less discomfort and morbidity than a classical open thoracotomy approach and has proven straightforward to learn and entirely successful.

Historical development of closure of the patent ductus arteriosus

The first successful ligation closure of a patent ductus arteriosus was performed in 1939 by Gross and Hubbard.[1] Since then, this procedure has become established as a safe and entirely effective therapy. Surgical options include ligation, division and clipping of the duct depending on the age and condition of the patient and the preference of the surgeon. The advantages given are low mortality and reliable PDA closure, but the potential morbidity of thoracotomy is important, especially in infants. Long-term post-thoracotomy pain is common,[2] and the risk of postoperative pulmonary complications represented by atelectasis and pneumonia is increased.[3] In addition, the incidence of thoracic scoliosis as a long-term complication in premature infants[4] is 20–30%. Until 1971, open surgical management via a left thoracotomy was the only therapeutic option. Subsequently, endovascular closure of the PDA was described,[5] and after numerous modifications of different devices, clinical trials were conducted[6,7,8] and have defined the results and limitations of this technique. The advantage is avoidance of any incision, but the main disadvantage remains persistent shunting, of the order of 27% at six week follow-up, which generally decreases to 15% at six months. In addition, this technique is applicable only for patients weighing more than 10 kg because the small size of the vessels makes the use of the device difficult.

Video endoscopic clip closure of the PDA

Patient selection

The authors have used this technique for all infants and children referred to their institution with PDA since April 1991 with the following exceptions:

- where PDA is part of a more complex congenital lesion requiring open heart surgery
- the size of the compressed duct must not exceed the length of the titanium clip (9 mm)

- a complicated ductus with either endocarditis, aneurysm formation or calcification; these cases typically present as adults
- a previous thoracotomy with pleural adhesions.

However, VATS closure can also be performed after an attempt at percutaneous catheter closure with the device in place and a persistent shunt (3 patients).

Instrumentation, positioning and port sites

The instrumentation required is:

- a video camera connected to a 4 mm diameter, 0° angled optic
- two 5 mm trocars
- an electrocautery hook for dissection
- two or three 60° angled hooks for lung retraction
- a titanium clip applier
- a suction device.

After induction of general anasthaesia and standard intubation, the patient is positioned on his or her right side, as for a posterolateral thoracotomy. A central line is placed via the jugular vein without an arterial line. Electrocardiogram monitoring, oxymeter and capnograph are routinely placed. The surgeon and scrub nurse are on the left side of the patient, the assistant on the right. The monitor is placed on the right side of the patient, facing the surgeon, with the cables also from the right side and clamped to the drape.

Two small incisions with a size 11 blade are made in the left hemithorax: the first incision is made just posterior to the scapula in the third intercostal space (for introduction of the videothoracoscope via the 5 mm trocar) and a second incision is made in the fourth intercostal space underneath the angle of the scapula (for introduction of the electrocautery hook via a 5 mm trocar). Two or three 60° angled hooks, 1 mm in diameter, are introduced directly through the third intercostal space in its middle part, just in front of the scapula, for lung retraction (Figs. 16.1, 16.2).

Figure 16.1 *Positioning of surgical instruments.*

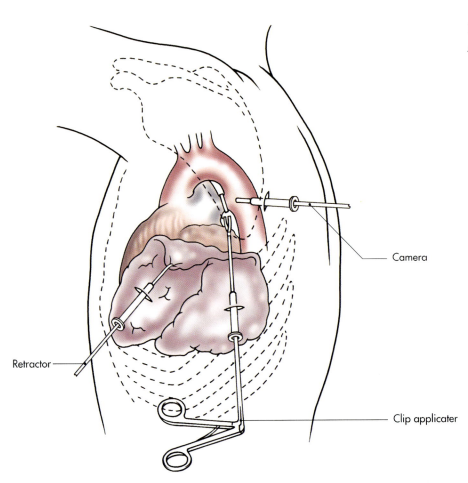

Camera

Retractor

Clip applicater

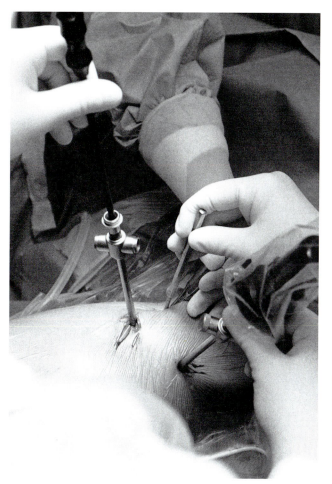

Figure 16.2 *Intra-operative view of the three access ports.*

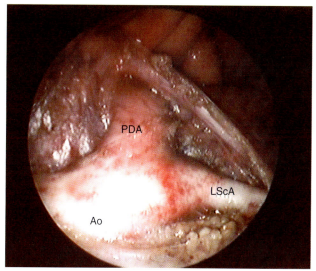

Figure 16.3 *Dissection of the pericardium on the pulmonary side of the PDA.*

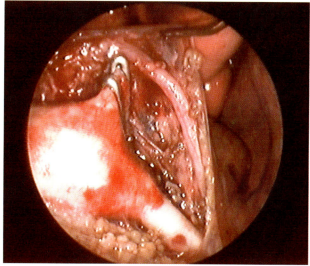

Figure 16.4 *Titanium clips in place on the ductus.*

Surgical technique

The upper lobe of the left lung is retracted inferomedially with the angled hooks, the PDA is identified and the mediastinal pleura is opened with the electrocautery hook. The PDA is dissected from the surrounding tissues and the aorta is dissected at its junction with the PDA. The pericardium is dissected on the pulmonary side to protect the recurrent laryngeal nerve from any traumatic injury (Fig. 16.3). It is essential to dissect on both sides of the PDA to place the clip adequately. The clip applier is then introduced without any trocar through the access of the fourth intercostal space. A first titanium clip (9 mm) is placed as distally as possible from the aortic junction on the pulmonary side of the PDA and a second clip is applied on the side close to the aorta (Fig. 16.4). After visual confirmation that both clips are well in place, the lung is inflated and a 2 mm diameter pleural suction catheter is placed before closure of the 5 mm skin incisions with sutures.

Postoperative care

Colour-flow Doppler echocardiography is performed in the operating room or in the recovery room before extubation to assess the completeness of closure of the PDA. If there is a persistent shunt, the patient is returned immediately to the operative room for reapplication of a new clip by VATS. Otherwise, if complete interruption is seen, extubation is performed and patients are placed either in the intensive care unit or in a regular paediatric room, according to the age and previous symptoms of pulmonary hypertension. The pleural suction catheter is removed a few hours after extubation, a routine chest X-ray is obtained, and a transthoracic echocardiogram performed before the patient is discharged. All patients are then regularly followed-up by their own paediatric cardiologist, who will perform a complete physical and transthoracic echocardiogram examination.

Results

Patients

The authors have used this technique since 1991[9] in over 340 patients. More than 30% were less than six months old and the mean weight for the entire series was 12.6 kg, with three patients weighing approximately 1 kg. The mean operating time was 20 minutes. Patients can be divided into three groups based on their age. Firstly, those less than six months old (30%), who required rapid closure of a poorly tolerated PDA associated with high left-to-right shunt and cardiac insufficiency. Secondly, those patients aged between six months and four years represent the most important group (54%) and underwent surgery within the classic period for optimal closure of an isolated, simple PDA. The third group (16%), aged 4–17 years, represents patients with a small ductus or late diagnosed patency.

Complications

There were no deaths, instances of haemorrhage or episodes of chylothorax and no transfusions were required. Six patients, early in the authors' experience, had a persistent PDA after the VATS procedure caused by insufficient dissection resulting in inadequate clip placement. For these patients, it was necessary to reintroduce the videothoracoscope and instruments in order to perform a better dissection and apply a new clip over the ductus and close it definitely. This complication has disappeared with experience. Recurrent laryngeal nerve dysfunction was noted also at the beginning of the authors' practice in six patients (five transient and one persistent). No complication or sequelae occurred in the last 300 patients. The authors believe that dissection must be sufficient in order to place the clip correctly, but not too extensive in order to avoid a transient left vocal cord paralysis.

Conclusion

The authors conclude that PDA closure by VATS provides the same results as thoracotomy with minimal morbidity and less residual shunting than an endovascular procedure. Therefore, this technique should be the one of choice for PDA closure in children.

References

1 Gross RE, Hubbard JP. Surgical ligation of a patent ductus arteriosus. Report of first successful case. *JAMA* 1939; **112**: 729–31.

2 Dajczman E, Gordon A, Kreisman H, Wolkove N. Long-term post thoracotomy pain. *Chest* 1991; **99**: 270–4.

3 Nomori H, Horio H, Fuyuno G, Kobayashi R, Yashima H. Respiratory muscle strength after lung resection with special reference to age and procedures of thoracotomy. *Eur J Cardiothorac Surg* 1996; **10**: 352–8.

4 Shelton JE, Walburg JR, Schneiderm E. Functional scoliosis as a long-term complication of surgical ligation for patent ductus arteriosus in premature infants. *J Pediatr Surg* 1986; **48A**: 855–7.

5 Portsmann W, Wierny L, Warnake H *et al.* Catheter closure of patent ductus arteriosus: 62 cases treated without thoracotomy. *Radiol Clin North Am* 1971; **9**: 203–18.

6 Rashkind WJ, Cuasco CC, Gibson R. Closure of patent ductus arteriosus in infants and children without thoracotomy. Proceedings of the Association of European Pediatric Cardiologists. Seventh Annual Meeting. Madrid, Spain, May 8–11, 1979; 17.

7 Hosking MC, Benson LN, Musewe N, Dyck JD, Freedom RM. Transcatheter occlusion of the persistently patent ductus arteriosus: forty month follow-up and prevalence of residual shunting. *Circulation* 1991; **84**: 2313–7.

8 Vieu T, Beaurain S, Angel C *et al.* Fermeture du canal arteriel par voie percutanée: comparaison des résultats et des coûts avec la fermeture chirurgicale. *Arch Mal Coeur* 1995; **88**: 1431–4.

9 Laborde F, Folliguet T, Batisse A *et al.* Video-assisted thoracoscopic surgical interruption: the technique of choice for patent ductus arteriosus. *J Thorac Cardiovasc Surg* 1995; **110**: 1681–5.

Minimally invasive cardiac surgery

J.I. Fann, M.F. Pompili, T.A. Burdon, J.H. Stevens and B.A. Reitz

17

Historical background and perspectives

Although coronary artery bypass grafting was performed experimentally in 1910 by Carrel,[1] it was not until 1953 that Demikov successfully grafted the left internal mammary artery to the left anterior descending artery in the dog.[2] In 1960, Goetz *et al.* performed the first human internal mammary artery to coronary artery bypass, using the right internal mammary artery as a conduit to the right coronary artery.[3] In 1964, Kolesov successfully grafted the left internal mammary artery graft to a branch of the circumflex artery in a human; he bypassed the left internal mammary artery to the left anterior descending artery two years later.[4-6] While these early feats directed at coronary revascularisation were performed on a beating heart without cardiopulmonary bypass, Favaloro presented the Cleveland Clinic experience in 1970 and recommended the use of cardiopulmonary bypass for revascularisation of left coronary artery branches but noted that bypass of the right coronary artery could be done safely without circulatory support in most patients.[7] Human mitral valve replacement using a mechanical prosthesis was first reported by Starr and Edwards in 1961.[8] Over the last 30 years, surgical treatment of mitral valve pathology has evolved to include valve replacement using improved materials and innovative and durable reconstructive procedures with low morbidity and mortality.[9-12] During this time, however, the operative exposure of the mitral valve via a median sternotomy remained essentially unchanged.

Introduction

Recent laparoscopic and thoracoscopic advances have altered the surgical approach to many general and thoracic diseases.[13-15] These less invasive surgical procedures have produced patients' benefit in terms of reduced morbidity and shorter hospitalisation, with consequently lower cost. Minimally invasive approaches to cardiac surgery[16-23] have developed more slowly, partly due to limitations in operative exposure and instrumentation, inadequate perfusion technology and inability to provide adequate myocardial protection and ventricular decompression.

In this chapter, the authors review the current status of minimally invasive cardiac surgery, with specific emphasis on approaches to coronary artery bypass grafting and valvular procedures.

The recent development of an endovascular system that achieves cardiopulmonary bypass and cardioplegic arrest has enabled the surgeon to perform various cardiac procedures in a minimally invasive fashion.[17,18,24-27,50,51] This new approach of port-access cardiac surgery with cardiopulmonary bypass and cardioplegic arrest is discussed in detail.

Initial applications of VATS to cardiovascular disease

A logical extension of the application of video-assisted thoracoscopic techniques to pulmonary and pleural diseases is the treatment of acquired and congenital cardiovascular disorders not requiring cardiopulmonary bypass.[28-30]

213

A VATS approach offers distinct advantages with less morbidity, possibly shorter hospitalisation and reduced cost. The reported morbidity of standard thoracotomy include scoliosis, breast deformity, winged scapula, shoulder weakness, reduced shoulder mobility and chest wall pain syndromes.[31–34] Pericardial drainage (Chapter 15) and interruption of the patent ductus arteriosus (Chapter 16) have been described earlier in this book. Burke et al. recently presented their paediatric experience at the Boston Children's Hospital with video-assisted thoracoscopic interruption of patent ductus arteriosus, vascular ring division, pericardial drainage and resection, arterial and venous collateral interruption, thoracic duct ligation, and epicardial pacemaker lead insertion.[28] Overall, there was less morbidity than with conventional thoracotomy, and the perioperative results were acceptable. Thus, thoracoscopic techniques can be safely applied to the treatment of certain cardiovascular disorders and may become an effective addition to the staged management of more complex forms of congenital heart disease.[28]

Coronary revascularisation without cardiopulmonary bypass

Although coronary revascularisation without cardio-pulmonary bypass was employed by a number of investigators in the past[5,6,35–37] and later abandoned by most surgeons as the technique of cardiopulmonary bypass with cardioplegic arrest improved, this approach coupled with the use of smaller incisions has been reintroduced as an alternative to the conventional method.[19,20,22,38–41] This is partly the result of newer pharmacologic agents which decrease heart rate and oxygen consumption and partly because of concern about the effects of cardiopulmonary bypass.

In the mid 1970s, Trapp and Bisarya presented a series of 63 patients who underwent coronary revascularisation without cardiopulmonary bypass, using a system of coronary artery perfusion proximal and distal to the anastomotic site.[36] Long-term results, however, were not available. Coronary revascularisation without cardio-pulmonary bypass has also been used in selected patients undergoing reoperative revascularisation.[42,43] Faro et al. reported a left thoracotomy approach to circumflex and left anterior descending artery revascularisation in seven patients with generally favourable results with graft patency

demonstrated in four out of five patients who underwent postoperative angiography.[42] Fanning et al. presented a series of 59 patients who underwent reoperative revascularisation without cardiopulmonary bypass, grafting the circumflex artery via a left thoracotomy and grafting the right coronary and left anterior descending arteries via a median sternotomy.[43] The operative mortality rate was 3.4%; of the 20 patients who were evaluated by angiography, 18 had patent grafts.

Since 1978, there have been over 2000 cases of coronary revascularisation without cardiopulmonary bypass performed in Argentina and Brazil.[38,40] Buffolo et al. presented 1274 such cases (most commonly to the left anterior descending artery and right coronary artery).[40] The operative mortality rate was 2.5%. Postoperative complication rates were generally less than those who underwent coronary revascularisation with cardio-pulmonary bypass. Specifically, the rate of pulmonary complications was 3.2% (compared to 9.7% for patients with cardiopulmonary bypass), neurologic complications was 1.1% (compared to 3.8%), and the incidence of arrhythmias was 5.5% (compared to 12.6%). Early patency rates of the left internal mammary artery graft in these patients were identical (93.4% patency) to those who underwent coronary revascularisation with cardio-pulmonary bypass (as seen in a sample of 30 patients in each group). Again identically, of the 6.6% which were failures, half were cases of stenosis and half of occlusion. Benetti et al. reported a 12-year experience with coronary artery bypass grafting without cardiopulmonary bypass in 700 patients.[38] Over time, the percentage of patients undergoing revascularisation without cardiopulmonary bypass increased, reaching 84% by 1989. The morbidity and mortality rates were low at 4% and 1%, respectively. Only 10% of the patients required blood transfusion, and 91% of the patients were extubated immediately postoperatively. In 54 patients undergoing coronary angiography within one month after the operation, graft patency approximated 90%.

Minimally invasive coronary revascularisation without cardiopulmonary bypass

To lessen the invasiveness of the conventional approach, Benetti et al. presented 30 cases of coronary revascularisation without cardiopulmonary bypass performed via a small fifth interspace thoracotomy.[19] There was no operative mortality. The left internal mammary artery was used as a graft in all cases; other conduits included a T graft with a radial artery anastomosed to the left internal mammary artery and sequential grafts to a diagonal and obtuse marginal branch. Calafiore *et al.* reported their experience with left anterior descending artery grafting without cardiopulmonary bypass via a limited left anterior thoracotomy in 155 patients with an operative mortality rate of 0.6%.[20] Nine patients (6%) developed graft failure requiring reoperation, and one patient underwent percutaneous transluminal coronary angioplasty for an anastomotic stenosis. Cooley successfully employed a similar technique of limited access myocardial revascularisation in eight out of nine patients.[21] Acuff *et al.* described a technique of minimally invasive coronary revascularisation without cardiopulmonary bypass that combines limited anterior thoracotomy and thoracoscopic left internal mammary artery harvest.[22] Because of the inability to reliably ligate the proximal side branches of the left internal mammary artery using a limited anterior thoracotomy without thoracoscopy, Acuff *et al.* preferentially employed thoracoscopy ensuring ligation of all side branches of the internal mammary artery in order to avoid a potential 'steal' phenomenon.

Multiple series have documented the relative safety and satisfactory graft patency rates of coronary revascularisation without cardiopulmonary bypass if performed properly by an experienced surgeon.[19,20,38,40,41,43] Advantages include decreased transfusion requirements, decreased incidence of low cardiac output syndrome, less time in the hospital postoperatively and lower overall cost. Furthermore, certain groups of patients — those with compromised left ventricular function, women, the elderly and those requiring a reoperation — may particularly benefit from this technique.[41] Along with the purported advantages of coronary artery bypass grafting without cardiopulmonary bypass, there are distinct advantages to a limited left anterior thoracotomy exposure.[20,40] As this technique is less invasive, the patients are more comfortable postoperatively, and the hospital stay is reduced probably because cardiopulmonary bypass has been avoided. The left internal mammary artery to left anterior descending artery anastomosis is facilitated by the proximity of the left anterior descending artery to the

anterior thoracotomy.[20,40] Theoretically, pericardial and mediastinal adhesions are less likely to develop, thereby potentially simplifying reoperations.

On the other hand, coronary revascularisation without cardiopulmonary bypass has limitations:

- it is technically more demanding
- it has a significant learning curve
- it may not be possible in a significant fraction of patients and
- it may yield results that are not as reproducible as with the conventional approach.[40]

Buffolo *et al.* excluded patients with left main disease and inevitably those with combined valvular and coronary diseases.[40] Also, the limited thoracotomy technique is restricted to those patients who have diseased coronary vessels that are accessible through this approach and whose internal mammary artery is adequate as a conduit, since vein grafts cannot be used as conduits.[21] Although occlusion of distal left anterior descending artery while performing the anastomosis has not been problematic in some reports,[20] there must be concern that the patient could develop haemodynamic instability or arrhythmias during the procedure. A technically satisfactory distal anastomosis depends on the size of the coronary artery and adequate exposure which is dependent on acceptable haemodynamics during cardiac retraction.[43] Narrow calibre left anterior descending and left internal mammary arteries thus contribute to the difficulty of this particular technique.

Minimally invasive coronary revascularisation with cardiopulmonary bypass

Operations on a non-arrested heart

Robinson *et al.* reported satisfactory outcome with coronary revascularisation in 16 animals and six patients with a minimally invasive approach utilising a left anterior mediastinotomy combined with cardiopulmonary bypass.[23] The internal mammary artery was harvested via the mediastinotomy with thoracoscopic assistance. Depending on the size of the heart and location of coronary disease as determined by angiography, either the third or fourth cartilage was excised. Although there was adequate exposure to permit grafting without cardiopulmonary bypass, for a number of reasons, they proceeded with cardiopulmonary bypass in all cases using femoral cannulation, no aortic cross-clamping, and hypothermic ventricular fibrillation.[23] Control of the coronary artery was achieved with either horizontal mattress silastic sutures or 7-0 polypropylene sutures placed circumferentially. The average cardiopulmonary bypass time was 64 minutes, and there was no operative mortality. One patient developed recurrence of angina four weeks after the procedure due to kinked and stenotic mid-left internal mammary artery graft, correctable by angioplasty. Putative advantages of this technique are that it is less invasive and that its design maintains many of the fundamental principles of open coronary procedures.[23] The anterior mediastinotomy method retains direct vision and conventional mean of anastomosis and instrumentation. Cardiopulmonary bypass and hypothermic ventricular fibrillation provided improved conditions for suturing compared to the approach with a beating heart.

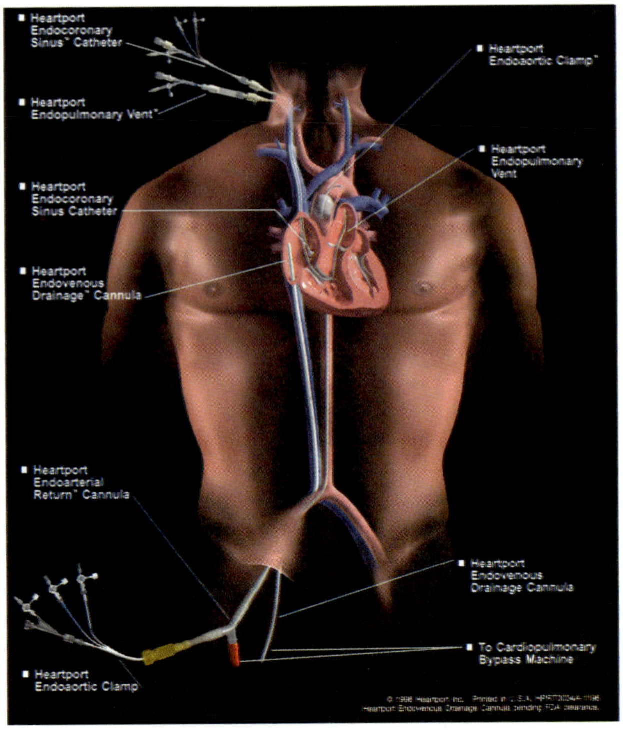

Coronary revascularisation with the port-access approach

In 1993, Peters proposed a method of minimally invasive cardiac surgery using femoral–femoral perfusion and a specially designed aortic balloon catheter passed into the ascending aorta to achieve cardioplegic arrest.[16] The endoaortic balloon catheter could provide aortic occlusion, delivery of cardioplegic solution and aortic root venting. This design was modified, providing a basis for an effective peripheral endovascular system for cardiopulmonary bypass with cardioplegic arrest with myocardial protection (e.g. Heartport* Endoaortic Clamp).[17] This system thus enables the surgeon to perform various open cardiac procedures using a less invasive approach and avoiding a standard median sternotomy.

The port-access system is based on a peripherally placed endoaortic clamp device that effectively achieves aortic occlusion, cardioplegia delivery, and left ventricular decompression.[17,18] This endoaortic device is a triple-lumen catheter with a distal inflatable balloon (Fig. 17.1). Proper positioning of the balloon component is important because misplacement can theoretically result in aortic valve incompetence with left ventricular distention, arch vessel

Figure 17.1 *Port-access cardiopulmonary bypass system. Femorofemoral cardiopulmonary bypass with augmented venous drainage is employed. The balloon occlusion catheter (endoaortic clamp) is inflated in the ascending aorta and cardioplegia is delivered in an antegrade fashion via the central lumen. The endopulmonary vent assists in decompression of the heart.* ©1996 Heartport Inc.

occlusion and an inability to achieve cardiac arrest. Fluoroscopy and transoesophageal echocardiography are useful in guiding endoaortic clamp placement.[44] Antegrade cardioplegia is delivered through a central lumen that extends to the tip; this lumen also serves as an aortic root vent after cardioplegia delivery. A second lumen is connected to a pressure transducer and monitors aortic root pressure. The third lumen is used for balloon inflation during aortic occlusion. A pulmonary artery venting catheter (e.g. Endopulmonary Vent*), is percutaneously placed through the jugular vein and passed into the pulmonary artery in order to further assist ventricular decompression.

Recently, Stevens *et al.* described the experimental use of the port-access system in coronary artery bypass grafting.[17] In a canine model, the internal mammary artery was accessed using thoracoscopic dissection. The endovascular cardiopulmonary bypass system was employed without

---

* Heartport, Redwood City, CA

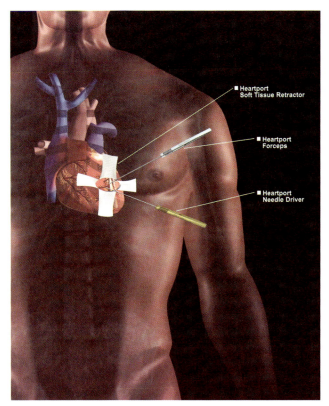

Figure 17.2 *A limited anterior thoracotomy incision is made at the fourth intercostal space with partial resection of the fourth rib. The left internal mammary artery is dissected under direct vision and with thoracoscopic assistance. After achieving cardioplegic arrest, the internal mammary artery to left anterior descending artery anastomosis is performed under direct vision.* ©*1996 Heartport Inc.*

difficulty, maintaining asystole and a still and bloodless operative field. After deflation of the endoaortic occlusion catheter, all animals were successfully weaned from cardiopulmonary bypass. This approach duplicates the advantages of traditional open-chest coronary revascularisation, while using a less invasive approach than median sternotomy. Multiple grafts are technically possible using this technique, because the arrested heart allows for better exposure of the lateral and posterior aspects of the heart.

Operative technique

The patient is positioned supine with the left chest slightly elevated. Technical considerations include double-lumen endobronchial intubation for single lung ventilation. An endovascular pulmonary artery vent catheter is inserted

using a jugular introducer sheath. A limited left anterior thoracotomy is made at the fourth intercostal space, and a segment of the fourth rib is resected. The left internal mammary artery is mobilised to the level of the first rib under direct vision and with thoracoscopic assistance. A soft tissue retractor (Heartport,•) is placed creating an 'oval port access'. A longitudinal pericardiotomy is made anterior to the phrenic nerve and the left anterior descending artery identified. After systemic heparinisation, the right femoral artery and vein are cannulated with a 23 or 21 Fr arterial cannula with a side limb (Heartport,•) and 28 Fr venous cannulae,* respectively. A 10.5 Fr endoaortic clamp is introduced via the side port of the femoral arterial cannula and its tip positioned in the ascending aorta under fluoroscopic and transoesophageal echocardiographic guidance.[44] Cardiopulmonary bypass is instituted and systemic hypothermia achieved. A centrifugal pump,† (Fig. 17.4) is used to augment venous drainage. Under fluoroscopic guidance, the balloon of the endoaortic clamp is inflated and antegrade cardioplegia delivered using the distal port of the endovascular balloon catheter (Fig. 17.3). An arteriotomy is made in the left anterior descending artery and the internal mammary artery is anastomosed to the left anterior artery in the conventional manner (Fig. 17.5, Fig. 17.6). The endoaortic clamp is removed and the patient weaned from cardiopulmonary bypass.

Results

The initial clinical trial included 10 patients who underwent port-access coronary revascularisation. The left internal mammary artery was harvested thoracoscopically; although the early experience was strictly through multiple thoracic ports, this technique evolved to a limited left anterior thoracotomy. Three patients required conversion to a open or median sternotomy revascularisation. All patients are alive at follow-up with a left internal mammary artery patency of 90%.[24] A multinational, multi-institutional study is currently in progress. The question of whether the port-access system provided adequate myocardial protection during aortic clamping was addressed by Schwartz *et al.* in a recent analysis of left ventricular function using the port-

•   Redwood City, CA

*   DLP, Inc., Grand Rapids, MI

†   Biomedicus, Medtronic, Minneapolis, MN

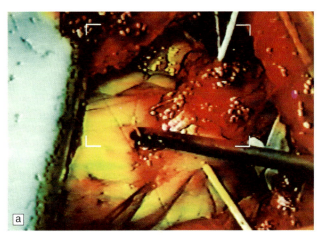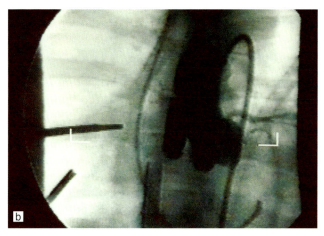

Figure 17.3 *(a) Operative view of left internal mammary artery bypass to left anterior descending coronary artery. (b) Fluoroscopic image showing contrast medium outlining the aortic root and coronary arteries after successful deployment of the endoaortic balloon clamp. (Note the transoesophageal echocardiography probe visible immediately to the convex side of the ascending aorta.)*

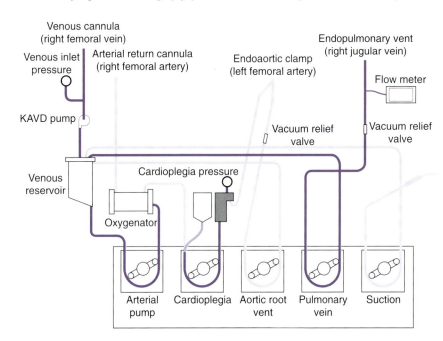

Figure 17.4 *Circuit diagram of the port-access cardiopulmonary bypass system. Femoral venous drainage is assisted by an in-line centrifugal pump. Aortic root and pulmonary artery vent lines each have an in-line pressure relief valve and are controlled by roller pumps. KAVD = kinetic assisted venous drainage. (Reproduced with permission, Stevens JH, Burdon TA, Siegel LC. Port-access coronary artery bypass with cardioplegic arrest: Acute and chronic canine studies. Ann Thorac Surg 1996; 62: 435–441.)*

access approach.[18] Based on indexes of left ventricular contractility, including maximal elastance, end-diastolic stroke work, preload recruitable stroke work, and stroke work–end-diastolic length relationship, no difference was detected between animals who underwent cardiopulmonary bypass using the port-access system and those undergoing conventional cardiopulmonary bypass (Table 17.1). By providing adequate delivery of cardioplegic solution with prompt cardiac arrest and myocardial cooling, the port-access system achieved equivalent myocardial protection compared to conventional methods.[18]

Mitral valve procedures

First-time and reoperative mitral valve replacement via a thoracotomy approach and hypothermic fibrillatory or cardioplegic arrest has been described.[45–8] Lin *et al.* reported two cases of mitral regurgitation approached through a limited right anterior thoracotomy with video assistance and femoral–femoral cardiopulmonary bypass.[45] The aorta was not cross-clamped and the mitral valve procedures were performed with hypothermic fibrillatory arrest. Both patients recovered and had an uneventful

Table 17.1

Effects of minimally invasive and conventional cardiopulmonary bypass (CPB) and cardioplegic arrest on myocardial contractile function

	Baseline before CPB	30 min after CPB	60 min after CPB	Significance*
M_w (erg cm^{-3} 10^3)				
Minimally invasive	143.2 ± 12.9	127.5 ± 17.8	122.3 ± 17.6	p = NS
Conventional	131.3 ± 21.9	122.5 ± 23.0	119.1 ± 22.0	
L_w (cm)				
Minimally invasive	4.8 ± 1.0	5.2 ± 1.0	5.4 ± 1.1	p = NS
Conventional	4.3 ± 0.7	5.0 ± 0.6	5.0 ± 0.6	
E_{max} (mmHg/cm)				
Minimally invasive	125.4 ± 58.7	143.0 ± 69.7	132.0 ± 84.9	p = NS
Conventional	107.3 ± 50.9	103.8 ± 59.8	101.4 ± 60.2	
PRWA (%)				
Minimally invasive	100	69 ± 16	60 ± 11	p = NS
Conventional	100	65 ± 18	62 ± 18	
SWEDL (%)				
Minimally invasive	100	89 ± 11	85 ± 10	p = NS
Conventional	100	93 ± 05	91 ± 04	

Values are mean ± standard deviation.

Slope (M_w), X-intercept (L_w), preload recruitable work area (PRWA), stroke work-end diastolic length relationship (SWEDL), maximal regional elastance (E_{max}).
Preload recruitable work area and stroke work-end diastolic length relationship are expressed as a percent of the pre-bypass values.
*Differences between groups tested by two-way analysis of variance for repeated measures. (Reproduced with permission. Schwartz *et al*.[18]

postoperative course. Thus, video-assisted thoracoscopy is a valuable adjunct in a minimally invasive approach to mitral valve surgery.

Using port-access technology, Pompili *et al*. performed mitral valve replacement in 15 dogs (11 acute and four chronic).[25] Via a 35 mm × 17 mm oval port placed in the left fifth intercostal space for direct exposure and access and a 10 mm port in the fourth intercostal space for the thoracoscope, the mitral valve and subvalvular apparatus were assessed and valve replacement carried out. The thoracic port was placed on the left because of the relative ease of mitral valve exposure via a left atriotomy in the canine model. A femorally placed endoaortic clamp was directed into the ascending aorta. After institution of femoral–femoral cardiopulmonary bypass, the endoaortic clamp was positioned and antegrade cardioplegia infused. Retrograde cardioplegia was instilled via a percutaneous coronary sinus cathether placed previously. After pericardiotomy and left atriotomy, mitral valve replacement

was performed with a mechanical prosthesis. After closure of the left atriotomy, de-airing manoeuvres were carried out and the animals were weaned from cardiopulmonary bypass. The aortic cross-clamp time averaged 68 minutes and the cardiopulmonary bypass time averaged 114 minutes.[25]

Operative technique

The patient is positioned supine. Technical considerations include double-lumen endobronchial intubation for single lung ventilation. With fluoroscopic guidance, a coronary sinus cardioplegia catheter (Endosinus catheter*) is placed in the coronary sinus via a jugular vein introducer, and an endovascular pulmonary artery vent catheter inserted using another jugular introducer sheath. A limited right thoracotomy is made at the fourth intercostal space between the mid and anterior axillary lines (Fig. 17.5). A segment of the fifth rib is resected and a soft tissue retractor placed. A 10 mm port is placed in the sixth intercostal space

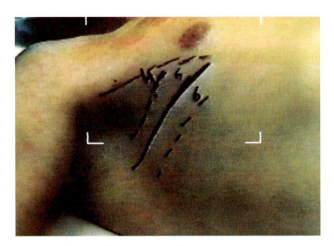

Figure 17.5 *Surface markings of incision for port access mitral valve surgery.*

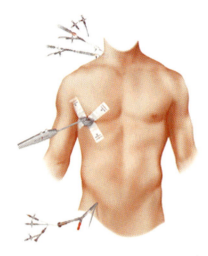

Figure 17.6 *A limited right thoracotomy is made at the fourth intercostal space and a soft tissue retractor placed to access the heart for mitral valve surgery.*

for placement of a thoracoscope. A longitudinal pericardiotomy anterior to the phrenic nerve is made under direct vision. After systemic heparinisation, the right femoral artery and vein are cannulated as described above. The endoaortic clamp is introduced and its tip positioned in the ascending aorta under fluoro-scopic and transoesophageal echocardiographic guidance. Cardiopulmonary bypass is instituted with augmented venous drainage. Under fluoroscopic guidance, the balloon of the endoaortic clamp is inflated and cold blood cardioplegia delivered in either an antegrade or a combination of antegrade and retrograde (via the coronary sinus catheter) fashion. After a longitudinal left atriotomy, the right atrium and the upper edge of left atriotomy are displaced upward using a retractor passed through a 5 mm port placed in the fifth interspace in the midclavicular line. The mitral valve and subvalvular apparatus are visualised, and the mitral valve replacement or repair carried out under direct vision and thoracoscopic guidance (Fig. 17.6). Prior to completion of atriotomy closure, de-airing manoeuvres are performed. The patient is rewarmed and weaned from cardiopulmonary bypass.

Results

The safety of port-access mitral valve replacement was documented experimentally by Schwartz *et al.* using

indexes of left ventricular contractility.[27] After port-access mitral valve replacement and weaning from cardiopulmonary bypass, the dogs had good return of left ventricular function at 30 and 60 minutes post-cardiopulmonary bypass. Preload recruitable stroke work returned to 96% and 85% of baseline at 30 and 60 minutes after conclusion of cardiopulmonary bypass. Transoesophageal echocardiography demonstrated normal prosthetic valve function as well as normal regional and global ventricular wall motion.[27] Thus, port-access mitral valve replacement can be safely performed with good myocardial protection and recovery of left ventricular function. In the initial clinical trial using the port-access approach, four patients underwent mitral valve replacement for rheumatic valvular disease via a right anterior thoracic oval port (or limited thoracotomy with a mean incision length of 10 ± 3 cm).[26] The mean cardiopulmonary bypass time was 138 ± 21 minutes and the aortic occlusion time was 92 ± 18 minutes. There were no operative deaths. Three patients had a satisfactory result and were well at short-term follow-up. One patient had a complicated postoperative course including chest wall haemorrhage with hypotension requiring exploration and tracheotomy for chronic respiratory failure. The results of a bi-institutional trial of port-access mitral valve procedures in the United States are forthcoming.

* Heartport, Redwood City, CA

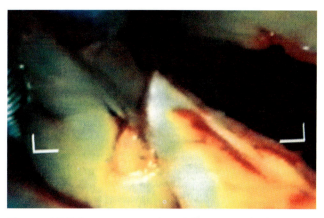

Figure 17.7 *Operative view achieved during mitral valve surgery. (Leaflet excision in process.)*

Aortic valve replacement using a minimally invasive approach

Cosgrove and Sabik from the Cleveland Clinic described a minimally invasive approach (10 cm right parasternal incision) to aortic valve replacement.[49] A right parasternal incision extending from the lower edge of the second costal cartilage to the upper edge of the fifth costal cartilage was made. The third and fourth costal cartilages were excised in order to provide adequate exposure, and the right internal mammary artery was ligated. After incising the pericardium, the ascending aorta and the right atrium were exposed. Femoral–femoral cardiopulmonary bypass was established. After aortic cross-clamp and cardioplegia infusion, the aortotomy was made and the aortic valve replaced in a conventional manner. The aortotomy was closed and de-airing manoeuvres performed. The patient was then weaned from cardiopulmonary bypass and the incision closed. At present, this minimally invasive technique is feasible, but further experience is necessary to evaluate fully this approach.

Conclusion

In an attempt to minimise the invasiveness of cardiac surgery, many surgeons have reported the relative safety of coronary revascularisation without cardiopulmonary bypass using a small anterior thoracotomy or mediastinotomy in selected patients. In spite of its real and potential advantages, including decreased transfusion requirements, lower incidence of low cardiac output syndrome, decreased hospitalisation and lower overall cost, coronary artery bypass grafting without cardiopulmonary bypass is technically more demanding, may not be possible in some patients, and may have less reproducible results. A novel endovascular system for cardiopulmonary bypass and cardioplegic arrest has been developed utilising peripheral cardiopulmonary bypass and a transfemoral placement of an endoaortic balloon occlusion catheter. This system provides for endovascular aortic occlusion, delivery of cardioplegic solution and left ventricular decompression. The port-access system enables the surgeon to effectively perform various cardiovascular procedures using a less invasive approach and avoiding a median sternotomy. Port-access coronary artery bypass grafting and mitral valve replacement have been performed experimentally and clinically with satisfactory outcome.

References

1 Carrel A. On the experimental surgery of the thoracic aorta and the heart. *Ann Surg* 1910; **52**: 83–95.

2 Demikhov VP. *Experimental transplantation of vital organs* (authorised translation from the Russian). New York: Consultant Bureau Enterprises, 1962: 200–7.

3 Goetz RH, Rohman M, Haller JD *et al.* Internal mammary-coronary artery anastomosis: A nonsuture method employing tantalum rings. *J Thorac Cardiovasc Surg* 1961; **41**: 378–86.

4 Kolezov VI, Kolesov EV. Twenty years' results with internal thoracic artery-coronary artery anastomosis (letter). *J Thorac Cardiovasc Surg* 1991; **101**: 360–1.

5 Kolesov VI. Mammary artery coronary artery anastomosis as method of treatment of angina pectoris. *J Thorac Cardiovasc Surg* 1967; **54**: 535–44.

6 Olearchyk AS, Kolesov VI. A pioneer of coronary artery revascularization by internal mammary–coronary artery grafting. *J Thorac Cardiovasc Surg* 1988; **96**: 13–18.

7 Favaloro RG, Effler DB, Groves LK *et al.* Direct myocardial revascularization by saphenous vein graft. Present operative technique and indication. *Ann Thorac Surg* 1970; **10**: 97–111.

8 Starr A, Edward ML, Mitral replacement: clinical experience with a ball-valve prosthesis. *Ann Surg* 1961; **54**: 726.

9 Fann JI, Miller DC, Moore KA *et al.* Twenty-year clinical experience with porcine bioprostheses. *Ann Thorac Surg* 1996; **62**: 1301–12.

10 Baudet EM, Puel V, McBride JT *et al.* Long-term results of valve replacement with the St Jude Medical prosthesis. *J Thorac Cardiovasc Surg* 1995; **109**: 858–70.

11 Deloche A, Jebara VA, Relland JY *et al.* Valve repair with Carpentier techniques: the second decade. *J Thorac Cardiovasc Surg* 1990; **99**: 990–1002.

12 Galloway AC, Colvin SB, Baumann FG *et al.* Current concepts in mitral valve reconstruction for mitral insufficiency. *Circulation* 1988; **78** (Suppl I): 97–105.

13 Landreneau RJ, Mack MJ, Hazelrigg SR *et al.* Video-assisted thoracic surgery: basic technical concepts and intercostal approach strategies. *Ann Thorac Surg* 1992; **54**: 800–7.

14 Mack MJ, Aronoff RJ, Acuff TE *et al*. Present role of thoracoscopy in the diagnosis and management of diseases of the chest. *Ann Thorac Surg* 1992; **54**: 403–9.

15 Begos DG, Modlin EM. Laparoscopic cholecystectomy: From gimmick to gold standard. *J Clin Gastroenterol* 1994; **19**: 325–30.

16 Peters WS. Minimally invasive cardiac surgery by cardioscopy. *Austral As J Cardiac Thorac Surg* 1993; **2**(3): 152–4.

17 Stevens JH, Burdon TA, Peters WS, Siegel LC, Pompili MF, Vierra MA, St. Goar FG, Ribakove GH, Mitchell RS, Reitz BA. Port-access coronary artery bypass grafting: A proposed surgical method. *J Thorac Cardiovasc Surg* 1996; **111**: 567–73.

18 Schwartz DS, Ribakove GH, Grossi EA, Stevens JH *et al*. Minimally invasive cardiopulmonary bypass with cardioplegic arrest: A closed chest technique with equivalent myocardial protection. *J Thorac Cardiovasc Surg* 1996; **111**: 556–66.

19 Benetti FJ, Ballester C, Sani G, Doonstra P, Grandjean J. Video-assisted coronary bypass surgery. *J Cardiov Surg* 1995; **10**: 620–5.

20 Calafiore AM, DiGiammarco G, Teodori G, Bosco G, D'Annunzio E, Barsotti A, Maddestra N, Paloscia L, Vitolla G, Sciarra A, Fino C, Contini M. Left anterior descending coronary artery grafting via left anterior small thoracotomy without cardiopulmonary bypass. *Ann Thorac Surg* 1996; **61**: 1658–65.

21 Cooley DA. Limited access myocardial revascularization. *Tex Heart Inst J* 1996; **23**: 81–4.

22 Acuff TE, Landreneau RJ, Griffith BP, Mack MJ. Minimally invasive coronary artery bypass grafting. *Ann Thorac Surg* 1996; **61**: 135–7.

23 Robinson MC, Gross DR, Zeman W, Stedje-Larson E. Minimally invasive coronary artery bypass grafting: A new method using an anterior mediastinotomy. *J Cardiov Surg* 1995; **10**: 529–36.

24 Reitz BA, Stevens JH, Burdon TA *et al*. Port-access coronary artery bypass grafting: Lessons learned in a Phase I clinical trial (Abstract). *Circulation* 1996; **94** (supp I): 1–52.

25 Pompili MF, Stevens JH, Burdon TA et al. Port-access mitral valve replacement in dogs. *J Thorac Cardiovasc Surg* 1996; **112**: 1268–74.

26 Pompili MF, Yakub A, Siegel LC *et al*. Port-access mitral valve replacement: Initial clinical experience (abst). *Circulation* 1996; **94** (supp I): I–533.

27 Schwartz DS, Ribakove GH, Grossi EA *et al*. Minimally invasive mitral valve replacement: Port-access technique, feasibility and myocardial function preservation. *J Thorac Cardiovasc Surg*, in press.

28 Burke RP, Wernovsky G, van der Velde M, Hansen D, Castaneda AR. Video-assisted thoracoscopic surgery for congenital heart disease. *J Thorac Cardiovasc Surg* 1995; **109**: 499–508.

29 Burke R, Chang A. Video-assisted thoracoscopic division of a vascular ring in an infant: a new operative technique. *J Cardiov Surg* 1993; **8**: 537–40.

30 Laborde F, Noirhomme P, Karam J *et al*. A new video-assisted thoracoscopic surgical technique for interruption of patent ductus arteriosus in infants and children. *J Thorac Cardiovasc Surg* 1993; **105**: 278–80.

31 Shelton JE, Julian R, Walburgh E, Schneider E. Functional scoliosis as a long-term complication of surgical ligation for patent ductus arteriosus in premature infants. *J Pediatr Surg* 1986; **48**(A): 855–7.

32 Jaureguizar E, Vasquez J, Murcia J, Diez Pardo J. Morbid musculoskeletal sequelae of thoracotomy for tracheosophageal fistula. *J Pediatr Surg* 1985; **20**: 511–14.

33 Dajczman E, Gordon A, Kreisman H, Wolkove N. Long-term post-thoracotomy pain. *Chest* 1991; **99**: 270–4.

34 Landreneau JR, Hazelrigg SR, Mack MJ *et al*. Postoperative pain-related morbidity: video-assisted thoracic surgery versus thoracotomy. *Ann Thorac Surg* 1993; **56**: 1285–9.

35 Favaloro RG. Saphenous vein autograft replacement of severe segmental coronary artery occlusion. *Ann Thorac Surg* 1968; **5**: 334–9.

36 Trapp WG, Bisarya R. Placement of coronary artery bypass graft without pump oxygenator. *Ann Thorac Surg* 1975; **19**: 1–9.

37 Ankeney LJ. To use or not to use the pump oxygenator in coronary bypass operations. *Ann Thorac Surg* 1975; **19**: 108–9.

38 Benetti FJ, Naselli G, Wood M *et al*. Direct myocardial revascularization without extracorporeal circulation. Experience in 700 patients. *Chest* 1991; **100**: 312–16.

39 Benetti FJ, Ballester C. Use of thoracoscopy and a minimal thoracotomy in mammary-coronary bypass to left anterior descending artery, without extracorporeal circulation. Experience in two cases. *J Cardiovasc Surg* 1995; **36**: 159–61.

40 Buffolo E, de Andrade JCS, Branco JNR, Teles CA, Aguiar LF, Gomes WJ. Coronary artery bypass grafting without cardiopulmonary bypass. *Ann Thorac Surg* 1996; **61**: 63–6.

41 Pfister AJ, Zaki S, Garcia JM, Mispireta LA, Corso PJ, Qazi AG, Boyce SW, Coughlin TR, Gurny P. Coronary artery bypass without cardiopulmonary bypass. *Ann Thorac Surg* 1992; **54**: 1085–92.

42 Faro RS, Javid H, Najafi H, Serry C. Left thoracotomy for reoperation for coronary revascularization. *J Thorac Cardiovasc Surg* 1982; **84**: 453–5.

43 Fanning WJ, Kakos GS, Williams TE. Reoperative coronary artery bypass grafting without cardiopulmonary bypass. *Ann Thorac Surg* 1993; **55**: 486–9.

44 St. Goar FG, Siegel LC, Stevens JH *et al*. Transesophageal echocardiographic monitoring of the endoaortic occlusion clamp: Preclinical and clinical studies (abst). *J Am Coll Cardiol* 1996; **27**: 190A. *et al*. AHA Circulation abstract.

45 Lin PJ, Chang CH, Chu JJ *et al*. Video-assisted mitral valve operations. *Ann Thorac Surg* 1996; **61**: 1781–7.

46 Michielon G, Doty DB. Hypothermic circulatory arrest for cardiac valve replacement reoperations. *Ann Thorac Surg* 1994; **57**: 1281–3.

47 Tribble CG, Killinger WA, Harman PK *et al*. Anterolateral thoracotomy as an alternative to repeat median sternotomy for replacement of the mitral valve. *Ann Thorac Surg* 1987; **43**: 380–2.

48 Kumar AS, Prasad S, Rai S, Saxena DK. Right thoracotomy revisited. *Texas Heart J* 1993; **20**: 40–1.

49 Cosgrove DM, Sabik JF. A minimally invasive approach for aortic valve surgery. *Ann Thorac Surg* 1996; **62**: 596–7.

50 Fann JI, Pompili MP, Burdon TA *et al*. Minimally invasive mitral valve surgery. *Seminars Thorac Cardiovasc Surg* 1997; **9**: 320–330.

51 Fann JI, Groh MA, Pompili MF *et al*. Port access multivessel coronary artery bypass grafting. *Op Tech Cardiac Thorac Surg* 1998; **3**: 16–31.

Editor's note to Chapter 17

In this chapter Fann and colleagues have presented the underlying principles of the Heartport Port-Access system together with their initial laboratory and clinical experience. They have successfully pioneered an approach to cardiopulmonary bypass which currently utilises small groin incisions but which could clearly progress with further development to a truly percutaneous approach. Many alternate descriptions exist for minimally invasive cardiopulmonary bypass procedures but these utilise variations on conventional cannulation and, where adopted, cardioplegic arrest is achieved in a standard manner by direct cannulation of the aorta following application of an aortic cross clamp. The Port-Access system is unique in providing a viable strategy to achieve aortic occlusion and cardioplegia infusion by percutaneous catheterisation.

Most groups reporting experience with the Port-Access system have reported good results for coronary surgery with Reichenspurner[52], for example, describing 42 cases undergoing successful bypass of the left anterior descending coronary in Dresden University Hospital. The approach has been criticised on the basis that only single vessel disease can be managed, but others have presented data describing patients undergoing multivessel bypass including a series from Ribakove[53] reporting 31 successful coronary bypass undergoing surgery in New York University Medical Center.

Experience with mitral valve surgery may be more variable. Mohr and colleagues from Leipzig University Heart Centre[54] reported their experience with 51 mitral valve cases operated on utilising the Heartport system and both naked eye and thoracoscopic visualisation via a right anterolateral access port. They described a relatively high operative mortality of 9.8% and significant morbidity. Their experience would seem to be at a variance, however, with the overall data for mitral valve surgery using this technique which included a collected mortality of 6.3% in over 250 patients at the time of their report.[55]

Of more concern is the risk of vascular injury and specifically retrograde dissection which appears to be associated with this system. This eventuality occurred in two of Mohr's cases and a further two of Reichenspurner's cases, suggesting an incidence of about 4.4% for this serious complication.

Those approaches to minimal access cardiac surgery which utilise conventional cannulation and bypass have the obvious advantages of convenience and familiarity. Using these approaches successful coronary bypass, valve surgery and repair of congenital intracardiac defects and tumours have been described.[56-60] Although there is currently a vogue for undertaking coronary bypass without the use of extracorporeal support this is clearly essential for all other procedures, and attempts to undertake these as minimal access operations may represent the end phase of current technology. The Port-Access system on the other hand is the beginning of a development process which should see progressive improvements in ease and simplicity of operation and safety. It takes no great stretch of imagination to envisage full percutaneous bypass with cardioplegic arrest allowing multivessel coronary bypass, aortic or mitral valve replacement and intracardiac repairs undertaken through small lateral port incisions.

Editor's additional references for Chapter 17

52 Ribakove GH, Miller JS, Anderson RV et al. Minimally invasive port-access coronary bypass grafting with early angiographic follow up: initial clinical experience. J Thorac Cardiovasc Surg 1998; 115: 1101–10.

53 Reichenspurner H, Gulielmos V, Wunderlich J et al. Port-access coronary artery bypass grafting with the use of cardiopulmonary bypass and cardioplegic arrest. Ann Thorac Surg 1998; 65: 413–9.

54 Mohr FW, Falk V, Diegeler A et al. Minimally invasive port-access mitral valve surgery. J Thorac Cardiovasc Surg 1998; 115: 567–74.

55 Chitwood WR. Discussion of article at reference 52. J Thorac Cardiovasc Surg 1998; 115: 574–5.

56 Gulielmos V, Knaut M, Wagner FM, Schüler S. Minimally invasive surgical technique for the treatment of multivessel coronary artery disease. Ann Thorac Surg 1998; 65: 1331–5.

57 Aklog L, Adams DH, Couper GS et al. Techniques and results of direct-access minimally invasive mitral valve surgery: a paradigm for the future. J Thorac Cardiovasc Surg 1998; 116: 705–15.

58 Cosgrove DM, Sabik JF, Navia JL. Minimally invasive valve operations. Ann Thorac Surg 1998; 65: 1535–1539.

59 Po-Jen Ko, Chau-Hsiung Chang, Pyng Jing Lin et al. Video-assisted minimal access in excision of left atrial myxoma. Ann Thorac Surg 1998; 66: 1301–5.

60 Pyng Jing Lin, Chau-Hsiung Chang, Jaw-Ji Chu et al. Minimally invasive cardiac surgical techniques in the closure of ventricular septal defect: an alternative approach. Ann Thorac Surg 1998; 65: 165–70.

Index